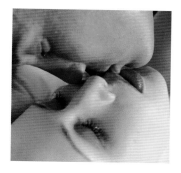

SEXUAL SUCCESS

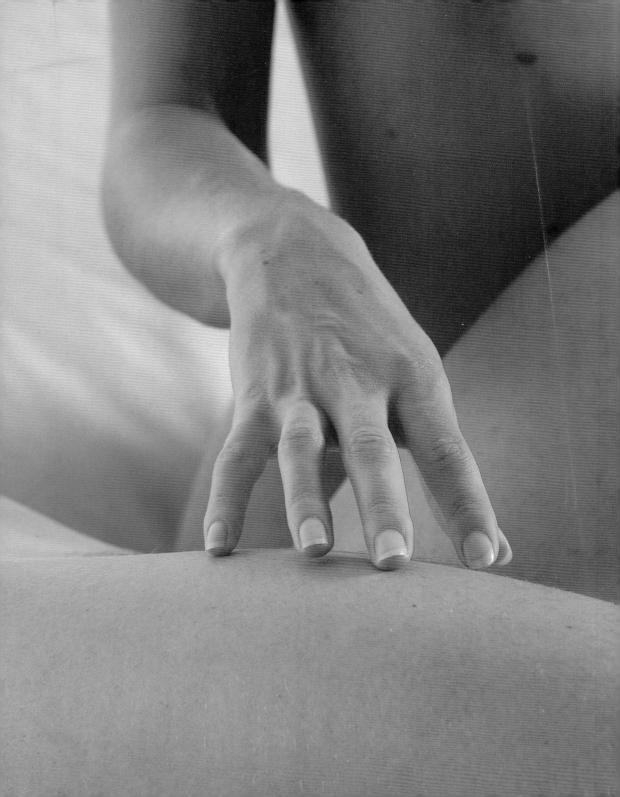

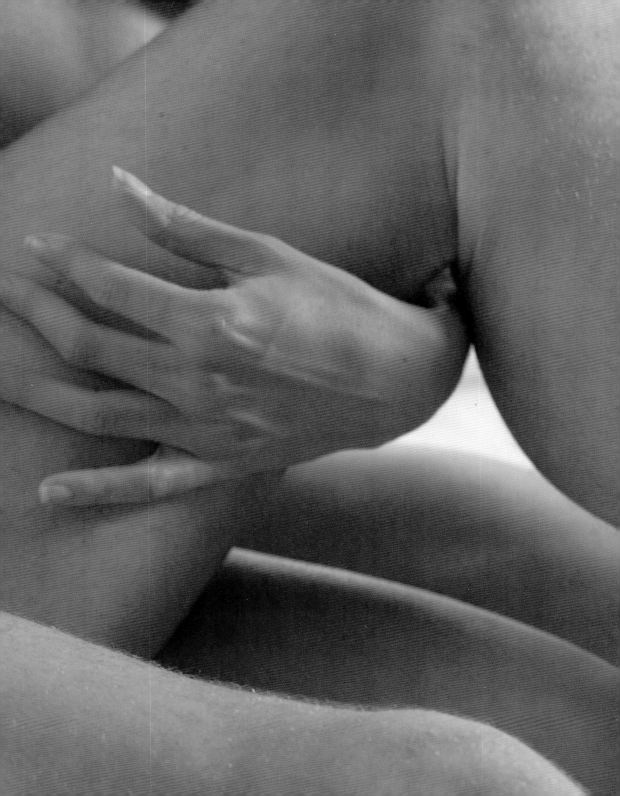

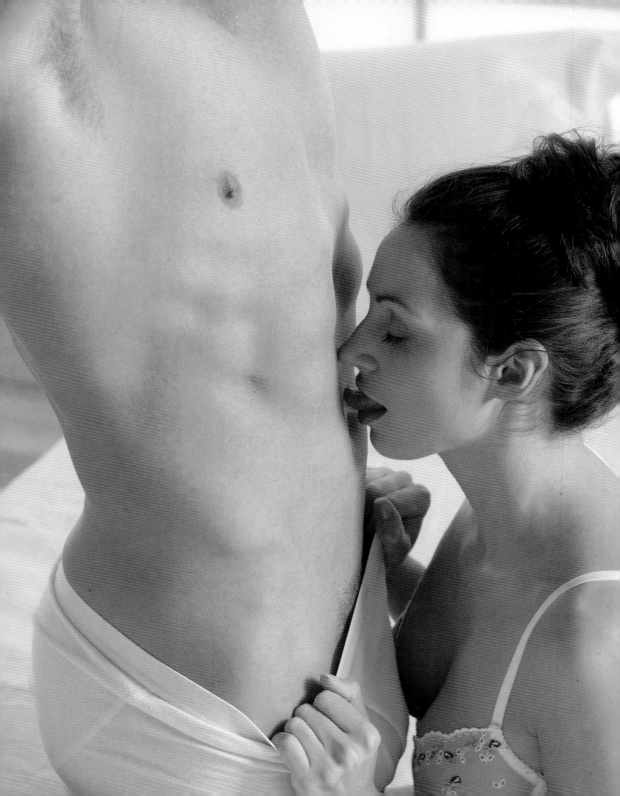

SEXUAL
SUCCESS

THE BEST-EVER PRACTICAL GUIDE TO IMPROVED SEX
AND LOVE-MAKING — WITH 500 PHOTOGRAPHS

Judy Bastyra

southwater

This edition is published by Southwater

Southwater is an imprint of Anness Publishing Ltd
Hermes House, 88–89 Blackfriars Road, London SE1 8HA
tel. 020 7401 2077; fax 020 7633 9499
www.southwaterbooks.com; info@anness.com

© Anness Publishing Ltd 2003, 2005

UK agent: The Manning Partnership Ltd, 6 The Old Dairy, Melcombe Road, Bath BA2 3LR;
tel. 01225 478444; fax 01225 478440; sales@manning-partnership.co.uk

UK distributor: Grantham Book Services Ltd, Isaac Newton Way, Alma Park Industrial
Estate, Grantham, Lincs NG31 9SD; tel. 01476 541080; fax 01476 541061;
orders@gbs.tbs-ltd.co.uk

North American agent/distributor: National Book Network, 4501 Forbes Boulevard,
Suite 200, Lanham, MD 20706; tel. 301 459 3366; fax 301 429 5746;
www.nbnbooks.com

Australian agent/distributor: Pan Macmillan Australia, Level 18, St Martins Tower,
31 Market St, Sydney, NSW 2000; tel. 1300 135 113; fax 1300 135 103;
customer.service@macmillan.com.au

New Zealand agent/distributor: David Bateman Ltd, 30 Tarndale Grove, Off Bush Road,
Albany, Auckland; tel. (09) 415 7664; fax (09) 415 8892

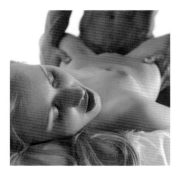

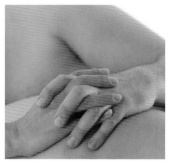

A CIP catalogue record for this book is available from the British Library.

Publisher: Joanna Lorenz
Editorial Director: Judith Simons
Project Editor: Katy Bevan
Copy Editors: Sarah Brown and Linda Doeser
Consultant: Marj Thoburn MBE
Designer: Whitelight
Photography: John Freeman – assisted by Alex Dow
Make-up Artist: Bettina Graham
Illustrations: Samantha Elmhurst
Production Manager: Steve Lang
Editorial Reader: Richard McGinlay

Previously published in two separate volumes, *Sensual Sex* and *Great Sex for Long-term Lovers.*

10 9 8 7 6 5 4 3 2 1

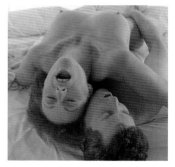

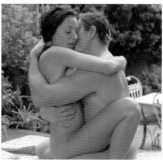

contents

foreword
8

introduction
10

attraction
14

body
26

seduction
44

orgasm
62

coitus
76

x-factors
106

erotica
124

shaking it up
142

divine sex
160

food for love
184

seasons
198

sexual health
218

glossary
246

bibliography
250

useful addresses
252

index
253

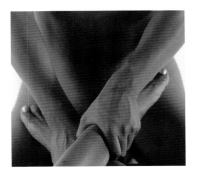

foreword

WHAT AN INTERESTING BOOK! We are all supposed to be experts, but I have certainly learnt a lot. This includes what coffee, Brussels sprouts and asparagus have in common, and a better understanding of anatomy. That the understanding of "why and where" improves skills and therefore motivation, and that sex is no different in this regard. Why smell matters; why post-coital is a part of seduction; and where the blissful sensation of orgasm comes from...

The advice starts at the beginning, with preening and cleaning, meeting places, chat-up lines that work (stick to the straightforward and avoid the search for the silver bullets: they are all dud), reading body language, and seduction. The book then gets down to the nitty-gritty of foreplay, finding the spot, coitus, oral and anal sex,

and a splendid array of erotica. The difficult areas of dysfunction, health and safety are not ducked and the referral list is comprehensive.

The entire book is presented in a non-judgemental way; refreshing in a society smothered by rules. Choose from the banquet the dishes you feel like today: this is not about right and wrong, but the sexual menu that changes from day to day.

We are surrounded by images of sex in magazines, on film and in advertisements, but so much of it seems to miss the point. Sex is a set of sensations, and both an emotional trip and an exploration of self. This book can help you reach parts you did not even know you had. Dip in and dip out, read it from cover to cover, read it separately or together.

BELOW | There are a myriad of ways to be intimate with your lover, many of which you will discover in this book.

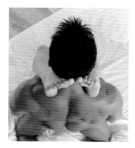

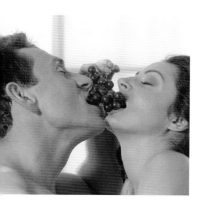

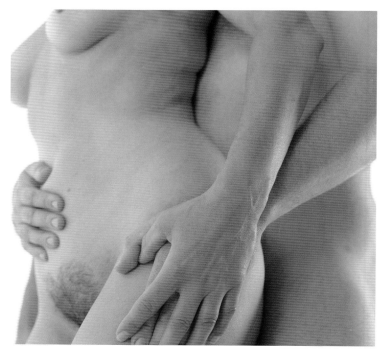

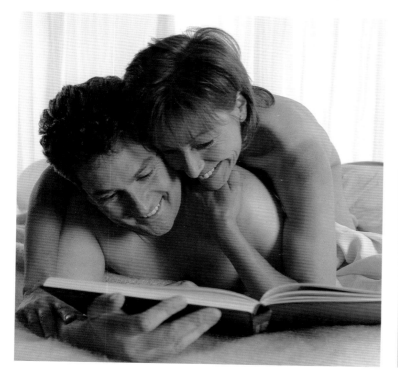

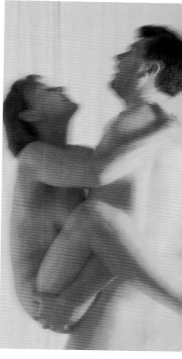

My experience is that people are becoming much more willing to discuss their sexual issues and are more likely to insist on a good sex life. Relate is perhaps best known for its relationship counselling. Less well known is that it has a long-standing sex therapy service as well. Sex therapy was developed in response to the realization that, in some cases, sexual problems were the source of the relationship difficulty. Of course, the reverse could be the case: poor emotional connections can cause poor sex. But in many cases, good sex can transform a relationship. And the beauty of it is that much of sex is behavioural: skills are needed and these can be taught and learnt.

This book presents and teaches the subject in an open, clear and affirming way, very much in keeping with a modern view, uncluttered by any inhibition or disapproval and sustained by the notion of sex as a gift that we can offer to each other.

For many, this will be a very personal read: curl up in your favourite place and enjoy a good cuddle before taking it further. A dose of sensuality can only be beneficial. Have a good time.

Ed Straw, Vice-President, Relate
(The UK's largest relationship support organization)

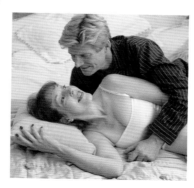

ABOVE AND BELOW | Enjoy a good read with your partner – it may open the door for discussion and then action.

introduction

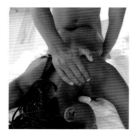

THIS PAGE AND OPPOSITE |
Good sex is at your fingertips.

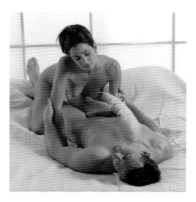

WRITING A SEX GUIDE has been a fascinating journey that has led me to call upon a wide variety of experts for advice, from bondage authorities to sex therapists, pornography entrepreneurs to medical professionals. A wide range of people have shared their most intimate experiences with me, and with their help I have produced an inspiring reference book that will provide some insight for people of all ages to help them to improve and spice up their sex lives.

Surprisingly, sex is still something we hardly talk about in our society. I mean *really* talk about. Despite the fact that we are living in a so-called "liberated society", so many of us are still so ignorant about the complexities of this very important part of our lives. I think it would be truthful to say that most of us could improve our sex lives and in turn make the rest of our lives more fulfilling. Communication and education are the two essential elements to make this possible. If I had any influence on our educational system I would ensure that all young people were taught about the art and skill of sex and not just the biological function and dangers. Sex is not just about the biological workings, it's about emotion, drive, experimentation, passion, love, friendship, care, tenderness and self-expression. You need to know your own needs as well as those of your partner. It really can be one of the most difficult subjects to discuss, and yet being able to communicate with each other about your needs and desires is a vital element to a successful sexual relationship. That's why communication crops up frequently within this book.

Without a doubt, sex is one of mankind's strongest appetites and within the sexual arena there is a whole menu of exciting and tempting things to try. Sometimes you are so starving, all you can think about is a quick fix. There is something wonderful about having a real hunger and having it satisfied quickly.

At other times you really want to take your time over a meal – choosing from the menu, the anticipation as you wait, and the climax of your main course, followed by a sweet dessert. You are immersed in a private world of pure indulgence. It's a whole different experience, this time long and languid, slow and sensual. You may not yet be satisfied, but you have set the scene for a continuing source of stimulation and pleasure.

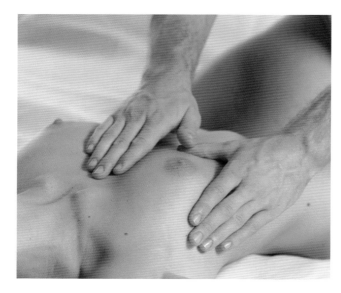

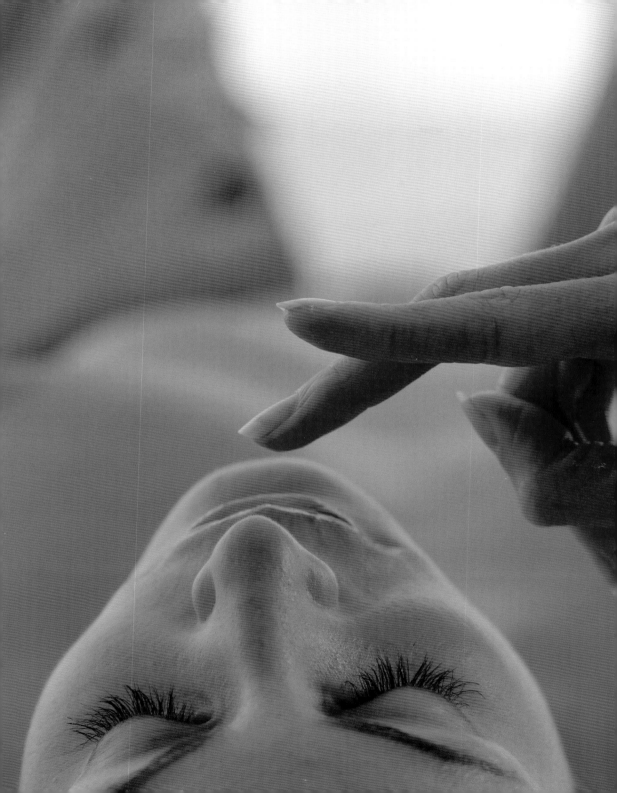

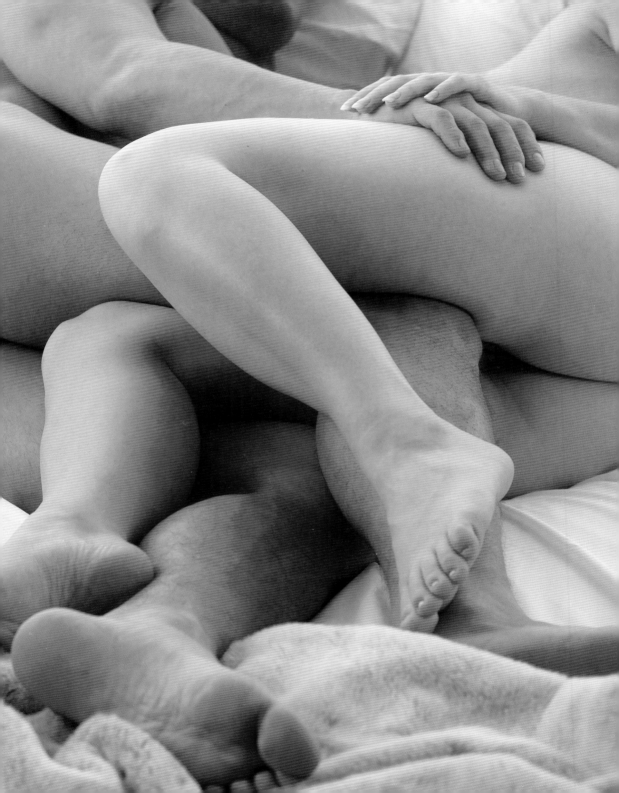

There's no fail-safe formula to successful sex. To some people, sex is just a functional activity for procreation, whereas for others it can be the life force itself. In this book I have attempted to cover as many different aspects and preferences as possible, from the very latest fads and phases in our Western society to the ancient Eastern teachings of the art of loving in the Kama Sutra, Ananga Ranga and Tantric sex.

This book is aimed at lovers, lovers of all the delights associated with sex and sensual pleasure. Hopefully, by dipping into it, and enjoying what you read, you will find something that you and your partner can use together to help make your sex life better.

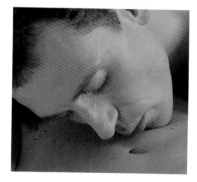

On a serious note, I would like to add a touch of realism. To have an outstanding sex life all the time is a dream that many of us harbour but few of us achieve. It is unlikely that even the most ardent lovers' sex life will be great 100 per cent of the time. But like most things it can always be refined and improved: sex doesn't remain static, it changes constantly with the seasons and the different influences in your life. That's what makes it so fascinating and exciting.

Sex doesn't just start and stop with the young: it usually gets better as you grow older. In fact it can help you live longer if you have an active sex life. You need to keep working at it throughout your life, just as you need to keep working at the rest of your relationship. Practice makes perfect. We are all students of sex, and even the greatest lovers have something to learn. Learning does not start and stop with a book. It begins with your partner and is a long exciting journey that you take together, venturing into each other's minds and sensuality. Your travels should take you both into uncharted territory, discovering what makes each other tick, and how to capture the essence of your loved one.

Bon voyage and bon appetit!

Judy Bastyra

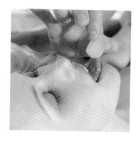

THIS PAGE AND OPPOSITE |
Touching doesn't just have to be with hands – use legs, lips and even the heat of your breath to touch and feel.

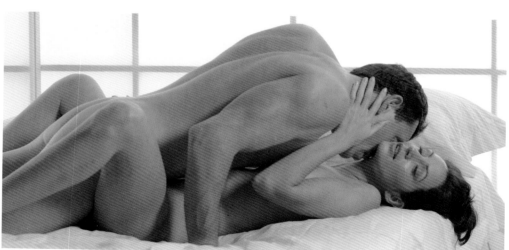

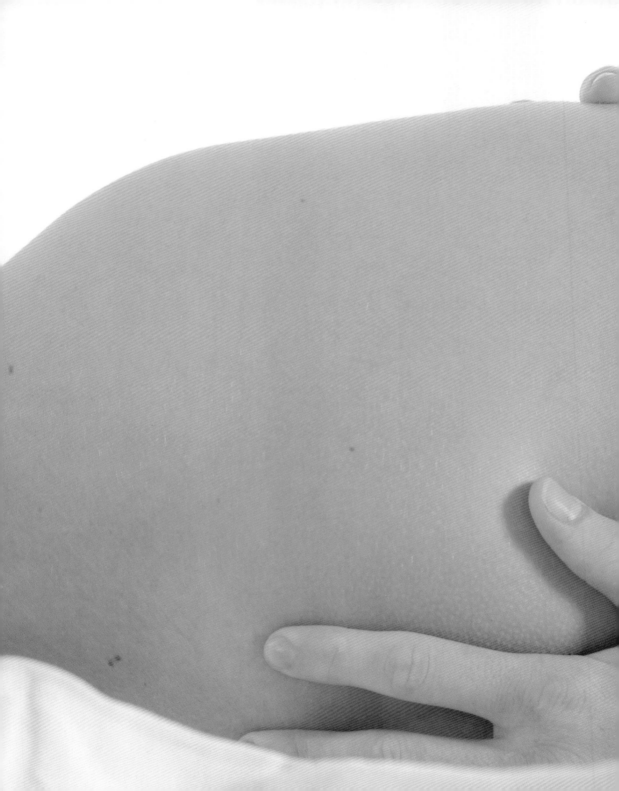

attraction

There is no accounting for the way individuals are attracted to each other. Although there are many theories, no one has managed to write a successful formula. Meanwhile, we are all susceptible to that certain indefinable special something, that *je ne sais quoi*, that creates a tingle when the right person comes along. When that happens, there are a few practical things you can do to give nature a helping hand.

first impressions

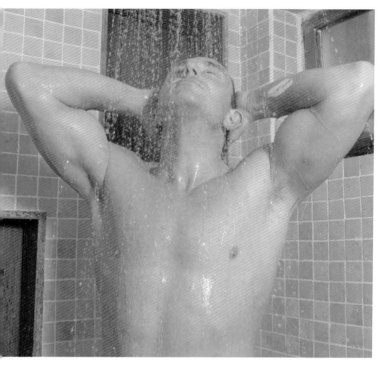

THE SOCIAL SCENE IN MANY WAYS matches the competitive environment in the workplace – too many people applying for the same job. So it's only common sense that the same amount of effort should be put into seeking your perfect partner as you put into finding your perfect job. For this you need preparation and a game plan.

First impressions are crucial, as you rarely get a second chance. People form their first impressions within four seconds of meeting, so appearances do count: hair, nails, teeth, smell, clothes, all the usual things. Women are usually better organized about this than men but it works both ways.

Nails, for example. It's not necessary to have weekly manicure sessions, but at least make sure that you give the undersides of your nails a really thorough scrub. There are few things more off-putting than unclipped and dirty-looking fingernails. Never mind where your hands have been: concentrate on where they are about to go.

Men, check that your beard, moustache or goatee is trimmed and tamed. Remember that women have sensitive skin. Scratchy facial hair not only gives them stubble-rash, but is also quite a turn-off. A recent survey has shown that 90 per

ABOVE | One of the main ingredients in a man's armpit sweat is androsterone, which helps to create that musty all-male smell – the same substance in truffles that makes pigs go crazy. However, it is best to continue washing until you find someone who loves you just the way you are.

RIGHT | Grooming is all important for men and women alike, although the latter tend to be more naturally conscientious.

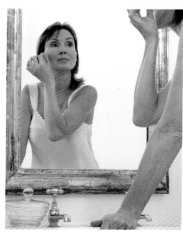

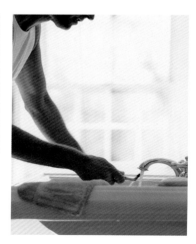

cent of women prefer clean-shaven men of any age. At the same time, take note of those unwanted hairs in the nose and ears. Check other areas such as your eyebrows. Hairs between the eyebrows can make a face appear severe, unapproachable, so undateable. A robust set of tweezers can solve this, and put you back in the running. Women, too, need the occasional battle with tweezers and the odd rogue hair.

Your teeth are important, as they will be checked out by anyone thinking of kissing you. If your teeth are stained from smoking or drinking coffee, then invest in some tooth whitener. Make sure your breath is inviting – carry mints with you. Bad breath is the *ultimate* turn-off.

the sweet smell of attraction

Make sure you have a shower before you go out, especially if it has been a hot day. There is nothing more attractive than meeting a man or woman who smells fresh and clean.

However, natural body scents have proved to be a big turn-on as relationships progress. Biologist Claus Wedekind of the University of Bern, Switzerland, published some interesting findings linking attraction with body odour and the immune system. In his study, a group of men were given plain T-shirts and instructed to wear them for two nights running without using artificial fragrance or cologne. The sweat-soaked articles were then given to a group of women for a sniffing session to rate the scents in levels of attractiveness. Both the men and the women were blood tested to discover the make-up of their major histocompatability complex (MHC). MHC is a brand of molecule, unique to each individual, which is involved in the immune system. Procreating with an individual with a different MHC results in offspring that inherit both parents' immune systems, and thus stronger immunity.

Wedekind's results showed that the women found the men's smell to be pleasant if the men had a different MHC from their own. This means that they were attracted to men who would produce stronger, more viable offspring with them.

No one can be certain whether people genuinely do fall for a particular individual purely because of their subtle scents, but have you ever said of someone, "It's not that they're particularly attractive, but there's just something about them…"?

exciting smells

Pheromones are specific hormones linked with smell, and everyone's pheromone profile is unique. The words "pheromone" and "hormone" come from the Greek *pherein*, meaning to carry or convey, and *horman*, meaning excite. These are mysterious chemicals which linger in the air, programming our brains with sexually stimulating information.

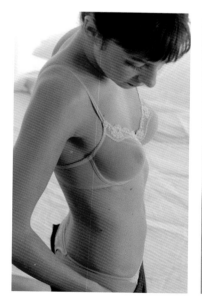

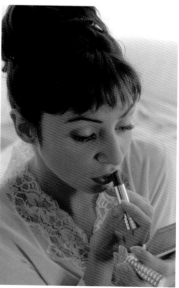

LEFT | Dressing and applying make-up for a date is an age-old ritual for women, but grooming shouldn't be ignored by men.

flirting

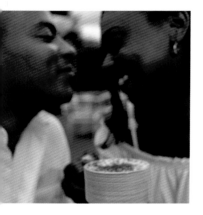
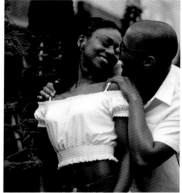
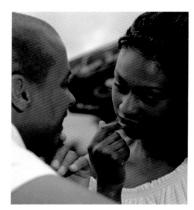

ABOVE | Flirting is a natural skill everyone can learn. Making body contact, and touching the face while maintaining eye contact, are classic ways of displaying interest in someone.

BELOW | Keeping eye contact while smiling is a great way to get someone's attention.

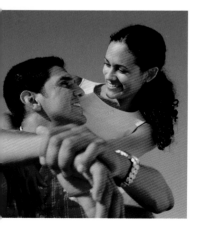

MANY THINGS ARE CHANGING in our society, but there are certain things that remain constant. One of those, fortunately, is flirting. Flirting is a fun and exciting game that comes naturally, but like any game, it takes practice, skill and determination.

the game begins

A lot of people find it difficult to attract members of the opposite sex. You may feel that you are too shy for flirting, or not confident enough to approach anyone who may interest you. It should be a comfort, therefore, to know that it doesn't matter how confident or outgoing the individual – everyone finds this tricky and there are some simple things you can do to improve your prospects. The best advice is to remember to be yourself.

Flirting begins once you've established eye contact. This is how the game begins. The eyes are said to be the windows of the soul and are the most powerful weapon in your arsenal.

Once you have noticed a person you think looks promising, try to catch his or her eye as he or she walks past. If your gaze is returned, try to hold on to the contact for a couple of seconds. For the more adventurous, this is a good time to use that charming smile (but please check that you don't have spinach between your teeth beforehand).

It is easy to affect someone's first impressions of you. It is important to smile, as it says that you are friendly and approachable. Your smile can completely alter your face. When you think of someone you love, you often imagine them smiling. Backing up a smile by saying hello is one step further. A wink is a really cheeky opener, if you are brave enough.

When you are in a large crowd, surrounded by friends or colleagues, you can seem quite unapproachable, especially to anyone who is not confident enough to penetrate your group and talk to you. If you have seen someone that you like the look of, then try to make it easy for him or her to approach you. Offer to go to the bar to get the next round of drinks, or go around topping up people's glasses at a party – anything that takes you away from the crowd and gives you an opportunity to sidle past him or her.

Sometimes, you might really like the look of someone you may be standing next to while waiting in line for the cinema or some other form of entertainment. Lines and queues are perfect opportunities for flirting, as you can easily strike up a conversation about the poor service, what film you are waiting to see or what time it is due to start.

women are natural flirts

Most women, for one reason or another, are more natural about flirting than men. Women tend to have a more flirtatious manner and will often flirt with both men and women. To add to the confusion, women who flirt are not necessarily doing it because they are attracted to whoever they are talking to, but more as a means of assessing how a person responds to them.

Austrian anthropologist Karl Grammer, the Director of the Ludwig Boltzmann Institute of Ethology in Vienna, conducted a study on 45 pairs of male and female strangers. They were secretly monitored through a two-way mirror to analyse how they interacted with one another. The majority of the women attracted male attention using flirtatious gestures and chatting easily, regardless of whether they later admitted to finding the men attractive. The subconscious flirting methods they used, such as nodding with encouragement, were merely a means of assessing the men's suitability. Grammer concluded, "You can predict male behaviour from female behaviour, but not the other way around."

Although this is an interesting insight into female behaviour, it is important to remember that this was a study of group interaction and not one to one. If, as a man, you are not sure whether a woman is interested in you when you are in a group environment, try to get to talk to her on her own. If she continues to flirt more directly at you alone, you could be in with a chance.

first moves

Once you have made eye contact and smiled, the next step is to take a deep breath and go over for round one – the chat. Remember, this is the 21st century and it's no use sitting idly twisting the straw in your drink and waiting for him (or her) to make the first move. It's up to you to get off your chair and introduce yourself. If you don't, someone else will beat you to it.

Your opening line is paramount. This will decide whether you end up pulling up a chair or doing the walk of shame. A study involving 1,000 women, conducted by leading psychologist

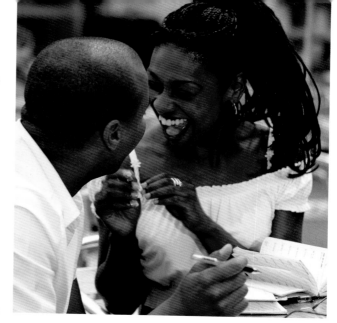

Chris Kleinke, showed that the straightforward approach is best. Charlene Muehlenhard of Texas University did a similar study on men with the same result, so keep it simple.

Kleinke's women's study showed that some of the most successful lines were simple and inoffensive openers, such as, "Do you want to dance?" or "Can I buy you lunch?" The least successful lines were those that were either smug or flippant, such as, "You remind me of a woman I used to date", or "Bet I can out-drink you!"

It's important to remember to give the object of your desire your undivided attention. This person is now *the* most fascinating you have ever met and they need to feel like it. Psychiatrist Danilo Ponce advises people to concentrate on personal attributes rather than material ones. He warns, "Don't compliment a woman's earrings – compliment her beautiful smile."

The most important thing to remember is that flirting is usually innocent and light-hearted. Try to avoid going into any situation with the thought that "this could be the one" at the back of your mind. Keep relaxed about it; at the end of the day, he or she is usually just another person looking for love. Enjoy the excitement of meeting a totally new person, keep an open mind and have fun.

ABOVE | Once you get to this stage, make sure you take the time to write future assignations in your diaries so neither of you forgets.

dating

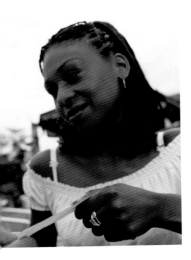

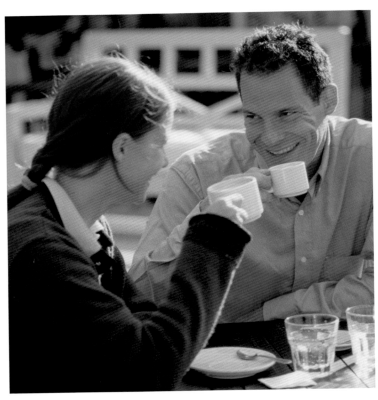

ABOVE | Don't fight over who pays – better to give in gracefully and then you can pay the next time.

RIGHT | Keep the conversation light, steering away from politics or subjects that you feel strongly about, until you know each other better.

A DATE IS AN OPPORTUNITY for you and your new acquaintance to get to know each other more fully, work out if you seem to be compatible and, perhaps more importantly, if you would like to see each other again.

Going on a date with a new person can be nerve-racking; it is exciting, but ultimately you each want to come across in your best light. Choosing where to go on a date relies a lot on the circumstances. If the decision has been left to you, try to find a place that is neutral and keep it relatively simple. You should aim to be in an environment where you can talk easily and that makes you both feel at ease. The cinema is not ideal as a first date, as you can't really talk to each other. However, it is a good option for a second date, especially if you have dinner afterwards as the film provides an ideal subject for discussion, helping you determine the depth of someone's character. It also provides insight into whether you have the same opinions about things, or if you can respect each other's differences.

meeting places

A daytime coffee or a drink after work is a good option for starters, as you can make it as short or long as you like. When going to a bar, remember to drink in moderation, as it's always a bonus if you can remember whether you would or wouldn't like to see him or her again the next day. It can also prevent you from making the mistake of sleeping with them on the first date, when you might not necessarily have done so had you been sober. (If you do choose to sleep with someone after the first date, then make sure that you are equipped to protect yourself using condoms.)

A walk in the local park is pretty romantic. The fresh air and natural surroundings can help you both feel comfortable and makes conversation flow more easily. Obviously you need fair weather, as shouting over gale-force winds with your freshly blow-dried hair flying around your head can really put a damper on proceedings, although it could provide comic entertainment if nothing else.

Alternatively, you could do something a little different, such as ice skating or bowling. Having an actual activity to do together is a fantastic option. While it provides a topic of conversation instantly, it also reduces the pressure to talk constantly, and can also be hilarious fun if a sense of humour in a partner is important to you.

The important thing to remember is to do something that you will both be comfortable doing. Imagine a really good evening or day out with your best friend, and mimic that. Where you both go should be a mutual decision so if, for example, you are a Formula One racing driver, a

blind date

Many single people have to go through a relentless trawl in search of their perfect mate. You don't have to go on television to get a blind date; these days there are a multitude of ways to meet people.

There are online dating agencies, holiday clubs and singles columns in newspapers and magazines. Why not choose a specialist publication you are interested in? You may find someone with like interests.

Speed dating is a refreshing addition to the singles scene, available at some special singles functions. Participants have the opportunity to date up to ten people in one evening. Each person is given a name badge and a score card before being paired up. After seven minutes, a bell is rung and the men move on to the next date. If there is a mutual interest, then the speed-dating organizers will give them each other's phone numbers.

Seven minutes may not be enough time to get to know someone, but they do say that most people gain an impression of a stranger within the first few minutes of meeting them.

day at the race track may make you look great, but could be a dull, or at worst uncomfortable, experience for them.

dating etiquette

There are certain things to consider before a date, such as who pays. The best option is to assume that you are going to pay half-and-half. If you are a woman, your date may be particularly chivalrous and insist on paying. You may be fine with this or it may make you feel uncomfortable, so the best way of dealing with it is to accept his generosity graciously and then suggest that next time you will pay – you shouldn't be made to feel that you owe him anything in return.

Keep the conversation light. There are some obvious no-go areas, such as discussing your ex-partners too much, or other potentially touchy subjects. Ideally, you want to give your date an idea of what makes you tick. The time to discuss more volatile subjects is when you get to know each other better, but for now, just keep it simple. It's always an idea to maintain an air of mystery; you want them to leave feeling like they have just touched the surface of you and would like to delve deeper. Don't be frosty – just don't give them too much personal information too soon. There will be plenty of time for that later.

BELOW LEFT | Some people are lucky enough to meet potential lovers at dinner parties hosted by friends.

BELOW RIGHT | Many people spend most of their days at work, so this shouldn't be excluded as a meeting place for like minds.

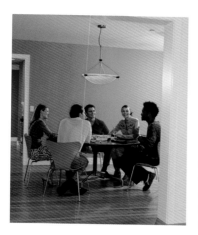

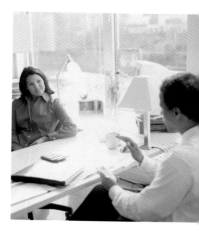

body language

BELOW | Body language, such as someone looking coy and touching their lips or chin with their fingers is a sure sign that he or she is attracted to you. Another positive indication that the attraction is mutual is when you feel comfortable casually touching one another or just being close.

MOST PEOPLE HAVE A RADAR that tells them when another person is interested, but some people are hard to read. This is when an understanding of body language is invaluable.

sexual signals

Women tend to use body language more than men, but many signs are used by both sexes. Men are notoriously bad at reading the signs, so a bit of study into what each gesture *really* means is crucial to get ahead in the dating game.

Charles Darwin said, "In the most distinct classes of the animal kingdom, with mammals, birds, reptiles, fish, insects, and even crustaceans, the difference between the sexes follows almost exactly the same rules; the males are always the wooers." Roughly translated, this means that the male will use all his sexual prowess in order to copulate, whether it's the peacock raising his elaborate fan and wafting it in the direction of the peahen, or a man dancing suggestively in the female's line of sight.

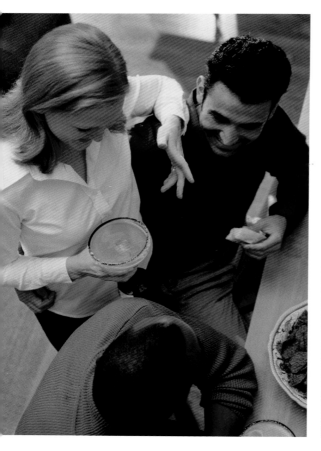

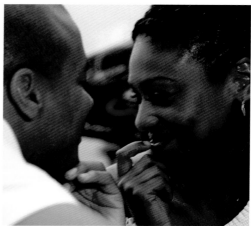

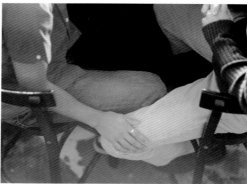

The females of the animal kingdom will, in turn, emit scents and signals to show either interest or lack of it. The peahen, for example, may coyly turn her back, and in some cases, so may a woman.

You should start reading body language even before the first approach. When talking to someone, watch how he or she sits, how he or she looks at you, and be aware of even the smallest gestures, because they all mean something. If you notice that you are, in fact, getting the opposite of these signs, it's time to stop talking and start walking so as not to waste your valuable time on a lost cause. You don't care; they weren't your type anyway, right?

BELOW | Feet directly pointed at you show positive interest.

BOTTOM | People watching. Use the signals in the box opposite and see how many signs you can recognize.

people watching

If the man or woman you are interested in displays some of these signals, you may be in luck. It is not a form of consent, but means you might stand a chance.

males and females – biting of lips, wetting of lips and showing the tongue, touching the front teeth.

males and females – gazing into the eyes with interest and dilating pupils.

females only – blinking more than usual, fluttering eyelashes and then looking up through them.

usually females only – twirling long hair around fingers.

males and females – he or she touches an arm, thigh or hand while talking.

males and females – matching your voice, speeding up and slowing down speech patterns in imitation.

males only – standing with legs apart, and often with hands on hips, he puffs out his chest like a cockerel.

males and females – pointing feet directly. This is a classic indication of interest.

males and females – mirroring movements; as one person leans back to sip on a drink, he or she does the same.

males and females – leaning forwards and decreasing personal space.

males and females – skin tones reddening slightly, particularly on the face.

males and females – exposing the palm of the hand while facing you, or cupping an elbow in one hand and holding the other hand out, palm up.

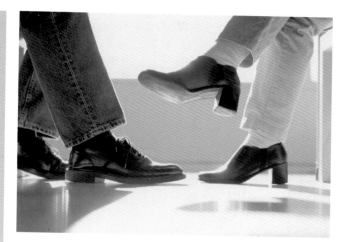

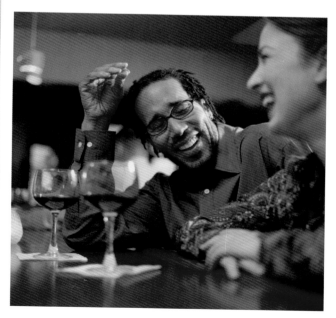

the next step

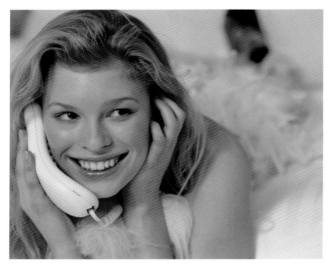

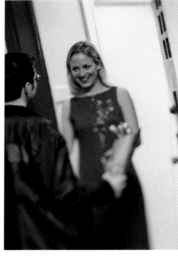

ABOVE | Making the next date. It can be difficult to get the correct balance between looking too keen and playing it too cool.

ABOVE RIGHT | Being given flowers – or even a single, perfect bloom – melts the heart of most people. A good tip, however, is not to buy them at the filling station.

SO YOU'VE MET SOMEONE you like, been out together and would love to see them again. But who should make the next move? If you are a phone person, a call the next day is always good, either to say thank you or to make sure they got home safely – both reasons are fairly innocuous and won't compromise you. If you want to play it cool, leave it for a couple of days before you pick up the phone, but not too long, as you may well freeze yourself right out of the picture.

If you are unsure of your reception and would prefer to protect yourself, a card or letter is always a good bet. With technology forging ahead, letters are fast becoming obsolete; a huge amount of correspondence is now sent through the computer and so for many people the only mail they receive is brown envelopes demanding payment. It is so exciting, therefore, to receive a crisp, hand-written envelope through the post. It's much more personal than a text message and you have the added advantage of the sensuousness of the whole experience, opening the envelope, feeling the paper, analysing the handwriting. Plus you can re-read it

as many times as you like. If you don't want to be too serious, a postcard is always good – a "thank you" card or "thinking of you" card or even a silly card about something you have in common.

You could send a bunch of flowers. Flowers are one of the traditional symbols of romance. But how often are men given flowers by women? It would certainly make a change. However, a red rose sent to his office could produce a few unwanted blushes and comments from his not-so-fortunate colleagues.

hi-tech approaches

If you are firmly fixed in the 21st century and prefer to use modern technology, you can always use your mobile phone (cellphone) or email to send a message. Mobile phones are all fitted with the text message service, which provides a great alternative for passing on short messages and greetings. Text messages have become common currency among the younger generation and can be less potentially embarrassing than a phone call. Sending a text does alleviate the heart-thumping sessions next to the phone, dialling the number, while at the same time praying the line will be busy. Simply write a few words, swallow and send. If you get a response, you can even propose another date to see each other again.

Some people think that sending an email or text message is a little cowardly and that the phone is always better, but it does let you think about what you want to say and you won't be flustered by his or her questions. Plus you can think of amusing one-liners, thus emphasizing what a fantastically interesting and witty person you are. It's certainly more casual than a phone call, definitely less embarrassing and can be flirtatious and playful. Statistics show that 42 per cent of people aged between 18 and 24 use text messages to flirt, 20 per cent of them have used a text message to ask someone out on a date and, horrendously, an unbelievable 13 per cent have ended a relationship by text message. Message received, over and out.

continuing courtship

Gifts such as chocolates or a topical book won't cost too much, and it's wonderful when you receive a gift to know that your date has been thinking about you and has taken the time and trouble to find something that they think you will like. Sometimes an inexpensive gift is more thoughtful than one that costs loads of money, but timing is everything. A naughty or suggestive present in the early stages of a relationship may not have the desired effect – so save it until later.

cyber sex

In a sense, technology has replaced and reinvented the love letter and other more creative forms of romantic communication. People today are so much busier with their careers that finding the time to get to know new people is often difficult.

Many potential couples begin (and end) their courtship by emailing each other. Some never actually come' face-to-face in the real world. Dating chat rooms have been set up specifically for people to meet other like-minded individuals.

tantalizing text

Shall I compare U 2 a ~0~'s day? U R mo luvlE & mo temperate.

Confused? This is the new language of love used by romantic text messagers. Some people use texting as a form of foreplay, making provocative suggestions, to keep their partners "simmering" before they meet. It's even possible to get texting dictionaries (dxnres) and Internet web sites provide translators so that you can type in what you want to say and you will receive an abbreviated version for your message. Here are some examples to get you started.

Hot4U – Hot for you
RUF2T – Are you free to talk?
PCM – Please call me
Un4gtebL – Unforgettable
IluvU (2) – I love you (too)
Sxy – Sexy
CU l8er – See you later
26E4U – Too sexy for you
ATB – All the best
LOL – Laugh out loud
MbRsd – Embarrassed
CU@ – See around
F2F – Face to face
ILYQ – I Like you
URA*- You are a star
URAQT – You are a cutie

However, it is important to remember that people are rarely who they say they are: the beauty of the Internet is that it lets people reinvent themselves into an idealistic version of who they really want to be. Some people are also opting for the Internet for sexual gratification, a process known as "outercourse". These chat rooms are for people who have the same erotic fantasies in common. Cyber sex can be relatively harmless, recreational fun if kept in context but there are a few pointers to remember to keep it that way. You should never give out your identity or address, and just keep the experience firmly where it should be... on the net.

BELOW | Some people like to send text messages to their date. They are quick and simple, once you have worked out the technology, and don't come across as being too heavy or serious.

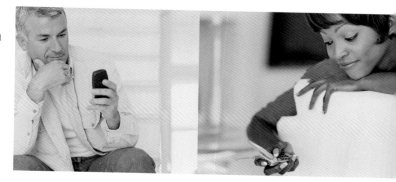

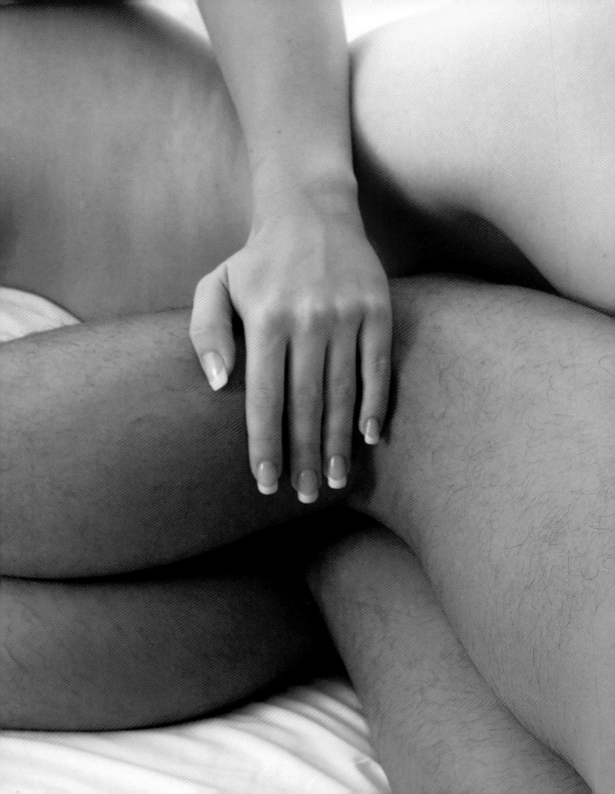

body

In order to achieve sexual harmony with your partner, you must have an understanding of both your lover's body and your own. Explore each other by touching and tasting different areas. After all, doing your sexual homework together is never going to be a chore.

the male body

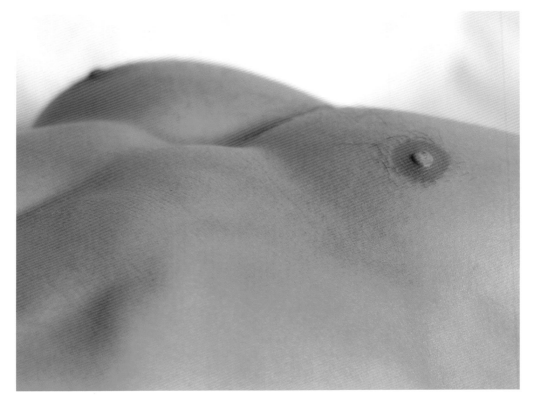

ABOVE | Many men love having their nipples played with. If they have been working out in the gym and have good pectoral muscles, lavish some time on that area to show your appreciation.

THE MALE BODY is a landscape that is well worth taking the time to explore. A body that is better known and understood will give improved and increased pleasure to its owner.

the penis

Forget dogs – the penis is man's best friend. Most men stroke and pet their penises at varying degrees of regularity. Some talk to their penises and even see it as a separate individual with its own identity and brain. So what is so special about it? Well, in some senses it does seem to have a mind of its own, especially during puberty, when it is liable to give a standing ovation at any given

opportunity. The subtle whiff of perfume from the new teacher, a hint of thigh from the woman on the bus, a pile of succulent melons in the supermarket – for young men these are trying times, a constant battle of mind over matter.

In spite of the apparent complexity and perplexity of its character, the penis is a remarkably simple organ in both structure and function. Biologically it only has two roles, those being the safe passage of urine and of sperm.

The penis has a variety of different components, all of which are made from erectile tissue, similar to that of the clitoris. In basic terms, there are four main parts making up the penis. The head, or glans, is the bulbous mushroom-shaped part at the end of the penis. The second is the shaft which makes up the length of the penis from the glans to the pubis (pelvic bones). The third is the urethra, which is the tube that runs through the shaft, and facilitates the passage of sperm and urine. Finally, the frenulum is the small piece of hypersensitive skin connecting the head to the shaft.

the glans or head

In the centre of the glans is the meatus, or urethral opening, which looks like a little slit. Sperm is ejaculated and urine expelled through this opening. The glans is the end point for a lot of nerves, making it one of the most sensitive areas on the penis.

In the uncircumcised man, the flaccid penis is covered with a thin membranous layer of skin called the prepuce or foreskin. When an uncircumcised man gets hard, this layer of skin slips back to display the glans and, during sex, it retracts further so that the glans is fully exposed. This dispels the myth that uncircumcised men have less sensitivity in that area compared with their circumcised counterparts. Circumcised or not, all the relevant areas are stimulated in exactly the same way. The only difference is that uncircumcised penises have to come outside to play first.

the shaft

The spongy erectile tissue that aids the stiffness of an erection is composed of three cylinders. The corpus spongiosum surrounds the urethra on the underside of the penis and expands at one end to form the glans. During erection and for a short time afterwards, the urethra is compressed so that it is not possible to pass urine, only semen. The other two vessels are called the corpora cavernosa, and lie at the top length of the penis.

When a man is sexually aroused, it is these three vessels which become engorged with blood, resulting in erection. Both the corpus spongiosum and the corpora cavernosa extend back inside the body towards the anus, underneath the prostate gland, to form the root of the penis, and are kept in place by ligaments.

the urethra

This is the tube that carries both urine and sperm down through the penis. The urethral sphincter muscles contract to allow either urine or semen to travel down the urethra, but not both at the same time.

the frenulum

This is located on the underside of the penis where the head meets the shaft in a puckering and folding of skin which tethers the foreskin to the head. It is an area of particular sensitivity, so it should never be ignored during lovemaking.

the corona

This is the ridge around the base of the glans where it meets the shaft. It is so sensitive that some say that light pressure around it can suppress orgasm and lengthen lovemaking. This is the area where smegma may collect, so wash regularly.

the testicles

Also called the testes (among many other less clinical names) the testicles are the most delicate and vulnerable part of the male body. Although they appear to be a pair, the testicles live in one sac which is called the scrotum. Externally, there is a very fine ridge around the centre of the scrotum called the median raphe. Inside, the septum divides the scrotum in two, so that the testicles each have their own compartment.

The job of the scrotum is to keep the testicles at the correct temperature for the production of sperm. This is a lower temperature than that of the rest of the body. You will probably have noticed that when they're warm, they hang lower and looser than when they're cold.

Each testicle is about the same size as an ovary, about 4cm/1½in long by 3cm/1¼in deep and 2.5cm/1in thick. Their main job is to produce and nourish sperm, but they are also responsible for producing the male sex hormones that control hairiness, muscularity and aggression. Each testicle produces nearly 150 million sperm every 24 hours, but after ejaculating several times it can take up to seven days to replace the sperm.

BELOW | The testes hang away from the body in one sac called the scrotum. Here the median raphe can be clearly seen.

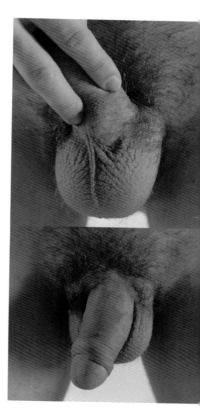

the anus

The anus is the tight, puckered hole located between the buttocks which, apart from its obvious function, can be seen as the gateway to the male G spot, the prostate. It is a tight muscle that many feel is impenetrable, but with the correct stimulation and enough lubrication, you can find it to be far more accommodating than you initially thought.

the perineum

This is the area of sensitive skin that covers the stretch between the anus and the testicles. It is often considered a flat, barren area with little purpose but to act as the frontier between the penis and anus. However, when you realize that it is located in an area of heightened sensitivity, it makes sense that here, too, is a miniature playground of pleasure, complete with its own delicious mixture of nerve endings, hot spots and endless possibilities.

sperm

The term sperm is often used to describe the milky substance produced when a man ejaculates. In truth, spermatozoa comprise only 10 per cent of this fluid, which is more correctly termed semen. In that 10 per cent, there are, on average, 200–500 million sperm, although the young adolescent male tends to produce more. This is owing to the production of androgen hormones, such as progesterone, during puberty. These hormones are also involved in the production of body and facial hair and the breaking of the voice.

BELOW | A man's body has many sensitive areas, both inside and out. All men should take time to explore their own bodies.

BELOW RIGHT | Male bodies come in all shapes and sizes.

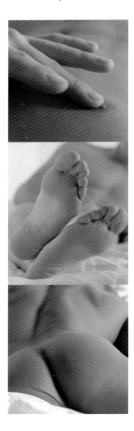

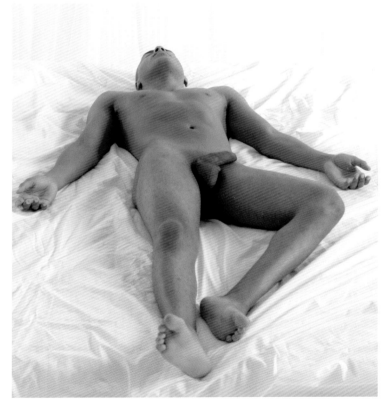

The remaining 90 per cent of the semen is composed of some 30 different substances and is referred to as seminal plasma. (Plasma is a fluid that carries solids suspended in it – in this case, semen carrying sperm.) These substances include calcium, cholesterol, fructose (a sugar that provides energy for the sperm) and lactic acid (a by-product of muscular activity). The amount of each substance varies in each ejaculate, depending on a number of different factors. For example, levels of lactic acid will increase after any form of muscular exercise. What has been eaten in the previous few hours also affects the chemical composition of the sperm and will have an effect on the taste too.

The production of semen marks the beginning of puberty and usually occurs around the ages of 12 and 13, when young males experience the emission of sperm during sleep – what is known as a "wet dream". This disposes of old sperm to allow for the production of new sperm. The emissions become less frequent as the boy starts to indulge in sexual activity.

semen – did you know?

• Semen is an eye irritant, so manual stimulation and oral sex need accuracy.
• Good for the skin, semen contains a lot of vitamins and minerals. Forget expensive creams and get your own private dispenser!
• Semen has a faintly metallic taste as it contains zinc.
• Per teaspoonful, semen contains around seven calories. For women watching their weight, there is no conflict between those love juices and that extra slice of pecan pie.
• Asparagus, Brussels sprouts and coffee all make semen taste unpleasant, while fresh mint, mangoes, green tea and confectionery all make for good-tasting sperm.
• Diabetics have sweet-tasting sperm owing to the excess amount of sugar in their bodies.

The quantity of semen produced varies from person to person. Most men ejaculate about one teaspoon of semen, although this amount can increase if a long period of time has passed since the last ejaculation. Extended foreplay and prolonged arousal time also increase the amount of semen produced, as reproductive glands, such as the prostate, are working harder.

The consistency and colour of semen is also variable. It is usually milky or pearly in colour but if it has been a while since the last ejaculation, then it may take on a slight yellowish tinge.

the big debate

For some reason men have it in their heads that women love huge penises. The reality is that a large penis can be difficult and even painful to accommodate. Remember, the average vagina is only around 10cm/4in in length. Although it is true that a small penis has its downside too, it is easier to accommodate by using different positions, fingers and sex aids, than a penis that is just too big. No matter how small or large, there's a solution for all eventualities. Anyone in a relationship having to deal with one or the other of these problems will know that half the fun is getting under the sheets and working out what to do about it.

erectile dysfunction

A quarter of all penises have a slight bend, either downwards or to the side, even when hard. Unless this causes pain or discomfort, it is completely normal. Some women report that a curved penis can heighten their experience and is easier to fellate.

Many men suffer other forms of erectile dysfunction, that is they are unable to keep an erection long enough to satisy themselves or their partner. As many as 10 per cent of the male population have erectile problems, many suffering in silence as only 5 per cent tend to seek professional help. If you think you may have an erectile problem, try not to keep it to yourself – consult your regular doctor, a urologist or a psychosexual counsellor who can help.

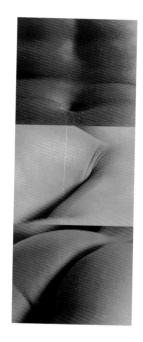

ABOVE | The landscape of the male body is often derided as holding fewer charms than the female physique – but beauty is very much in the eye of the beholder.

the internal male sex organs

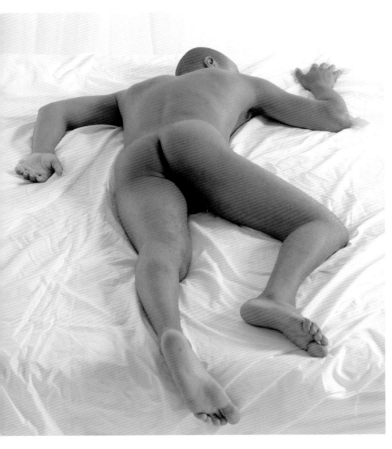

ABOVE | What's inside is just as important as the stuff you can see.

THESE ARE THE PARTS that you can't see from the outside, but understanding them is crucial to getting to know your own body.

the epididymis

This is a canal that leads from each testicle to the vas deferens. It is in the epididymis that sperm learn to swim before they make their long and perilous journey along the vas deferens and past three different glands on their way to the urethra before being ejaculated.

the vas deferens

"Vas" is Latin for vessel and "deferens" means bringing. The vas deferens are the ducts that transport the sperm up from each testicle to the penis through the epididymis. Sperm then travels through the vas deferens, which can be felt under the skin of the scrotum running up towards the groin. Most men have two, and some have three. The vas deferens is the part that is cut when a man has a vasectomy. Sometimes when a vasectomy doesn't work, it's because a man has three vas deferens and the surgeon has missed the third one.

As the vas deferens don't have any hormonal function, having a vasectomy does not affect a man's virility or the production of sex hormones and is often a good solution to the matter of long-term contraception.

the seminal vesicles

These glands are responsible for secreting seminal fluid that makes up the majority – about two thirds – of the semen. The fluid contains fructose, which provides the sperm with loads of energy for their arduous journey, and prostaglandins, which help break down the mucous lining of the woman's cervix to ease the way for them.

the bulbourethral glands

Also known as Cowper's glands, these pea-sized glands secrete most of the pre-seminal fluid that escapes from the penis before orgasm. The clear fluid protects the sperm from the acidic environment of the urethra.

the prostate gland

This little gland is about the size of a walnut. It is responsible for about a quarter of the fluid that makes up the ejaculate. It is located about 5cm/ 2in inside the anus on the front wall of the rectum, just below the bladder. The prostate gland is also known as the male G spot as, if it is stimulated, it

the male sex organs

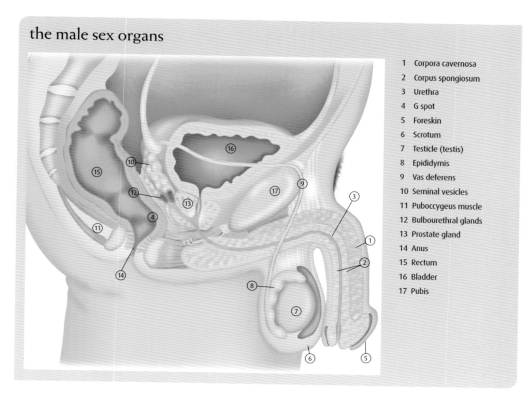

1 Corpora cavernosa
2 Corpus spongiosum
3 Urethra
4 G spot
5 Foreskin
6 Scrotum
7 Testicle (testis)
8 Epididymis
9 Vas deferens
10 Seminal vesicles
11 Puboccygeus muscle
12 Bulbourethral glands
13 Prostate gland
14 Anus
15 Rectum
16 Bladder
17 Pubis

produces a much more intense orgasm for the man. At the beginning of the 20th century, quite a few women used a steel device that was sold at the time to massage their husband's prostate during intercourse. During World War II, military medics gave prostate manipulation to soldiers who hadn't been with a woman for months to relieve them of pelvic congestion. This is called milking the prostate. Many men still feel shy about having their prostate touched, as the only route to it is via the anus. However, once they've overcome this hurdle, they will wonder how they could have missed it.

the puboccygeus muscle

Known as the PC muscle, this helps support the pelvic floor and is responsible for the fierce contractions that are felt during orgasm. It is well worthwhile keeping it in trim by flexing regularly.

the rectum

The anal sphincters are the two powerful muscles that control the entrance to the anus. The rectum is the passage through which the faeces are expelled, although, in fact, they just spend a very short time there, as they are stored further up inside the colon.

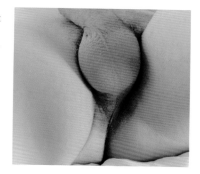

LEFT | The Leydig cells in the testes secrete testosterone and androsterone, male hormones which regulate hirsuteness and aggression, among other things.

sexploration and health

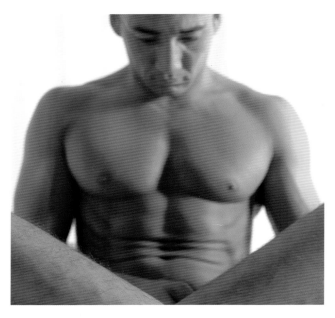

ABOVE | Take some time, in private, to become familiar with your own body.

could be described as inseparable. However, men may not have examined themselves properly from different angles using a mirror, so why not try it? There are quite a few parts you might have overlooked and you may discover areas of sensitivity that you have previously ignored.

Lie on your back, bend your legs and put your feet flat on the bed. Separate your knees, so you can get a good view of your sex organs. Using a hand-held shaving mirror with a magnifying side and a regular side, look at all the different parts. As well as being informative, this procedure is also something that you should get into the habit of doing to check that everything is in good health.

cleanliness and health

Keeping your foreskin clean and smegma-free is essential to a successful sex life. If you wouldn't want it in your own mouth, then you can't expect anyone else to put it in theirs – or anywhere else. While washing, cradle your testicles in your hand and massage them to check for bumps and abnormalities. Explore your sensitive areas, such as the perineum and anus.

Prostate cancer is the most common form of cancer in males between the ages of 15 and 34 and, for unknown reasons, is four times as likely to occur in white males than it is in black males. The good news is that it is very easy to identify through self-checks and, over the last couple of decades, advances in therapeutic drugs and improved diagnostics have boosted the survival rate, making prostate cancer often completely curable if caught and treated early enough. Most tumours are discovered through self-examination. They usually present as an enlarged painless lump that can vary from the size of a pea to that of an egg. Other abnormalities may include an enlarged testicle, feelings of heaviness or sudden collections of fluid in the scrotum. Aches in the lower abdomen or groin, or enlarged or tender breasts can also indicate a problem.

COMPARED TO WOMEN, very few men tend to have hang-ups about their bodies. Having said that, there is one part of the male body that often causes concern – the penis. Very many men are obsessed with their penis and there are very few who haven't, at one time or other in their lives, worried about whether it is long enough, thick enough or hard enough.

The penis can be a tremendous source of anxiety to men. If it doesn't shape up in the sack, they can feel very embarrassed. Women, on the other hand, don't have to worry about things like that. They can always have sex as long as they are well lubricated.

It is more than likely that most men have examined their penises extremely thoroughly. Certainly, they know how they work and which part is the most sensitive as they often touch themselves. The first thing a male infant discovers on his body is his penis and from then on they

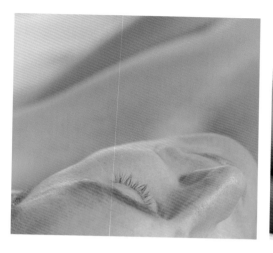

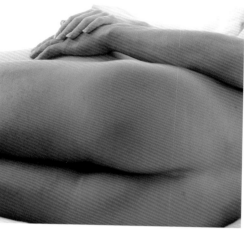

measuring up

The average erect penis is about 15cm/6in long. Ninety per cent of penises are between 13cm/5in and 18cm/7in. The smallest functioning penis stood tall at a proud 1.5cm/⅝in, and the largest soared at 30cm/12in.

When measuring your penis, always make sure that it is, first and foremost, erect. Then gently angle it down, so that it is perpendicular to your body. Use a regular ruler (metre rules are not usually necessary) to measure from the pubic bone at the base of your penis to the tip. Measuring the underside of the penis will give you a better result than measuring the top side.

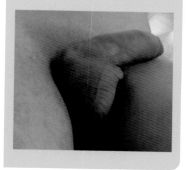

self-examination

It is best to try testicular self-examination (TSE) after a warm bath or shower, as the heat will relax the scrotum, making it easier to feel the full area. The National Cancer Institute recommends that all men, not just those in "at risk" groups, do the following at least once a month:

● Standing in front of a mirror, use both hands to check for swellings or abnormalities on the skin of the scrotum. Placing your index and middle finger under your testicle and your thumb on top, roll the testicles between your thumbs and fingers. If one seems bigger than the other, this is perfectly normal – don't panic.

● The soft, tube-like structure behind the testicle is the epididymis, which carries and collects sperm. Find this and become familiar with how it feels so that you don't mistake it for an abnormal lump. Cancerous lumps are most commonly located at the sides of the testicle although they sometimes appear at the front.

It is imperative that you contact your doctor should you find any lumps or bumps that you are concerned about. Many men feel embarrassed about a stranger handling their genitals but testicular cancer is a harsh reality. A lump does not automatically mean cancer, but it is better to be safe and most doctors will congratulate you for your preventative actions.

ABOVE LEFT AND RIGHT | The more familiar and comfortable you are with yourself, the more at ease you will be with others. Self-examination should not be considered as vanity, but as a necessary precaution against illness.

the female body

THE GEOGRAPHY of the female genitalia can be a source of much confusion and frustration to both men and women. Compared to the male genitalia, where what you see is pretty much what you get, it takes a greater basic understanding of the structure to find your way around the female body. An improved understanding of how everything works and where it is located greatly improves the love life of most couples.

the labia

The vulva is the outside part of the female genitalia that the eye can see. The protective folds, or lips, that make up the vulva are called the labia. The outer labia, or labia majora, are usually covered in pubic hair. The inner labia, or labia minora, are a lot thinner, less fleshy and much more sensitive, as they are rich in nerve endings. They contain numerous oils and sweat glands, which help to keep the vulva hygienic and healthy. Inner labia vary in shape and size. In some women, they are small and hidden from view. In others, there is more skin and sometimes the folds of skin protrude beyond the outer labia, which is perfectly normal.

the mons pubis

The pubic mound, or mons pubis, is the mound of fatty tissue that protects the pubic bone during sex. Also known as the Mount of Venus, this area has many nerve endings, and at puberty, becomes covered in pubic hair.

BELOW | There is much more to the female body than meets the naked eye.

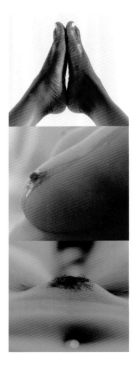

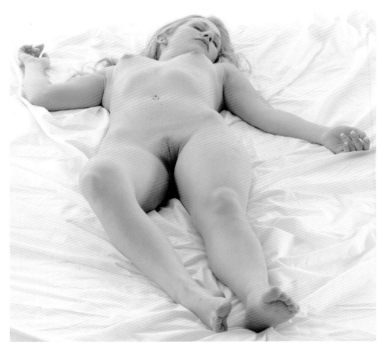

the clitoris

The magic button, die Kitzler, le cli cli or the clitoris – all women have one. On close inspection, the head, or glans, of the clitoris can be seen underneath the clitoral hood. Recent research has shown the clitoris to be a much larger organ than the part that can be seen externally.

Clitorises vary in shape and size from woman to woman, but in all women they are the only organ in the body whose sole purpose is to provide sexual pleasure. The clitoris is located just below the pubic bone so it can be gently manipulated and stimulated through intercourse, although this is often dependent on the sexual position. The head is only about the size of a pea but has between 6,000 and 8,000 nerve endings, which is why some women find direct stimulation too intense. Under the hood, the erectile tissue that makes up the rest of the clitoris forks off towards the back of the pelvis. The surrounding protective clitoral muscles are also extremely sensitive and their contraction aids a woman's sexual response.

On the 1 August, 1998 Helen O'Connell, a urology surgeon at the Royal Melbourne Hospital, noted that the clitoral nerve system extended further than the visible tip of the clitoris, causing a media frenzy of speculation about the mystery of the giant female sex organs, some subsequent reports claiming that the clitoris was over 5 m/15 ft long.

The reportage of Ms O'Connell's article, in spite of its inaccuracies, was the first time it was acknowledged that there was more to the clitoris than meets the eye. Anatomists now state that the clitoris is made up of three parts: the glans, the shaft and the crura.

By pulling back the clitoral hood, you can clearly see the glans, which is comprised of erectile tissue that enlarges during arousal. Under the hood is a flexible cord known as the shaft, which feels rubbery to the touch. The majority of the clitoral structure is inside the body but the head, or glans, is clearly visible from the outside too. The third part of the clitoris is a wishbone-shaped structure comprising two crus, or crura, located where the shaft of the clitoris divides. It is made of two extending wings of erectile tissue, the crura. You cannot see them, as they are internal structures, but they also contribute to sexual arousal and orgasm. In total the clitoris is about 9cm/3½in long. The two crus are covered by the inner labia but stretch back through to the muscles of the perineum between the vagina and anus.

The clitoris and the penis are one and the same structure in the first eight weeks of foetal development. However, although the clitoris is made up of erectile tissues, it does not form an erection but it does swell and engorge with blood.

the bulbs of vestibule

These bulbs lie on either side of the vaginal opening within the labia minora, are surrounded by muscle tissue, and fill with blood during arousal and contract during orgasm. It is thought that these bulbs facilitate intercourse by stiffening the walls of the vaginal opening, thus making entry of the penis easier.

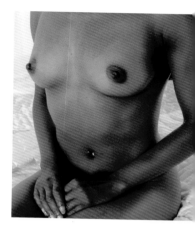

ABOVE | Sometimes inhibition can be a hindrance to learning about your own body.

the female sex organs

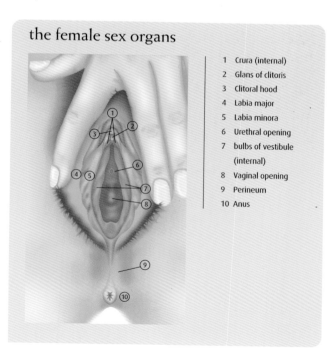

1   Crura (internal)
2   Glans of clitoris
3   Clitoral hood
4   Labia major
5   Labia minora
6   Urethral opening
7   bulbs of vestibule (internal)
8   Vaginal opening
9   Perineum
10 Anus

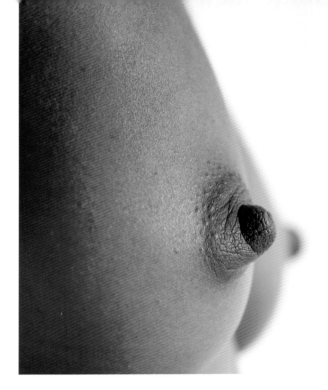

the anus

The tight muscular opening to the rectum, the anus, is a very sensitive area that some people like to incorporate into their lovemaking. But beware, permission should always be asked first, and hands, fingers, dildos and anything else should be thoroughly cleaned before they are put back into the vagina after being in the anus.

breasts

Whether you own big, voluptuous bosoms or a smaller more compact pair, you will know that breasts are the ultimate toys for most men, regardless of shape and size. Gameboys, football and Formula One all take a back seat in male priorities when set against a pair of breasts.

The breasts are composed of a mass of milk gland tissues that lie in a bed of fat and are attached to the muscular wall at the front of the chest. The milk ducts from the glands lead to milk sinuses, which are collecting areas, found just behind the nipple. Fibrous tissue runs between the ducts, providing the breasts with their firmness and structure. Breast size is wholly dependent on the amount of fat and glandular tissue, which is to some extent hormone-controlled and may vary throughout a woman's life.

A lot of people assume that larger breasts are better than smaller ones. Breast size and shape is inherited from both your parents. Women with large breasts often complain that people stare at their chests and feel that they are judged initially solely on their breast size, rather than their personality and intelligence, while other women have based their careers on the size of their chest. Either way, women must resist the pressure to look like everybody else – learn to love your assets, whatever their size.

Breasts are important to women psychologically, as they are a symbol of fertility and ability to feed offspring. Women can suffer huge grief if they must have a breast removed or if they reach adulthood without developing breasts. Plastic surgery is now available, with some degree of success, although it is important to weigh up the problem against your quality of life before taking any radical steps.

ABOVE | It is very common to have one breast larger than the other. Around 40 per cent of women have breasts of different sizes, but variations are generally minor. One breast tends to grow faster than the other and by the age of 20 they are usually fully formed.

urethral opening

For a long time people thought that women's urine came out of the vagina but in fact it comes out of a tiny hole just below the clitoris, called the urethral opening. The vaginal opening is found further below this, and is covered by a thin membranous layer called the hymen. This only partially covers the vaginal opening to allow for the flow of menstrual blood. The hymen is usually broken, either through exercise or using tampons, long before a girl loses her virginity.

the perineum

The flat area between the bottom of the vulva and the anus, the perineum, has a multitude of nerve endings that are very sensitive to touch. Some women like this area to be gently massaged during sexual arousal. The perineum is quite supple, making it possible for a woman to feel her partner's penis if she presses this area gently during penetration. Midwives recommend massaging the perineum with a mild oil, such as almond oil, to improve elasticity before childbirth.

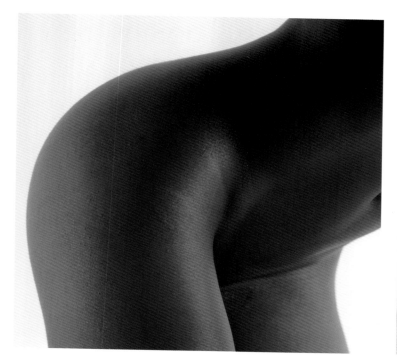
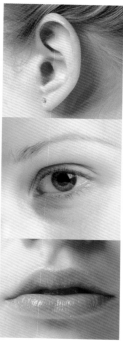

It is important to be measured for the correct size bra at a reputable store, especially if you are on the large side, to gain good support. Too many women wear the wrong size foundation garments. Take some time to become familiar with your breasts and learn to love them, using moisturizing cream to care for the thin skin that covers them.

The odd hair on the nipple is completely normal. If it is a real problem, your doctor can advise you on electrolysis or other hair-removal techniques, but the odd one here or there just needs plucking with your tweezers.

Inverted nipples, those that turn inwards instead of outwards, can be a cause for concern as they look different from those of other women. This condition affects about 10 per cent of women and is, in most cases, not a problem. During arousal or breast-feeding, the inverted nipple usually pops out. If breast-feeding is a problem, consult a doctor or midwife who will be able to advise you on how to rectify the situation.

the nipples

The term nipple only actually describes one part of the pigmented area of the breast. The protruding bud in the centre is the nipple. The surrounding circular area is the areola, the colour of which depends on the woman's skin colour, but in most cases it is pink, brown or black. Again, the size varies from woman to woman, but some are as large as 12.5cm/5in in diameter. The small nodes scattered on the surface of the areola are called the tubercles of Montgomery and are perfectly normal. The nipple has up to 20 milk duct openings which are active during the later stages of pregnancy and throughout the breast-feeding period. These ducts are directly linked to the brain and so the suckling of a baby or the attentions of a partner can have a very profound emotional effect on a lactating woman. The nipple is one of the most sensually sensitive areas on both men and women, and some women claim to be able to reach orgasm from nipple stimulation alone.

ABOVE | Total arousal starts with the senses: the taste of skin mingled with good wine, the sound of breathing against soft music, the sight of face and body in a candlelit room. Satisfaction involves sight, hearing, taste and smell as well as touch sensations.

the internal female sex organs

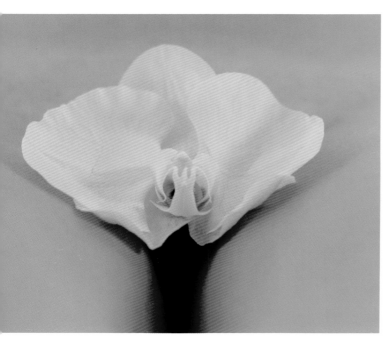

American sex researchers found that the vaginal walls are also responsible for the secretion of the love juices that are released during arousal. These juices lubricate the movements of sex, minimizing friction, which might be painful. Some women secrete more juice than others, and some even climax with the same liquid ferocity as men.

the cervix

Commonly known as the neck of the womb, the cervix connects the vagina and the uterus via a narrow tunnel that runs through the cervix and into the opening of the uterus. During intercourse the cervix drops down to help the sperm travel up the canal, into the uterus, on its way to the egg. The cervix is sometimes blocked with a mucous plug to protect the uterus from infection. This mucus thins during ovulation to allow sperm to enter the uterus. In the last stages of labour, the cervix has the ability to open wide enough to allow the passage of the baby.

It is important that women are aware of their cervixes and problems that may occur. Regular Pap or smear tests are vital in sexually active women.

the uterus

Also called the womb, the uterus is about the same size as a woman's clenched fist. It is composed of several layers of tissue and muscle. The inner lining, or endometrium, builds up over a month and then sheds during menstruation, keeping the environment clean and regenerated. The myometrium lies next to the endometrium and comprises powerful muscular tissue that contracts during both labour and orgasm. As oestrogen levels dwindle away during the menopause, the uterus decreases in size.

the fallopian tubes

The fallopian tubes link the ovaries to the uterus, branching out to lie symmetrically next to the outer wall of the uterus. They are about 10cm/4in

ABOVE | The female sexual organs, especially the vulva, have often been described as a flower. Women artists such as Georgia O'Keeffe and Judy Chicago have used the flower as a metaphor for the female pudenda in their work.

THESE ARE THE PARTS of a woman's body that are not immediately visible, but understanding them is crucial for health and sexual satisfaction.

the vagina

Vagina in Latin translates to mean sheath. True to its name, the main purpose of the vagina is to fit snugly around the penis, encouraging the safe passage of sperm to their final destination. The average vaginal canal is between 7.5cm/3in and 10cm/4in in length, although it is sometimes slightly longer in women who have had children. The muscular tissue inside the vagina allows for expansion and contraction, as it has to be able to open wide enough for a baby's head to pass through. During sexual excitement, the walls of the vagina balloon and extend, as well as contracting around the penis during orgasm.

in length and, at one end, they have finger-like projections which stroke the surface of the ovaries in order to pick up an egg before drawing it down the tube. If fertilization occurs, the first stage usually develops in the fallopian tube.

Until fairly recently, women needed at least one healthy tube to have a baby, although now microsurgery to unblock the tubes and IVF have helped to overcome these problems.

the ovaries

The ovaries are small, pinkish-white organs that lie in the pelvic area. They are about 3cm/1¼in long and 2cm/¾in wide and contain around 100,000 eggs each (formed before birth), but release only one a month, during ovulation. The ovaries are also responsible for the release of oestrogen and progesterone, hormones that play a vital role in the menstrual cycle.

the pelvic floor muscle

This is the powerful pubococcygeus muscle that supports the pelvic floor and the reproductive organs. During orgasm it contracts. By keeping your pelvic floor muscles well exercised you will reap the benefits in the bedroom, as deliberately contracting them during sex induces a pleasant "milking" sensation around your partner's penis.

Maintaining strong pelvic floor muscles also helps with childbirth and a speedy recovery. Pilates classes teach women to exercise their pelvic floor muscles, although there are numerous exercises that can be done independently. The beauty is that you can do them any time, anywhere and no one can tell what you're up to. To test your pelvic floor muscles try to stop your flow of urine for ten seconds and then continue. If you can achieve this, your pelvic muscles are quite strong; if not, a few minutes' exercising a day may save problems later.

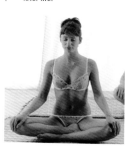

BELOW | Regular exercise of the pelvic floor muscles will be a benefit now, as well as in later life.

the internal female sex organs

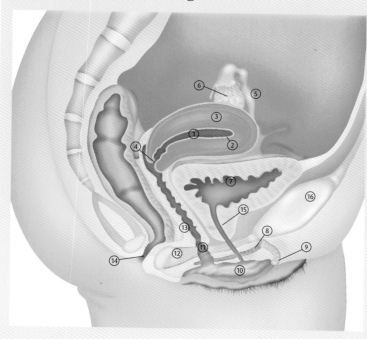

1   Uterus
2   Endometrium
3   Myometrium
4   Cervix
5   Fallopian tubes
6   Ovaries
7   Bladder
8   Crus
9   Clitoral shaft and glans
10 Labia majora and minora
11 Vagina
12 Pubococcygeus muscle
13 G spot
14 Anus
15 Urethra
16 Pubic bone

sexploration

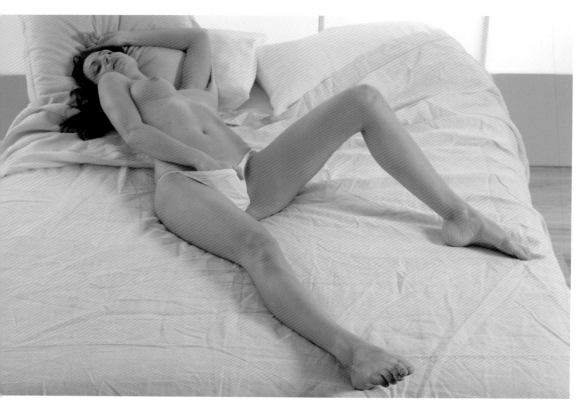

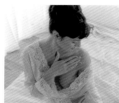

TOP | It is a natural progression to explore and take things further.

ABOVE | Look after your skin by using body moisturizers.

IT IS AMAZING how many women are unaware of where their organs are and how they work. This is where some intimate personal inspection with a small hand-held mirror in a quiet, undisturbed room becomes invaluable.

By asking your partner to join you, you can also introduce him to your personal playground, not only educating you both, but setting the perfect scene for some fun. Not only will this benefit you in understanding more about yourself as a sexual person, but it is also an excellent exercise that can help you to recognize the signs and symptoms that may indicate health problems in the future.

mirror image

An empty house and some free time provide the perfect opportunity to introduce yourself to yourself. Stand in front of a full-length mirror for a long time and look at your naked body. Acknowledge your unique sexiness. Notice the creases, the lines, the roundness and touch of your skin.

Compliment yourself on your attributes and concentrate on what looks good. Instead of grimacing at the parts you are not so keen on, try to view them in a positive light. A round protruding belly, for example, can either be seen as fat and unattractive, or a sign of femininity and fertility. Move your body around, sitting, kneeling and standing. Watch how your body moves and how your muscles and tendons work together. Gently touch your nipples, run your forefingers around them, pinch them gently between your forefinger and thumb, gradually increasing the pressure to see if you enjoy the sensation.

Grab the trusty hand-held mirror and find a comfortable position to sit. Spread your legs, with the mirror angled so that you can clearly see and examine yourself. You will need to separate your labia in order to access your clitoris. To see your clitoris more clearly you may also need to pull back the clitoral hood, but remember this is a sensitive area, so handle with care.

Move your hands and fingers around your vaginal area, working out which areas are more sensitive than others. Don't ignore your anus and perineum, as for some women these are really exciting hot spots. Soon you and your delicate sexual organs should be thoroughly acquainted and you may then feel that you want to take the relationship a step further.

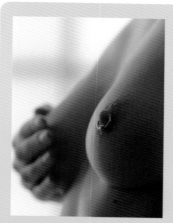

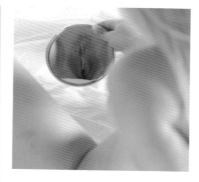

LEFT | Get that mirror out and have a look.

BELOW | Get to know how you like to be stimulated by trying it out for yourself.

breast checking

Lie flat or stand with one arm raised above your head. With your opposite hand, use the pads of your fingertips to massage the breast area, using small circular movements to check for any bumps or other abnormalities.

Put your raised arm back by your side and, using the opposite hand again, check the armpit area for lumps or swellings. Then repeat the whole process on the opposite side.

If you do find something *don't panic*. Visit your doctor for advice and remember that not all lumps are a sign of something sinister: often they are just fatty tissue deposits, but it's better to be safe than sorry.

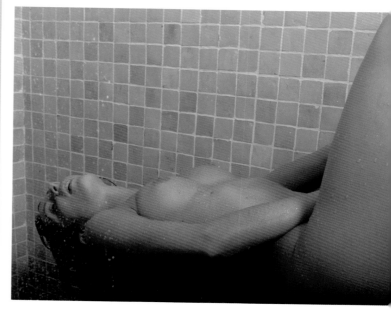

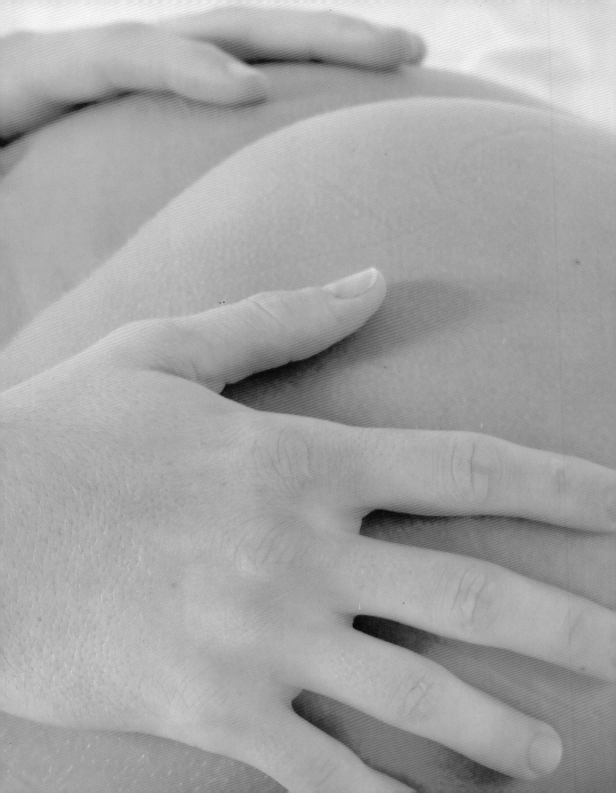

seduction

Seduction is the subtle art of exploring the chemistry that exists between you and then using it to the best possible advantage. It includes romance, persuasion and temptation, and doesn't stop after the first thrills of a relationship. The art of seduction also includes the post-coital afterglow – the comfort of lying together after sex – as well as recognizing that you may want to seduce a member of the same, rather than the opposite, sex.

the importance of seduction

A BOOK ON SEXUAL TECHNIQUES focuses a great deal on the physical aspects of sexual relationship, making it easy to ignore other essential elements such as romance and seduction. But sex is not just about the physical. Unlike most animals, humans have sex not just for procreation, but for relaxation, comfort, recreation and love.

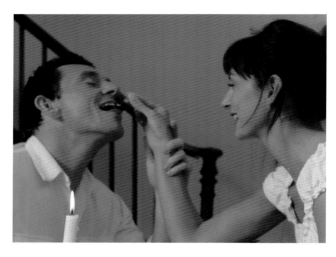

As the most complex organisms in the animal kingdom, humans need to have the erotic epicentre of the body – the brain – stimulated when preparing themselves for sex. Forget the clitoris, the G-spot, the penis and the prostate; if you're not in the mood, you're not in the mood, and this is controlled by the brain.

The true foundations of sensuality, sexual enjoyment and fulfilment are laid in the brain; the attic of your body rather than the basement. Preparation, anticipation and relaxation all start in the head, making mental stimulation an essential component of foreplay.

irresistible temptation

Dating, romancing, courting and flirting may seem a bit old-fashioned to some people, but even the most hardened cynic melts when a certain tune is played on the radio, igniting an old memory of a past relationship or a particularly memorable episode of a present one.

It is at the stage of the relationship, when you are in love, that the senses are at their most heightened; the sky seems bluer, flowers seem to smell sweeter, everything tastes better and even jokes are funnier. Great memories are made during this period of getting to know one another. Smells are particularly evocative: the scent someone uses, the aroma of freshly baked bread when you first went shopping together, even the smell of a certain brand of coffee can all have an effect. Let's face it, the thrills and delights of sex are about much more than physical pleasure alone, however wonderful that may be.

Romance doesn't have to be all flowers, teddy bears and soppy letters, but at the beginning of a relationship, it is the grounding from which all your other memories with that person will blossom. It is a sad fact that the better you get to know someone, the more complacent you are likely to become about romantic gestures, so the scope for these gestures is quite limited.

ABOVE AND RIGHT | In the first stages of a relationship you think of little else but each other. Senses are alive with anticipation and you lavish each other with romantic and thoughtful gestures.

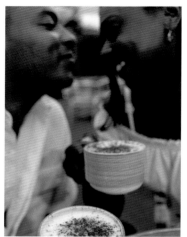

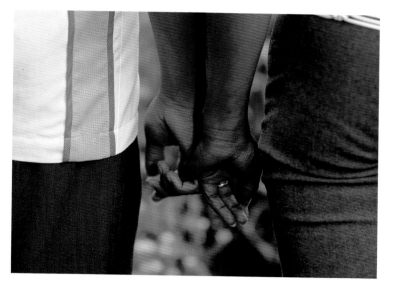

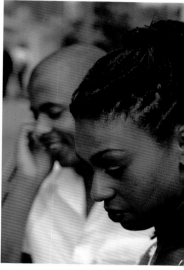

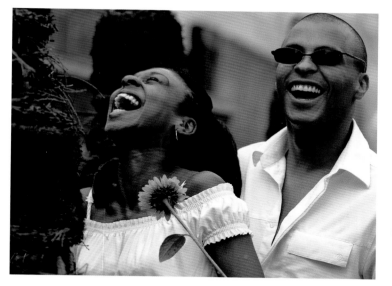

ABOVE LEFT | In the first flush of mutual attraction, simply touching hands or intertwining your fingers can send shivers of delight through you.

ABOVE RIGHT | Don't make the mistake of ignoring your date – they deserve your full attention.

LEFT | Giving a small token such as a flower may seem old-fashioned, but shows that you care.

Romancing can start before you have even become established partners, let alone had sex, with phone calls, text messages, notes, letters and emails. Small, thoughtful gestures often have a far greater impact than large, lavish ones. Show that you are getting to understand your new partner and potential lover, that you listen to what they say and that you care about what they want and like by buying the CD that you heard them mention, or an interesting book, her favourite flowers, his favourite beer, or some other small token just "because it reminded me of you".

kissing

rubbing noses

Although Europeans have been kissing for a couple of thousand years, it's believed that the practice may well have originated in India. Vedic Sanskrit texts from about 1500BC describe the custom of rubbing and pressing noses together. This type of greeting, often called "Eskimo" kissing, is also associated with the Inuit and with Pacific islanders. The lips don't actually touch; what is really happening is that each person literally inhales the odour of the scent glands on the cheeks of the other person. Animals do it all the time. Have you ever noticed that cats often rub their faces against their human pals as well as their feline friends?

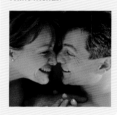

YOU CAN USUALLY TELL what sort of lover someone will be by the way they kiss. After all, kissing is usually your first moment of real sexual contact. While kissing, you literally get to taste and smell what is on offer. Kissing is not a universal custom; many remote cultures hadn't a clue about it until Europeans arrived and showed them what to do.

The tongue and lips are two of the most sensitive erogenous areas of the body, packed with nerve endings. When you kiss with passion, it releases a chemical in the brain similar to those engendered by extreme sports, such as skydiving or parachuting. Called neurotransmitters, these chemicals attach to pleasure receptors in the brain, resulting in euphoria, fluttering in your belly and a feeling of elation. Even if there isn't a grand passion when you kiss, it may still create an enjoyable physical sensation.

There's a whole repertoire of kissing you can try out while you explore your lover's erogenous zones. Not all passionate kisses have to involve tickling each other's tonsils. An almost imperceptible brush of the lips can be just as exciting.

lip sync

Most people like the idea of kissing someone with smooth and shapely lips, a generous smile and good teeth. Bad teeth are one of the ultimate turn-offs. Lip size doesn't indicate whether someone is a good kisser or not, but some mouths are just so kissable. It could be the shape, the smile or the fullness of the lips or even the way the person wets their lips with their tongue.

A survey carried out on kissing showed that women like kissing better than men and enjoy the whole long, lingering embrace, without it

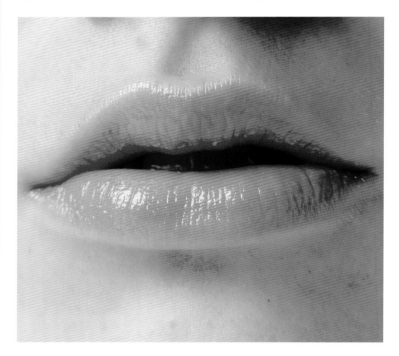

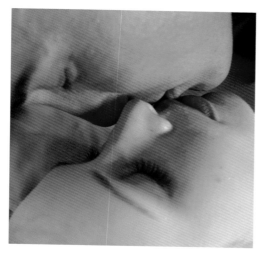
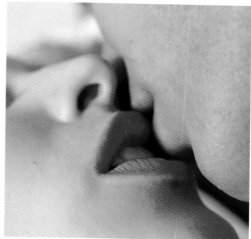

necessarily leading to anything else. In fact, some women have said that they find kissing the most erotic part of sex and have often had an orgasm just from a passionate session of kissing.

Men, on the other hand, do enjoy kissing but seem to see it as a necessary part of the ritual required to get to intercourse. Of course, lots of men, especially British and American men, hate public displays of affection. Mediterranean men seem to love kissing in public, though. They kiss their wives, mothers, girlfriends, kids, fathers and male pals with equal fervour. They even kiss three times on the cheek in greeting, instead of two.

Apart from the mouth and cheeks, there are loads of other places on the body that are just begging to be kissed – eyelids, nose, ears, neck (delicious), armpit (yes really), insides of wrists, fingertips, backs of knees, ankles, soles and toes, and lots more places in between. The best way to find out is to go on a kissing tour of your lover, working your way around the whole body.

kissing asides

What differentiates an average kisser from an exemplary kisser? That's the million dollar question. A relaxed mouth and an open mind are good places to begin. As to where to go from there, here are a few suggestions:

French kissing Gently caress the inside of your partner's mouth with your tongue. As he or she responds, you can quicken the pace and intensity, going for a fuller thrust.

chicken kisses Great for relaxation and moments of tenderness. Purse your lips and then plant a light kiss, a little like a peck, but at the rate of about three a second. It's between a kiss and a tickle really, but feels good. A good nose wrinkler.

silent but deadly Some of the sexiest kisses are the silent ones, lips and eyes closed, caressing each other's hair, face and neck with your hands.

stereophonic kiss Moan or slurp while you're kissing. Some people adore the sound and sensation of the inside of their ears being kissed – the sloshing sound really turns them on.

talking kiss Hold your partner's face between your hands and kiss different parts of their face, first each eyebrow, then eyelids, nose and so on, and between each kiss say something erotic. Describe what you are going to do to them, how you want them to kiss or lick you, where, and what position you want to try.

nibbling Don't bite, it hurts. Nuzzling, on the other hand, is delightful.

callcards Don't. Love bites are not exciting.

butterfly kiss Tried and tested. Use your eyelashes to brush against your partner's face or body.

ABOVE | A kiss has so many facets: security, love and comfort, as well as passion.

BELOW | Exploring the many different ways to kiss your new partner, from deeply passionate to lightly teasing or blowing, is a totally thrilling experience.

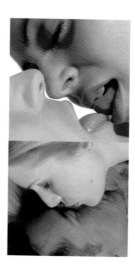

foreplay

REMEMBER THOSE TIMES growing up, before penetrative sex was *de rigeur*? Those steamy sessions in the car or cinema, the way you stroked each other's hands, walking along totally absorbed and wrapped up in each other? Those emotions and sensations were very exciting, in some ways better than sex itself. Foreplay is like looking through a keyhole and seeing how you will both fit together as lovers. It's a means of exploring each other physically and sensually, setting guidelines and maybe even boundaries, likes and dislikes, wants and needs. You are learning and working out ways to relax and please one another.

Asking what feels good and what your partner wants is the only way to fulfil both yourself and your partner sexually. When you indulge in foreplay, imagine you are a tourist on a body tour, asking directions to various destinations. Many people begin by caressing in a way that they would like to be caressed themselves, which is a good starting point as long as you are flexible enough to adapt to the preferences of your partner.

RIGHT | Take the time to undress each other slowly if you can bear the anticipation.

BELOW | Stroke and kiss using bold and confident movements and you will arouse your partner to fever pitch.

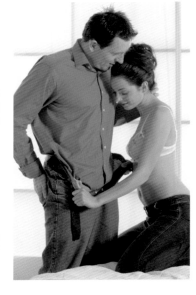

talking dirty

The idea of talking dirty fills some people with disgust. Others love it and actively incorporate it into their sexual repertoire. Still more people think that they might quite like it but would feel rather silly doing it.

Talking dirty doesn't necessarily mean putting your mouth up against your partner's ear and shrieking a string of four letter expletives. You can start with some encouraging oohs and ahhs when he or she is doing something particularly pleasurable to you. When you feel comfortable with this, progress to whispering things like, "You make me feel so sexy when you do that," or, "You taste so good." Fundamentally, talking dirty is an excellent form of sexual communication, in which you actively praise your partner for what he or she is doing.

If you feel stupid saying that this or that feels great, remember how you feel when he or she says it to you. The likelihood is that you don't cringe, but feel good that you are the source of so much pleasure. If you speak a foreign language, you might lose your inhibitions talking dirty in French or Spanish.

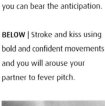

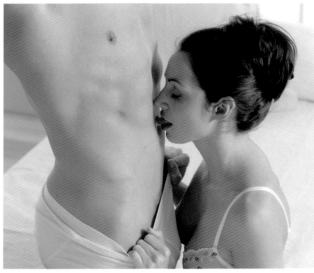

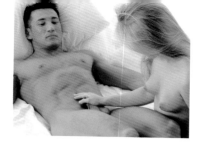

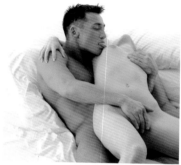

tried and tested

Foreplay doesn't have to start in the bedroom but can begin hours before. It could be a knowing look at a party, a naughty text message while you are at work or even an unexpected note in your pocket saying, "You're going to get some tonight."

As foreplay is in many ways the most exciting part of sex, it's fun to prolong it for as long as possible. Your partner and you should take time over this opportunity to indulge each other, caressing each other's bodies and enjoying the time you have together. You and your partner will enjoy sex so much more if the body is fully aroused, and moist, before coitus.

Start with the undressing. All too often, couples see clothes as an awkward barrier that must be removed quickly. However, it's very sexy to watch your loved one remove his or her own clothes. If you're feeling cheeky, put some music on and treat your partner to a long, slow, sexy striptease. He is guaranteed to adore it and she is bound to find it highly amusing, especially if he uses a hat at the end. It's also erotic to remove each other's clothes, taking it in turns to remove an item.

Kissing can set the pace for the type of lovemaking you both want to indulge in. Try a slow, loving kiss, caressing each other's mouths

with your tongues, or a more passionate, frenzied kiss where you are slightly rougher and more urgent with each other. Small kisses all over your lover's body will make them go wild with desire.

Try not to go straight for each other's genitals, but explore other parts of each other's bodies – fingers, toes, armpits and belly buttons – first. Really tantalize each other with massaging hand strokes and tender licks and kisses. Eventually you may end up stimulating each other almost to orgasm, until you cannot stand it any more, and then one thing can lead to another, if you are ready.

Foreplay should not just be a means to an end, but enjoyed for the pleasure it gives in its own right. This includes emotional foreplay as well as sexual. Touching, undressing and small kindnesses throughout the day are just as important as your wrist action.

The strokes and techniques you and your partner prefer are as individual as you are and will vary, depending on your mood, what sort of day you have had, and even the weather. Take some tips from the sections on masturbation in this book for more detailed instruction. The secret to good foreplay is simple. Take your time, and don't rush yourself or your partner. If you take half an hour to massage your partner's inner thigh, don't expect reciprocation. You should enjoy doing it as much as he or she enjoys receiving it. It will be your turn to be pleasured the next time.

tantric sex

These ancient teachings appreciate the differences in arousal times between men and women and aim to harmonize these differences by focusing on the female right to reach sexual arousal and teaching men to curb their passion.

One of the main teachings is the retention of the male orgasm, which according to Tantra weakens the life energy with each ejaculate. Men are taught to moderate their breathing and draw orgasmic energy towards the brain, thus allowing for a greater sense of spiritual realization. Extended foreplay is at the forefront of tantric loving, encouraging strengthened emotional connection through holding, caressing and eye contact.

ABOVE LEFT | Of course, touching each other's genitals is not off-limits, but bring your other senses, such as sight and taste, into play as well.

BELOW | Who could possibly have guessed that the film *The Full Monty* would have got quite so many hats off the hatstand?

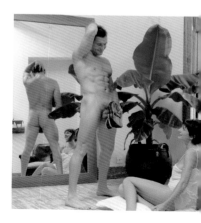

erogenous zones

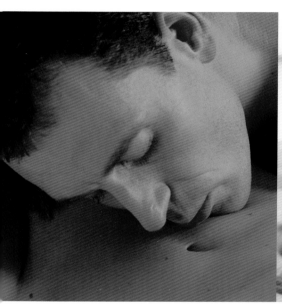
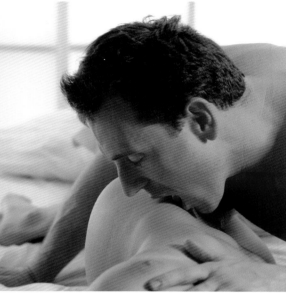

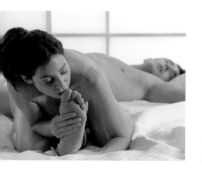

HOW OFTEN HAS YOUR partner absently stroked the back of your neck while watching television, sending electrifying spasms through your body? For a truly sensual experience, take yourself on a body voyage, concentrating more on the journey than the destination. Consider your partner's body as a luscious and varied landscape with an array of areas yet to be explored.

With sex it's all too easy to concentrate on the obvious: the testicles, clitoris, penis and breasts, but these make up a relatively small proportion of the bigger picture. It's often the less obvious areas that yield the most heated results. Touching and caressing all of each other's bodies can produce feelings that are not just sexual. The right touch can make you feel warm all over and reaffirm the deep-rooted feelings of love and care that you have for one another. Focusing on other parts of the body during foreplay shows that you find your partner sexy all over and not just at the hotspots.

the navel

The skin around the navel is a lot thinner, making it an extremely sensitive area. Belly buttons have taken on a new lease of life since they have begun to be decorated with tattoos and navel rings or studs. Some people are a bit squeamish about their belly buttons, but others enjoy having their navels caressed by a soft tongue. It may make them giggle a bit, but after all, this is meant to be fun.

the toe job

This is one of those things you either love or hate. Some people find the idea of placing a set of toes anywhere near their lips revolting, whereas others find it a real turn on. If cleanliness is an issue for you, then why not treat your partner to a pre-toe-job pedicure? Providing he or she is not too ticklish, the pedicure process can be very relaxing. Alternatively, encourage your partner to have a bath and a good scrub beforehand and then

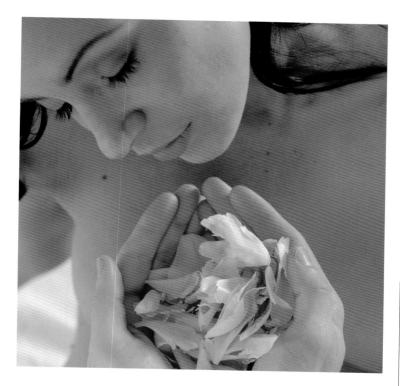

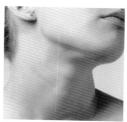

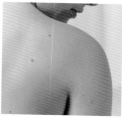

ABOVE | Stroking your partner's neck creates a tingling feeling of warmth along the spine.

ABOVE LEFT | Smell is one of the most powerful senses. Use the beautiful fragrance of flower petals or scented candles to create the mood.

BELOW | The male nipple is a sensitive erogenous zone that responds to a delicate touch.

moisturize their feet. It's surprising how you can begin to see feet as a seriously sexy zone, once you start to take care of them. It will start to look as if all those foot fetishists can't be wrong.

instep

For those who can bear to have their feet touched without collapsing in hysterics, the instep of the foot is a sensitive, nerve-rich area that can be licked and stroked. Many people love to have their feet massaged and pampered and the feet can also be used as an interesting and different way to stimulate other areas, but make sure they're warmed up first.

back of neck

There is something strangely comforting and at the same time sensually delightful about having the back of your neck stroked. It sends a mixture of warm and thrilling shock waves along the entire length of your spine, leaving you feeling energized and loved. This is a very relaxing and loving place to caress your partner, as it has a mysterious link to his or her sensual centres.

armpit

No one is suggesting that you bury your face in your partner's armpits just as he or she leaves the gym, but think just how sensitive your armpits are. They are a veritable minefield of nerve endings and after a bath or shower they respond well to some gentle caressing and tingling licks.

fingers

The fingers are an understandably popular focus of attention, not least because the tips are so sensitive. During a romantic meal you may feed each other, licking and sucking the juices from fingers and wrists. The act of sucking fingers is so erotic because it is loaded with innuendo.

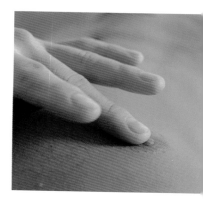

sensual massage

RESEARCH HAS SHOWN that the art of massage and touch has therapeutic effects on people, both physically and emotionally. The skin is the largest organ in the body, feeding the brain with information on our external environment, and if it is caressed gently and lovingly, then the brain will also relax and unwind. After a stressful day, massaging your partner allows you some time to wind down and enjoy each other's company.

Being massaged in a brightly lit room with blaring rock music may appeal to some, but for true sensuality it is better to dim the lights or even use candles, prepare some aromatic oils and put on some relaxing background music.

Have a warm, not hot, shower beforehand and make sure the room is warm enough. Both you and your partner must be comfortable, so the bed or the floor are usually the best places for a massage. Massaging in front of – but not too close to – an open fire is also extremely sensual, as the warmth and flickering light from the flames, combined with the soft crackle of burning wood, ignite the earthy and primal instincts in you.

basic technique

The secret to a good massage is to maintain a constant confident touch, using flowing unbroken strokes. Experiment with different pressures and

BELOW | Although massage is not necessarily a precursor to sex, it can set the scene and get you in the mood.

BELOW RIGHT | Gentle breast massage is a wonderfully sensual experience for both of you during foreplay.

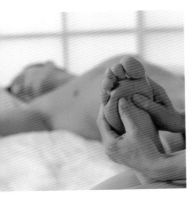

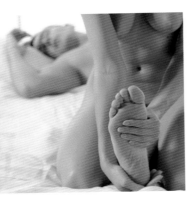

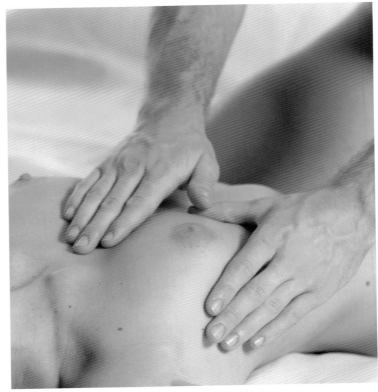

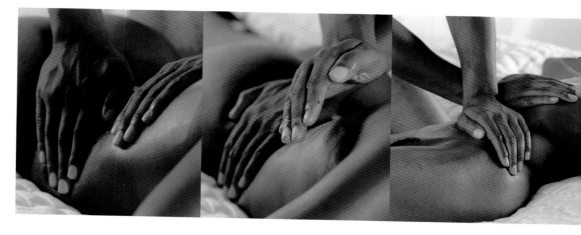

speeds, exploring a range of different techniques and communicating with each other as to what feels most delightful.

To lubricate the areas that you intend to massage, pour some blended oil in your hands, rubbing them together to warm them up. Apply enough oil so that your hands glide smoothly over the surface of your partner's body, but remember that a little goes a long way.

circle strokes

These stretch out the muscles, releasing tension from the soft tissues. They are best applied to broad surfaces, such as the back, thighs, chest and belly. Place both hands on the body, flat and side

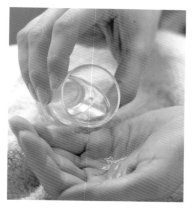

by side. Lead with your right hand and move them in a clockwise direction, using a constant, fairly gentle pressure.

fanning strokes

These strokes also release tension from the soft tissue and are ideal on the back, as it is a large broad surface. To fan upwards, place both hands flat at the base of the spine on each side of the spine. Glide them both up, concentrating pressure in your palm before fanning out to the sides of the body. From here, mould your hands around the sides of your partner's body and drag them down to the base again.

kneading strokes

These are ideal for fleshy areas, such as the buttocks and thighs, releasing tension from the larger muscles. Imagine that you are kneading dough by squeezing a portion of flesh in your fingers and then rolling it from one hand to the other and back again.

percussion strokes

Rapid strokes that create a vibrating sensation help to improve skin tone and circulation to nerve endings. Hacking involves a series of chopping movements, with alternate hands concentrating on the same area. The wrists must remain relaxed, so the action is bouncy rather than stiff.

ABOVE | With circle strokes, keep both hands next to each other, so your right hand will have to pass over the left.

BELOW LEFT | Warm some oil in your hands to avoid the shock of a cold touch.

BELOW | Percussion strokes can be fun, but be gentle.

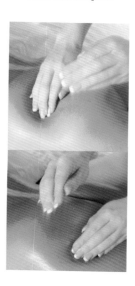

post-coital

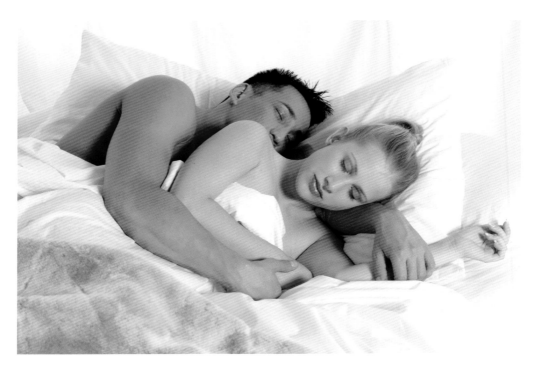

SEDUCTION DOESN'T STOP when the sex does. After sex is a time for cuddling, snuggling up and also sleeping – a time of lying together, perhaps talking, and certainly still enjoying each other's bodies. You continue to make love by caressing each other. The orgasm isn't the end of the process: touching is the ultimate way to complete the act of making love.

On the other hand, there is the thorny question of men who fall asleep immediately after sex. Most women find it exasperating if their partners roll over with their backs towards them and start snoring because, for them, the moments after sex are particularly precious and loving, when, lying in their partner's arms, they feel most relaxed and contented. It seems that it isn't simply physical tiredness that overcomes men just after they have

had an orgasm, although undoubtedly this is a factor. There is also a mental and emotional response. For a short while, men enter a euphoric, almost dangerously happy, fulfilled and vulnerable state. They are physically spent and their hormonal system is temporarily shut down. All their basic instincts, including by this time sexual impulses, are in abeyance and the feeling of relaxation is complete and overwhelming. If she chooses to, a woman could consider that his falling asleep is an indication of total trust.

Of course, there are no absolute rules and many men don't fall asleep and do like to talk after sex. Some light a cigarette, others switch on the radio. Naturally, it is usually in the early stages of a relationship that men make the most effort to please their partners after sex. Falling asleep

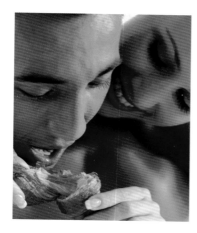

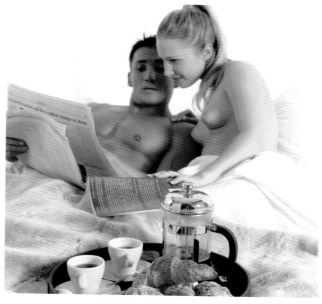

immediately is more typical of a long-term relationship because a man feels secure enough to do so. Women behave slightly differently. Some will fall asleep quickly or may not feel like talking, but most like cuddling up. Whatever happens, lying together in the "spoons" position or falling asleep in each other's arms can give you both a feeling of closeness, security and peace.

enjoying the afterglow

According to the *Kama Sutra*, lovemaking hasn't finished until the man has rubbed sandalwood ointment on to his partner's body. They should then eat sweetmeats and drink fresh juice, while enjoying the moonlight and an agreeable conversation. Finally, as the woman turns her face towards the moon, the man gives her a lesson in astronomy, pointing out the different planets.

Perhaps stargazing is not such a fabulous idea, but eating after sex is truly divine. You can have breakfast, lunch and dinner in bed and it's easy to prepare a delicious selection of fruits, chocolates, savoury nibbles and wine or champagne

beforehand to enjoy post-coitally. And if you have no veranda, there's no moon and it's freezing outside, how about taking a bath together? Put some lovely scented lotion in the bath, create an atmosphere, perhaps put candles around the bathroom, and slide in. Make time in your busy lives for some special time together.

Many women are able to enjoy more than one orgasm and men may also want to go in for another session. All men require some recovery time – even very young, fit men usually need about 20 minutes before trying again. This time of lying together, talking and enjoying each other's bodies can sometimes lead to a surprise, especially if the woman starts licking her partner's penis, and, of course, repeating penetrative sex is not the only option.

ABOVE LEFT | Sharing something to eat after sex is a deliciously sensuous experience and may even refuel your energies for more.

ABOVE RIGHT | Making love, then enjoying a lazy breakfast in bed reading the weekend newspapers is one of life's greatest pleasures.

BELOW | Enjoy a long and indulgent bubble bath together, prolonging the intimacy of touch after you have made love.

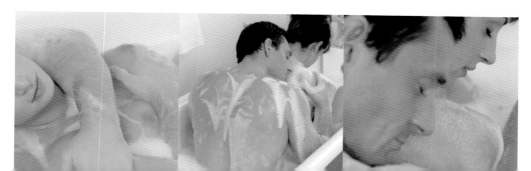

pillow talk

COMMUNICATION IS KEY even in the shortest relationships – it is important that you let the other person know what you are expecting. This is not just to avoid misunderstandings, but also in order to get what you want.

What are your sexual preferences? Are there things you really don't like your partner doing, but are unwilling to mention in case they feel criticized? Are there things you would love your partner to try, but are still too embarrassed to mention? Is there something slightly perverse that you would like to do during sex, but are afraid to broach it in case you seem a little weird?

Being intimate and speaking about your innermost feelings is generally difficult for both men and women. In an ideal world, we would be able to tell each other everything but, in reality, few people actually do, especially if there is a problem, until they have to deal with the subject. It takes time, sometimes years, to build up trust

within a relationship and to discuss your innermost fantasies, fears and needs. Over this period, you can begin to know by verbal and body language what your lover enjoys or dislikes at certain times because you know them very well.

sexual communication

A good place for intimate chats is obviously the bedroom or lying cosily together on the sofa. The best way to tell your partner about your likes and dislikes is by affirmation – "I love it when you touch me there," or "It feels better this way." Direct criticism can be very intimidating and upsetting, so it is best avoided, but describing what you didn't like in previous sexual relationships may be constructive: "I felt embarrassed when my previous lover used to talk dirty when we were making love," or "The way my previous wife bit me each time she had an orgasm was really irritating." However, intimate disclosures about previous partners can

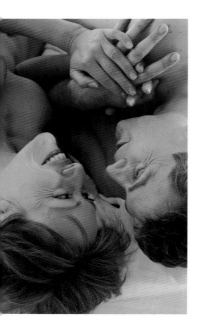

BELOW | Communication is the essence of a mutually satisfying sex life. It can be heartbreaking if you have a problem that can easily be resolved but you are afraid to discuss it with each other.

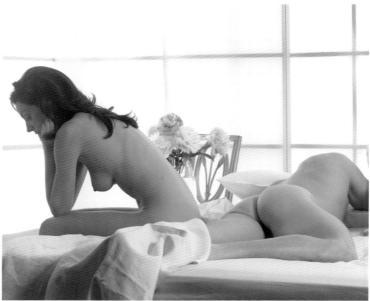

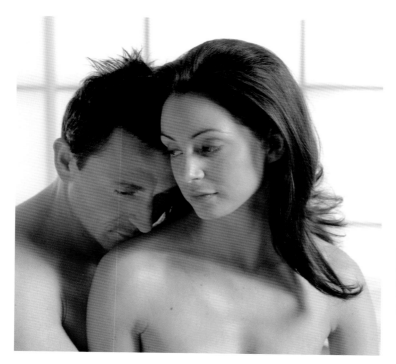

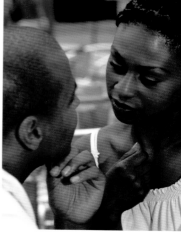

also upset current ones and a long list of differently skilled lovers is not recommended. Apart from anything else, it is likely to be interpreted as a comparative scale. You have to gauge your partner's response and act accordingly, remembering to build on the positive aspects of your relationship.

Theoretically, the longer you are with someone, the easier it should be to discuss your needs. However, all sexual relationships change over time and just because the sex was vigorous during the first year doesn't mean it will be during the tenth. Continuing communication and co-operation is vital, especially when you have to deal with problems. If left unresolved, problems can eat into the relationship, creating rifts between you. If the problem is shared, however, then she won't feel resentful or frustrated and he won't feel upset and to blame – or vice versa.

Some serious issues, such as bisexuality, might come out as a bolt from the blue at a later stage in a relationship, and that can be quite devastating

for the uninformed partner, if the subject has never been broached before. Besides the nature of the discovery, a major secret can seem like a betrayal. There are no instant solutions for the big sexual surprises, but it is important to be aware that professional support is available and if you are faced with something really challenging, you should seek advice to help you get to grips with the implications for the relationship. As always, it is far better to confront issues as they arise, rather than to let them fester.

If you are treating each other badly in general, then your sex life will probably be dire. There is no drug in the world that will cure a relationship problem like this as you get older. One of the most successful ways of keeping an intimate relationship flourishing is by being best friends. You may end up having sex only once a week or twice a month or much less frequently, but being respectful, loving and open with one another is the key. Honesty really is the best policy.

ABOVE | Sex is just an extension of a relationship. Communication is the key. So make sure you are clear about what you need and expect for yourself.

gay sex

RIGHT | Best friends can be lovers as well.

BELOW AND BELOW RIGHT | Giving and receiving pleasure and relishing each other's sexuality is at the heart of all relationships between couples, whatever their sex.

THIS BOOK IS written primarily from a heterosexual point of view, but what do you do if you find you are attracted or seduced by a member of the same sex? It is worth noting that gay sex, both male and female, is not so very different from so-called straight sex – the relationships have many of the same problems, the partners have many of the same feelings and the sexual techniques are pretty similar. Society's attitude, however, is still quite mixed and this can impose additional pressures on gay partners.

coming out

Telling the family often poses a problem. Not everyone's family consists of middle-class liberals with a pansexual view of the world. In fact, it will probably take time for most parents to come to terms with the fact that their child is gay.

Although some families are truly homophobic, most will ultimately support their kids. The first reaction is often, "I'm never going to become a grandparent," then, "What about AIDS?" But

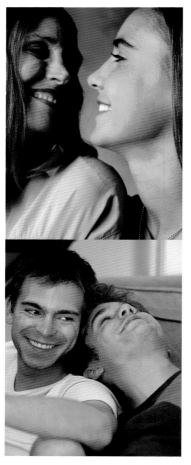

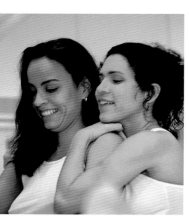

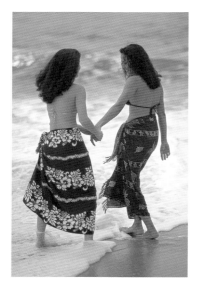

overall, the most common worry is, "Where are they going to meet someone who will help them have a stable and happy life?" If you can't manage to tell your family face to face, it's often a good idea to write to them. Reassure them that whatever your sexual preferences are you are still the same person they know and love. It's no big deal. There are support groups that can help families through this tricky stage.

Whether you are still at school, college or in the workplace, check the organization's policy on privacy before telling anyone – friend, teacher or fellow staff. In some instances, they may be legally obliged to tell someone else. Before you know it, a confidence could become a juicy story – people in groups are natural gossips, whether they mean to be or not.

Never come out when you are high or drunk – you may regret it the next day. Public announcements embarrass everybody. Outing someone else is, at the very least, bad manners and could cause grief and pain to a number of friends and relations. Great sensitivity is required for mature people coming out to their partners or children, as this is bound to be traumatic for all parties. Seeking advice before you approach the subject is recommended and again, there are lesbian and gay helplines with a wealth of experience in how to handle this delicate situation.

how to look after yourself

Whether you are gay or heterosexual, safer sex is the name of the game. You can acquire sexually transmitted infections (STIs) from kissing, petting and oral sex, as well as from intercourse. If you are into multiple partners, it's essential for your sake and theirs to use protection.

what gays do in bed

Gay or heterosexual, the body's erogenous zones are exactly the same and, in both cases, are not confined to the genitalia. Both gay women and men love to kiss, cuddle, massage, stroke, pet and kiss each other's erogenous zones, including nipples, arms, toes, fingers, ears, face, neck and genitalia. They masturbate each other and may indulge in fantasy, sometimes cross-dressing. Women may use strap-ons for vaginal or anal sex or insert fingers or hands. Men may have anal sex and non-penetrative sex. Gay men and women are just as likely or unlikely to indulge in S&M as heterosexual men and women. In other words, couples like to give pleasure to their partners, whatever their sex, and explore and enjoy their own sexuality.

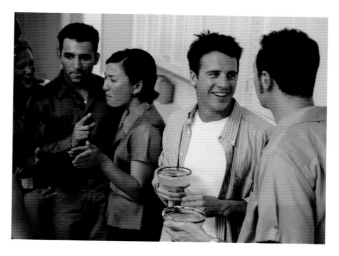

how do you know if you are gay?

The jury is still out on whether people are born with a genetic package that predetermines sexual preference or whether it's possible to be "turned into" a gay man or woman by your parenting and/or environment. The argument is still raging about nature and nurture:

"I first knew when I was a teenager and was more aroused by the men's underwear advertisements than the women's."

"I first became aware of being a gay women when I was kissed by the high school heart-throb and realized that I was more interested in the art teacher."

"I'd never enjoyed sex with my husband and thought it was just one of those things. When we split up after the children had grown up and I met Joan, it was as if someone had switched on a light in my life."

"I kind of knew that I had gay tendencies as a boy, but my parents were so religious that it just wasn't acceptable. I had some therapy before I married and then was happily married for several years. My wife and kids have been through hell since I came out, but as the years go by, we are managing to support one another and rebuild our family life."

ABOVE | Gay relationships have much in common with heterosexual ones.

BELOW | Meeting other gay people is easier today with gay clubs and the Internet.

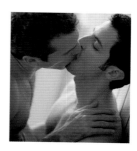

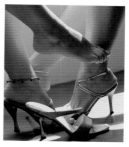

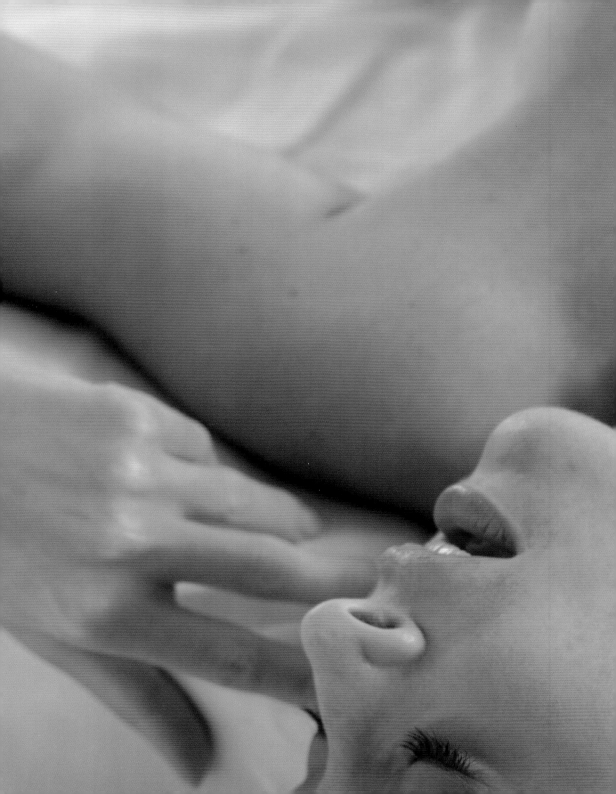

orgasm

Orgasms last seconds or minutes. They trigger divine sensations throughout the body, starting in the pelvis and genital area and sending overwhelming waves of delight rushing through you. They can make you feel relaxed, energized or exhausted, ecstatic, overjoyed or tearful, but always absolutely wonderful – and the even better news is that they are also good for you.

the big o

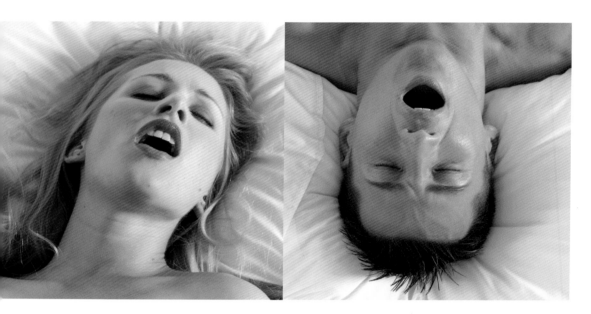

ABOVE | For both men and women, there are different ways of reaching orgasm, producing different sensations – all of them delicious.

IT IS SOMETHING that fascinates us and that we aspire to – the ecstatic shiver that we feel at the end of making love. *La petite morte* (the little death), as the French call it, is the extreme pleasure. You can have orgasms by yourself through masturbation or together with your partner.

For a man, orgasm is a relatively simple process. He becomes aroused, is stimulated to the point of no return and ejaculates, although there are techniques, notably Tantrism, for achieving orgasm without ejaculation. For women, orgasm has always been more controversial and complicated. Sigmund Freud, for example, while not denying that there was such a thing as a clitoral orgasm, believed that the most satisfying orgasm for a woman was a vaginal one, experienced through penetration by the penis. But then, how much did Freud really know about how women feel and what they experience? Since it is estimated that only around 30 per cent of women can have orgasms through intercourse alone,

Freud's insistence has made many women, who need extra clitoral stimulation to reach a climax, feel like failures. More recently, sexologists have recognized that when women have orgasms, they are as a direct result of clitoral stimulation.

more than one way…

Your orgasm will unleash different sensations according to the different methods used to reach it: masturbation, oral sex or penetration. It is often said that orgasm through masturbation, for example, is more intense than orgasm with a partner, because we ourselves know the best means of delivery. Equally, many women say that they need to feel a penis, fingers or a dildo inside them during orgasm because it makes it a more body-intense experience.

There is no one way of having the ultimate orgasm. Some men need only look at a naked woman; some women, especially during ovulation, climax while fantasizing, or even by being involved in an intellectual discussion. Everyone is different and you must explore, by yourself or with your partner, the most satisfying and exciting methods of achieving your orgasms.

different strokes

There is evidence that both men and women can experience orgasm in other parts of their bodies, not simply around their genital and pelvic areas. People who have suffered nerve damage to their genital area develop orgasmic feelings in other areas of their bodies. Some women can have an orgasm only through nipple stimulation, some men only through fellatio. Women have reported orgasms while giving birth, and breast-feeding women may experience sexual sensations as suckling induces similar uterine contractions and nipple erections to those of orgasm.

all in the head?

Orgasms also have an important psychological dimension. The brain has been described as the most important erogenous zone in the entire body. Warm, loving and positive emotional and psychological feelings towards your partner and towards making love set you directly on the path to reaching orgasm.

However, many negative emotions, such as anger at your partner or even depression over your finances, can put a damper on reaching orgasm. If either partner is having problems attaining orgasm, forget it for a while. Do other things instead, such as lots of kissing and caressing. If you get the most important element of your relationship right, being best friends, your orgasms will flow from there. Communication on both sides is necessary for mutual delight.

BELOW | What may bring a man to orgasm the quickest (rhythmic thrusting) is not necessarily the best method for achieving female orgasm. Sex is not always an intuitive practice but can be learned together.

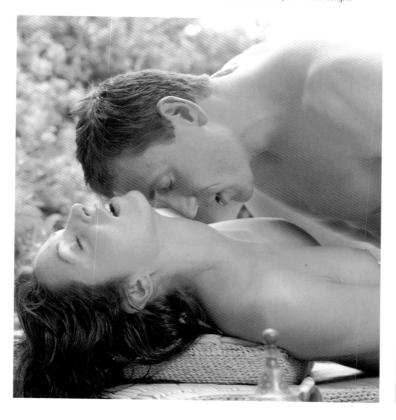

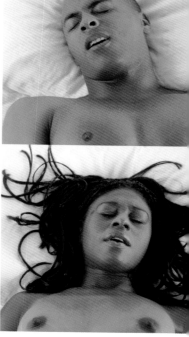

the science of orgasm

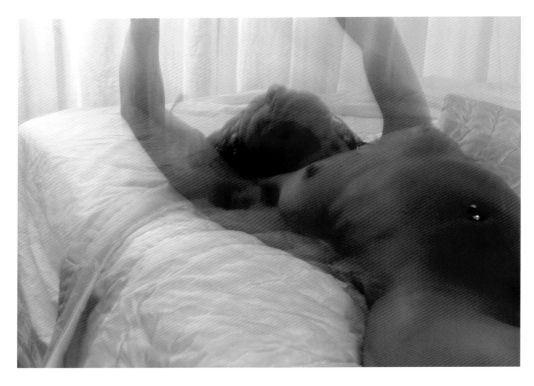

ABOVE | Orgasm is not essentially a shared experience. Most people disappear momentarily into their own worlds, which can lead to feelings of separation. A kiss and a cuddle can easily rectify this when you come back down to earth.

WHAT ACTUALLY HAPPENS during orgasm is different for each gender. However, while individual male and female responses and intensity may vary, the science of the process is the same for all men and for all women.

women

When a woman's clitoris is stimulated and she becomes aroused – the excitement phase – blood rushes to the pelvic area and her vagina becomes moist. The vagina expands and lengthens, the clitoris and breasts swell and the nipples become erect. In the plateau phase, the vaginal lips puff up further, parts of the vagina wall swell with blood and the opening to the vagina narrows. The woman's heartbeat increases, her muscles stiffen

and a pink flush may appear over her body. At this point the clitoris sometimes disappears; if the woman's partner is in the middle of stimulation, this can be a little disconcerting. Just before orgasm, the inner labia (lips) change colour.

At orgasm, the third phase, the muscular tension and engorgement of blood vessels reach a peak. When the orgasm happens, feelings of warmth and delight emanate from the body. The vaginal walls contract rhythmically for a few seconds and tension is released. The number and intensity of the contractions vary. Stimulation of the G-spot can induce female ejaculation of a liquid similar to male prostate fluid. The muscles of the uterus also contract, pulling up the sperm to help them find their way to the right place.

In the fourth phase, resolution, the genitals return to normal. This phase can sometimes last for up to half an hour.

men

The blissful sensations of orgasm come, in part, from the seminal fluid exploding into the urinary passage deep in the prostate gland. Most men experience orgasm as sensation and ejaculation.

When a man becomes aroused, his penis stiffens, his heart rate increases and his muscles tighten. The most obvious sign of the build-up towards orgasm is in the penis and testicles: the veins start to bulge, the colour of the glans (head) becomes darker and the testicles rise up towards the body. Once the penis is standing at its biggest, the ridge around the head becomes extra sensitive and the man has reached the point of no return. He will then orgasm, in up to eight contractions, at around one-second intervals.

enhancing orgasm

Women are capable of having multiple orgasms, but some don't realize that they can just keep on going. Multiple orgasms come in a series of waves, one after the other.

Sequential orgasms are slightly different and come on and off after a few minutes. For both, you simply have to keep stimulating the clitoris. If it is painful to do so after orgasm, which it quite often

is, try stroking the vulva area or other parts of the body, or more penetration instead. Many women have difficulty reaching orgasm through penetration alone and need extra stimulation of the clitoris by finger or a vibrator. Try pushing your clitoris against the penis or pubic bone.

Some men say that having their testicles stroked at orgasm heightens the sensation; others love it when their nipples are sucked. The nearest a man will ever get to a multiple orgasm, though, will probably be when he's a teenager and can ejaculate several times in a row. If a man has a second orgasm within a couple of hours, the sensations can be much more intense. There is no proven medical explanation for this but one reason may be that his senses have been heightened by his first orgasm.

For men, extended sexual pleasure has to be mastered. The longer the foreplay, the more intense the orgasm. The ancient art of Tantric sex teaches men how to peak and plateau without going to orgasm immediately. It also teaches men to orgasm without ejaculation and, by moving the energy away from the penis and testicles, to have a whole body orgasm. In the meantime, try the squeeze technique. Just before orgasm, place your thumb on one side of the base of the penis and the tips of your index and middle fingers on the other side, then squeeze. This stops the blood flowing to the penis and slows everything down.

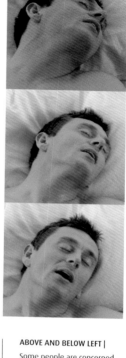

ABOVE AND BELOW LEFT |
Some people are concerned about what they look like and how they behave during orgasm. But the best orgasms are those where you throw inhibition to the wind and succumb to ecstasy.

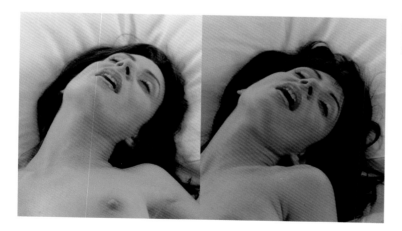

find the spot

THERE HAVE BEEN MANY CLAIMS for the miraculous orgasms that are possible from the stimulation of various areas of the body and many publications have been sold extolling their virtues, although there is no clinical proof that any of them exist.

g spot

This sensitive area, discovered by a Dr Grafenberg, is supposedly located in women on the roof of the vagina, about 5cm/2in up on the outer wall, on the tissue that surrounds the urethra. Many women say that the orgasms from G spot stimulation are really spectacular, while others report only discomfort. To stimulate this patch, insert a finger into an aroused vagina (it may be easier if you squat down). You can buy vibrators specially made for G spot stimulation. It is said to be easier to have multiple orgasms with G spot stimulation and you may experience a full body sensation. You may feel that you need to pass water when you touch this spot, so watch out – and empty your bladder first.

The male G spot is his prostate gland which, when stimulated, can produce the most wonderful orgasms, sometimes even if his penis isn't being touched. The nerve pathway from the penis to the brain runs through the rectum and a nerve centre is located beneath the prostate, so the sensations are powerful. A lubricated finger inserted into his anus – avoid long fingernails – will find the walnut-sized prostate gland about 5cm/2in up, towards the belly button. Caress this and his orgasm will be intensified.

afe zone and u spot

The AFE (anterior fornix erotic) zone is on the opposite wall of the vagina to the G spot. It is bigger, easier to access and more sensitive than

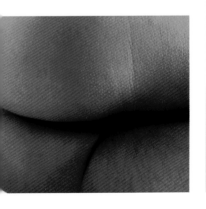

BELOW | There seems to be a spot for every letter of the alphabet, with new discoveries every day. However, they all appear to be located around the same area as the G spot, the good news being that if you miss the G spot you've a host of other potential targets.

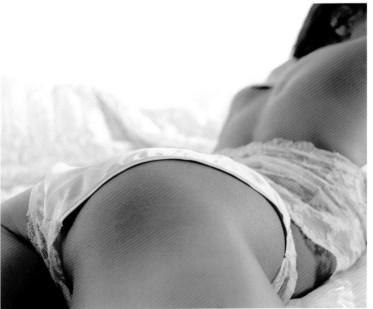

the G spot. Apart from manual stimulation, the woman can mount the man and work his penis to find the spot. Another recently hyped erotic zone is the U spot, a tiny area of external tissue above the opening of the urethra and right below the clitoris. Any stimulation here needs to be very gentle as a urinary tract infection will put a stop to any fun. The fact is that this whole area has so many nerve endings that all of it is an erogenous zone, so you can make up your own special spots.

simultaneous orgasm

This is said to be the ultimate goal of lovemaking. If it happens, then simultaneous orgasm is fantastic. However, not many couples manage it, so don't let yourself be disappointed. in fact, there are reasons why it may not be such a good idea. What about watching your partner orgasm? Isn't that the most erotic thing in the world? And if both partners are concentrating on their own orgasm, there can be a sense of dislocation in which both feel momentarily separated from the other.

faking it

It's not only women who fake orgasms. An increasing number of men are doing it too, as a result of pressure, expectation and lack of confidence. If a partner fails to orgasm, it is not a good idea to insist that you help them have one. You may be projecting your own fears on to them and seeking reassurance that you are a good lover. Just let it be for a little while. If a relationship falls apart, it is more likely to be for other emotional reasons than from difficulties in obtaining orgasm.

problems with orgasm

Anorgasmia is the inability of women to achieve orgasm, even with stimulation. It may have a physical cause, including illnesses, such as advanced diabetes, or if you are on certain medication, have hormone deficiencies or anorexia. It is also caused by a rare condition called vaginismus, an involuntary spasm of the muscles surrounding the vaginal opening. The spasm makes it very difficult, or even impossible, for a penis to enter. If you think you have a

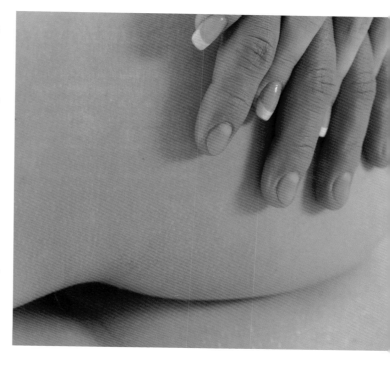

physical problem, check with your gynaecologist. For the majority of women who can't orgasm, it is generally for a psychological reason. A number of cultural, social or relationship issues may be involved – anxiety, control issues within a relationship, past sexual abuse, or a fear of being penetrated. It can also have roots in your religious or moral upbringing. Remember, too, that reaching orgasm may just take time at the beginning of a relationship, especially if a woman is extra anxious to make everything work out well.

Men sometimes suffer from the reverse problem – premature ejaculation. This, too, may have physical causes and you should check with your doctor if it is a recurring problem. This is also true of repeated failure to maintain an erection. However, more often than not, both these problems are occasional and can be resolved with patience, understanding and a little imagination within the context of a loving relationship. Anxiety often plays a major causal role.

ABOVE | No spot is a magic button and orgasms don't happen to schedules, so don't neglect loving caresses as well as powerful stimulation or you may create anxiety and defeat your purpose.

BELOW | Explore every nook and cranny of your bodies to find your pleasure spots.

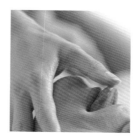

men and masturbation

IN THE PAST, standard dictionaries defined masturbation as "self-abuse". Today, it is more accurately defined as "self-pleasuring". Around 95 per cent of men masturbate, a statistic that has probably not changed over the years. Sex experts believe that masturbation is an integral part of a healthy lifestyle. It is a sexual practice that is now recognized as both normal and beneficial.

ABOVE | The shower is a popular venue as it offers privacy and no need to clean up after oneself.

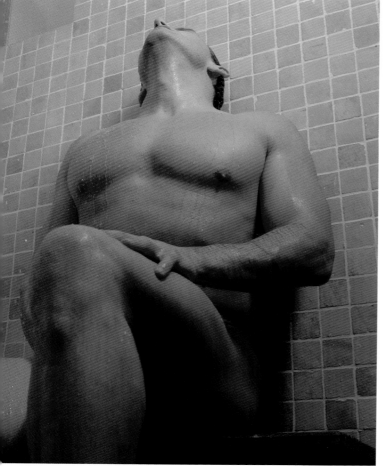

Men are inclined to masturbate more frequently than women. Some men masturbate two or more times a day and some a few times per month. It's possible that men masturbate more than women because, biologically, they need to "clean the tubes" more often, removing old semen so it can be replaced with new. Whatever the reason, masturbation forms an integral part of the average male's routine, whether he is conscious of this or not.

light relief

All too often, masturbation is done with only the end point in mind, the orgasm. It is tempting to creep between the sheets, sit on the toilet or have a quick pull elsewhere to relieve sexual tension. This is fine, but in order to get more from your orgasm, it's worth taking time and practising the art of masturbation to prolong the delicious sensations that lead up to climax. This will result in a more intense orgasm, as well as training for those long-distance sessions with your partner.

Like sex, masturbation can be divided into two categories, the "quickie" and the long, drawn-out sensual session. Instead of concentrating solely on the penis when masturbating, try to explore other areas such as your nipples, chest, thighs, perineum and buttocks. If you have never tried stimulating your anus, give it a go. No-one can see you.

Masturbation is a great opportunity to let your imagination run wild. Different people have different fantasies and the content of yours is personal and not something you should feel ashamed or embarrassed about. Everyone has fantasies and they may be the absolute pinnacle of depravity. Often what gets your rocks off in your head would have the totally opposite effect in reality.

There is no right or wrong way to masturbate. Some men prefer a strong gripping movement, others prefer a lighter touch. Many men prefer to confine stimulation to the head or glans alone. This may involve a pulling action, which stimulates just the head and frenulum area. Other men incorporate the shaft into their technique. Whatever works for you wins. The idea of this book is not to preach on about correct technique, but to encourage a little extra variety and new discovery.

The techniques described here have been tried and tested. They are merely a guide, however, as teaching a man to masturbate is comparable to preaching to the converted. It is interesting that masturbation is still one of the hardest topics to discuss in a relationship, so leaving this chapter open on your girlfriend's pillow may be helpful.

calligraphy grip

Hold your penis in the same way that you would a pen, with your thumb nearest you and your forefinger furthest away. Stroke your penis up and down in this way, stimulating your frenulum and glans. If you want more contact, simply wrap the rest of your fingers around to form a fist and use your thumb at the top to stimulate the head.

turn and twist

Grip the top of the head like a water tap and twist as you would if turning a tap on or off. This may be better with some lubrication and stimulation of the shaft with your other hand.

the mattress massage

This involves lying on the mattress and rubbing your penis up and down the fabric. You can spice this up with cushions strategically placed along your penis to increase the pressure and friction.

prayer pumper

Put your hands tightly together as if in prayer. Add some lubrication and then insert your penis into the groove formed at the joining of your wrists. Using your pelvis, thrust into your hands, adjusting the depth of your penetration.

san francisco shuffle

Hold your penis in a similar way to the calligraphy grip, using either a fist or your thumb and forefinger. Stroke up and instead of going back down, go over the top of the head, maintaining contact, and down the other side, so that the top

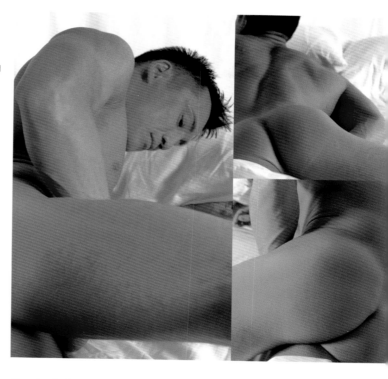

of your hand is closest to your stomach and your thumb is pointing away from your body. Then reverse the direction.

dressing up

For this one, all you need to do is experiment with different fabrics and textures by placing socks, gloves and other garments over your penis. Different fabrics will provide a variety of sensations; just be sure to get permission from your girlfriend before using her gloves.

Fabrics have different textures that will stimulate your nerve endings in different ways. The cool chill of silk for example, will induce a sensation similar to water, whereas the harder, rougher and warmer feel of leather, combined with its distinctive smell, is a completely different sensory experience. Experimentation is the key here and soon you will become more aware of what fabrics and textures turn you on.

ABOVE | There are as many positions and places for masturbation as there are men on the planet.

BELOW | The television is a great source of stimulating material to inspire a session of self-pleasuring.

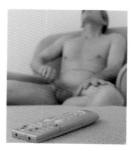

women and masturbation

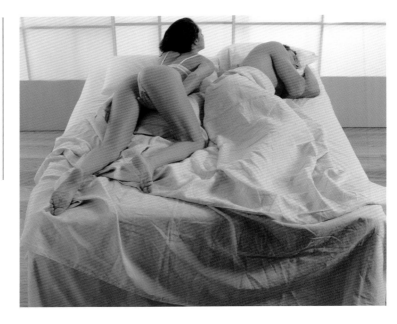

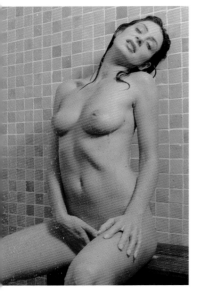

FOR YEARS IT WAS SEEN as dirty and depraved to pleasure yourself, especially if you happened to be a woman. It was not until 1972 that the American Medical Association declared masturbation a normal sexual activity.

Although today some women find it hard to approach the subject of masturbation, the truth is that the majority of women are doing it. Recent statistics show that 82 per cent of women masturbate, a statistic that is increasing with time. Are more women masturbating now? Probably not, they are just more inclined to admit to it.

For many women, masturbation is the only means of getting sexual fulfilment and orgasm and it is thought that a woman is three times as likely to orgasm through masturbation than through penetrative sex. A huge number of women find it difficult or even impossible to climax with a partner through penetrative sex alone and need clitoral stimulation.

cliterati

Emily Dubberley, journalist and sexpert on masturbation says of the orgasm, "It's like one of those water balloons that just slips through your fingers when you try to get hold of it, or a bar of soap in the bath. Try to grab on to it too hard and it just flies away." Because there wasn't enough masturbation material for women on the Internet, she founded cliterati.co.uk, so if you are not feeling imaginative enough to think of something yourself, look up the site for some raunchy inspiration.

setting the scene

Most men can masturbate almost any time, anywhere, with pleasing results, but for women it is often more complex. Masturbation is a fine art that involves all the senses to set the mood.

It's often worth doing some preparation beforehand to get you in the right frame of mind. Solitude is a must. Turn off your pager, unhook the phone and feed the dog, making sure that you give yourself a window of distraction-free time, unless you are excited by rushing and perhaps the possibility of being discovered.

There is no set place that leads to a more orgasmic experience. Wherever you feel comfortable is ideal, but it's sometimes fun to seek variety and try different positions, from lying on your front in bed, standing in the shower or jumping into the back seat of your car. Any literature or visual aids should be ready to hand.

techniques

There is no correct or incorrect technique – the important first step is to explore your body and find out what goes where in your pleasure zone. It's also important to experiment with touch and caress to find out what you like and what does it for you, as preferences vary greatly from woman to woman.

Many women like to fantasize as they play with themselves. If you are a fantasizer, this is an opportunity to let your mind wander into the impossible, sordid or even dangerous. It doesn't matter, your mind is totally secure and you should never feel guilty about what turns you on. Fantasy and reality are two different worlds.

Using lubrication can often help to get things moving a bit more smoothly. You can use water-based lubricants, which are usually odourless and tasteless, or even your own saliva. Some women produce more love juices than others and feel that lubrication is not necessary. Either way, it evokes a different sensation and experience, so experiment.

crossed clitoris caress

Using your third and fourth finger, caress your clitoris and the surrounding areas in a cross-like movement, moving from north to south and then east to west, with your clitoris as the central point. Change the direction and pressure until you discover your most sensitive spots.

passion pinching

Gently squeeze your clitoris between your thumb and forefinger or middle finger and lift it slightly, squeezing at the same time. Roll it between your

fingers, starting slowly and then picking up momentum. Again, experiment with different paces and pressures. For women with super-sensitive clitorises direct contact may be too intense. If this is the case with you, try to keep the clitoris covered with a layer of the inner labia, avoiding direct stimulation.

circular cyclone

This is an old favourite that, once perfected, will guarantee orgasm. Place your forefinger and middle finger just over the top of your clitoris and rub in a circular motion over your clitoris, varying the size and frequency of the circles. Because you are stimulating just above the clitoris, you can use a bit more pressure.

figure of eight

Another favourite that is fairly self-explanatory. The top of the eight concentrates on the clitoris and the bottom incorporates the vulva and labia. Use a smaller circle for the clitoris and larger, more sweeping circles for the bottom circle. Use forefinger and middle finger or whichever two fingers feel more comfortable.

tri-digit fidget

This one uses three fingers. Use your fourth finger and forefinger to hold back the inner and outer labia folds, leaving your middle finger free to concentrate on clitoral stimulation. With your free hand you could use a vibrator.

victory roll

With your middle finger and forefinger in a V shape, rub up and down your vulva with the clitoris in the middle. This stimulates the sides of your clitoris and the inner labia. By varying the width of the V, you can experiment with the different sensations.

tapping

Spread your labia to fully expose the clitoris. With your index finger, lightly tap the tip of your clitoris. This is not for everyone and some may find this sensation too much, but it adds variety and spice in combination with other techniques.

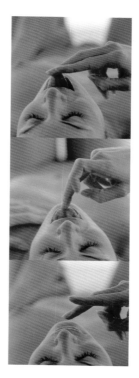

ABOVE AND BELOW | If you do not have any lubricant handy, use your saliva to lubricate yourself when masturbating.

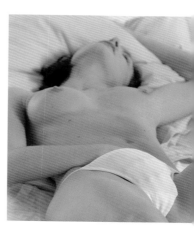

doing it together

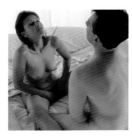

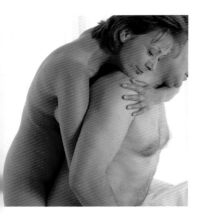

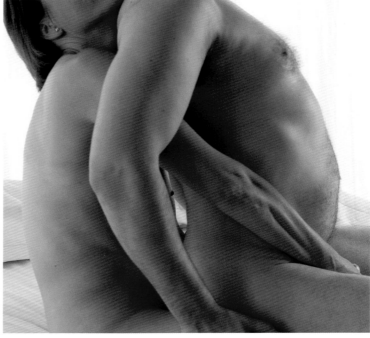

TOP | Watching each other masturbating can be a learning experience.

ABOVE AND ABOVE RIGHT | Sharing the experience of masturbation is simply another form of intimacy, which can be deeply erotic and exciting. It does not replace the pleasures of penetrative sex, but actually enhances them.

FAR RIGHT | Body shapes can fit together in many different ways.

THE ART OF PLEASING yourself is often considered a solo activity that should remain behind closed doors. Many people, especially women, still cling to the taboo of masturbation and hence find it too difficult even to discuss with their partner, let alone do in front of them.

Broaching the subject of masturbating in front of each other can be tricky, but the benefits can be well worth it. Some people, both men and women, find it difficult to climax through penetrative sex. This can lead to a variety of problems, many of which stem from the dreaded fake orgasm. There is simply no room for deceit in a healthy sex life.

The majority of people continue to masturbate in relationships for a variety of reasons, none of which are solely due to sexual dissatisfaction with their partner. Many couples, particularly young

ones, enjoy mutual masturbation as a safer means of exploring each other and enjoying each other without penetration.

spectator sport

There is also the option of pleasuring yourself while your partner is closely involved. Masturbation can result in some of the most intense orgasms and it seems only reasonable that these experiences should be witnessed. Most people would jump at the chance of watching their loved one having a great time and sharing the experience.

Take the opportunity of watching your partner to observe how they like to be touched. Try laying your hand over your partner's as they stimulate themselves. That way you will become attuned to the rhythm he or she finds most pleasurable.

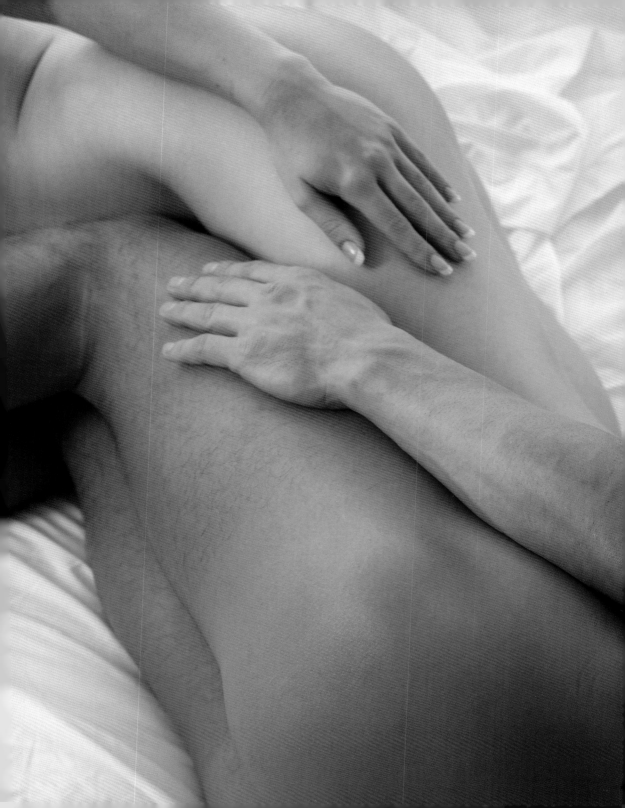

coitus

For really good sex you need to have a repertoire of different positions to keep your lovemaking interesting, stimulating and truly satisfying. Although more than 600 sexual postures have been recorded – some very weird and wonderful – most of them in fact stem from six basic positions.

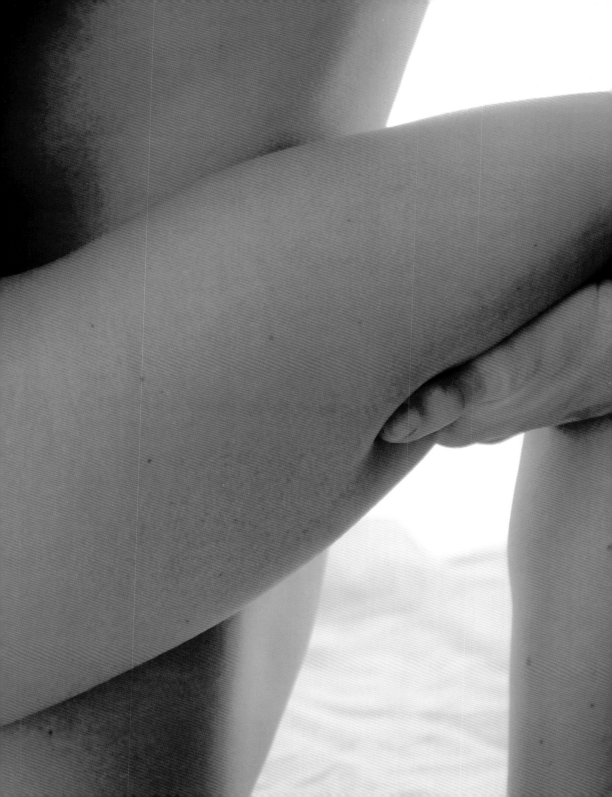

how to do it

EVERYONE HAS AN OPINION and preference on sexual positions. Some are spoons subscribers, while others are doggy devotees. The quest for the ultimate position is a little like letting a child loose in a chocolate factory. We all know there's plenty to choose from, starting with the well-tried and tested missionary position and progressing to something that any acrobat would be proud of. Some positions even look downright painful and others defy the imagination. However, regardless of the complicated twists and tangles your pals may boast of, there are really only six basic positions: man on top, woman on top, side by side

RIGHT | Making love while facing provides infinite opportunities for touching and exploring each other's bodies.

BELOW | Looking into your lover's eyes and watching their face during sex is one of the pleasures of the woman or man on top position.

(spoons), sitting or kneeling, rear entry (doggy) and standing. All the rest are, in effect, variations on these six.

It certainly makes for a more interesting sex life if you vary your positions and, although this doesn't need to be done with military precision, it can be great fun experimenting with something new. Some positions allow deeper penetration, while others let you stimulate different areas of each other's bodies during intercourse. There's a position for every type of passion. Each can be adapted to suit individual needs, regardless of height and weight differences, penis width and length, mobility, age and flexibility. All it takes is a little imagination, practice and enthusiasm (and of course, the magic ingredient, humour).

Physical and verbal communication with your partner is paramount. As you learn each other's likes and dislikes, you'll be able to anticipate when to change positions or lead where necessary. It's always a great turn-on if one of you suggests a new position, saying, "I've read about this one. Shall we give it a go?"

ringing the changes

Most of us are creatures of habit and usually opt for only two or three sexual positions because they are tried and tested favourites. However, familiarity is said to breed contempt and could lead to bedroom boredom. Trying new positions may seem strange at first, but really does add spice and adventure to your sex life.

This is not to suggest that you should swing from the chandeliers like an urban Tarzan. Know your limitations and don't attempt any positions that are too physically strenuous for you. The posture you choose must be comfortable for both you and your partner or you'll end up in a frustrating, unsatisfying and possibly painful tangle. If a new position doesn't quite work, don't worry. You may discover something amazing on the way that would reinvent this chapter.

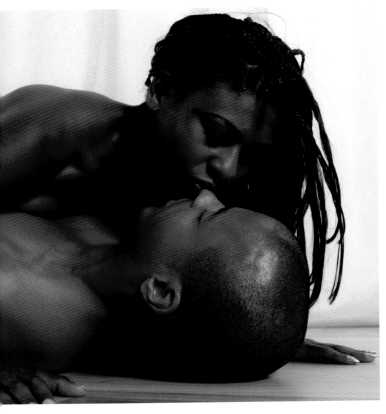

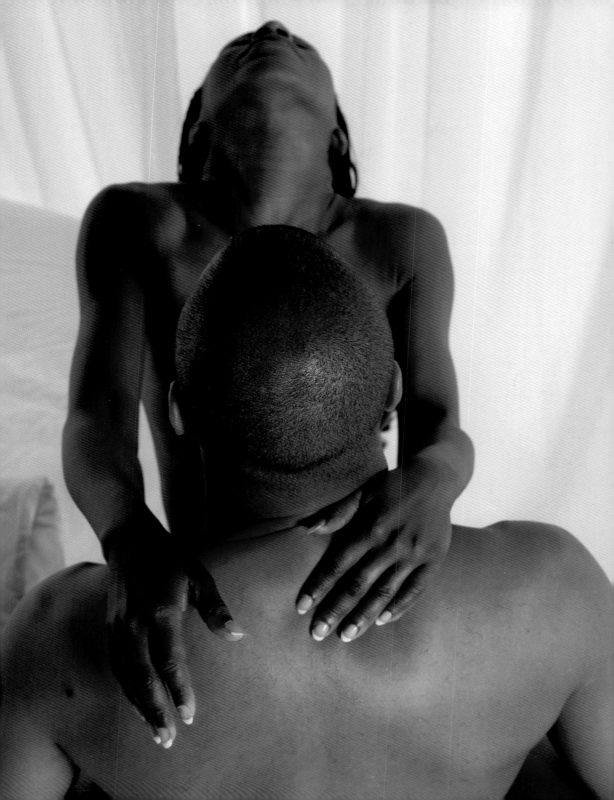

man on top

THIS WAS THE POSITION said to have been promoted by nineteenth-century missionaries as they travelled the world and discovered other cultures enjoying multi-positional and uninhibited sex. It was decided that the position of man dominant on top of woman was the only acceptable one and so attempts were made to impose it on anyone having sex.

Perhaps because of this history, the position has got rather a bad name. Images of bored women looking at their watches over their partners' shoulders or deciding on a new colour for the bedroom ceiling are all associated with the missionary position. It is also a position that people, particularly women, may resort to because

they are not very confident about their bodies. Their stomachs are flatter lying supine, and because it is a fairly standard position, there are no worries about being shown up for physical inflexibility, having your breasts dangling or worrying about showing a large bottom. Most people try this position for the first few times when having sex with a new partner, and when they feel more confident, move on to more challenging positions.

Having said all this, the missionary position is one of the most intimate; where your bodies converge and meld into each other, where you can kiss, caress and have your skins touching, and where you can have long, lingering sex.

BELOW | The missionary position is a very natural and easy position for sex, so it is a favourite for both a speedy romp or a prolonged session of love for couples of all ages.

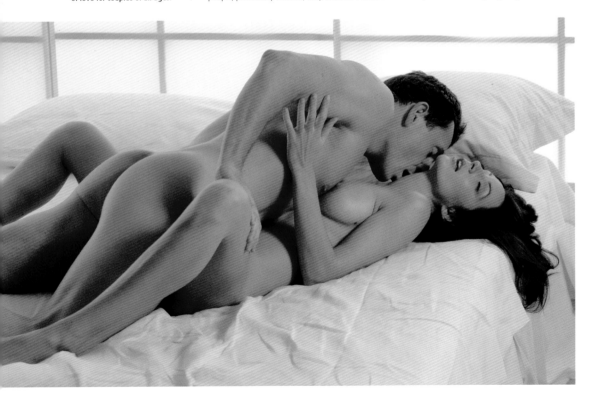

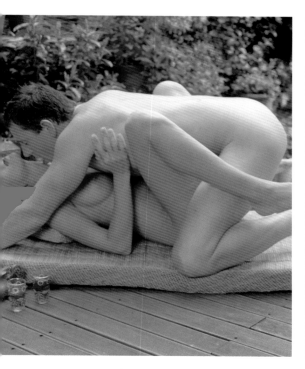
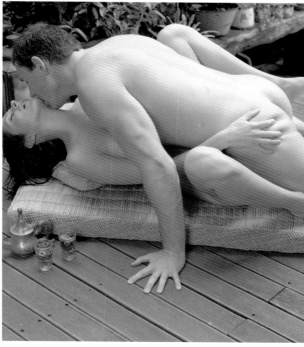

basic man on top

This is the classic man on top position. To begin with, his legs are usually positioned in between the woman's legs, which are both slightly splayed out. The woman can put her hands around her partner's neck and the man, resting on his elbows, can cup his hands around her head.

This is a great position for kissing and caressing each other, nibbling at each other's ears, whispering lovely things and then having long, slow sex. You can place your hands under each other's bottoms and rock to and fro, as this helps with clitoral arousal.

For the woman, once you are aroused, part your legs and let him in. At the same time, caress his testicles and the shaft of his penis before he enters you. Stroke his back and work your way down with your free hands to play with his anus.

For men, you are more able to control the rate of your thrust and, therefore, when you come in this position. Slow entry and almost total withdrawal of your penis will drive her mad: place the tip of the penis just inside the vagina and withdraw it, repeating this slowly or quickly. This creates a wonderful feeling and heightens sexual tension. However, be careful if you are highly aroused, as you may come too soon.

The main problem with this position is that it is not so good for clitoral stimulation, because the penis is often not at the best angle. If the woman arches her back, he can penetrate even deeper.

PLUS POINTS You can watch each other's faces, both as a guide to what excites your partner most and to arouse your own feelings still more.
It is a very versatile position that can be adapted to all kinds of places besides the bed or sofa.

MINUS POINTS A small, light woman can be quite squashed by a heavy partner, even if he takes most of his weight on his hands or elbows.
It is not very comfortable for either partner to make love in this position following a large meal.

ABOVE | Having sex *al fresco* is wonderfully liberating. However, do make sure that you have total privacy to avoid the risk of being overlooked or offending other people.

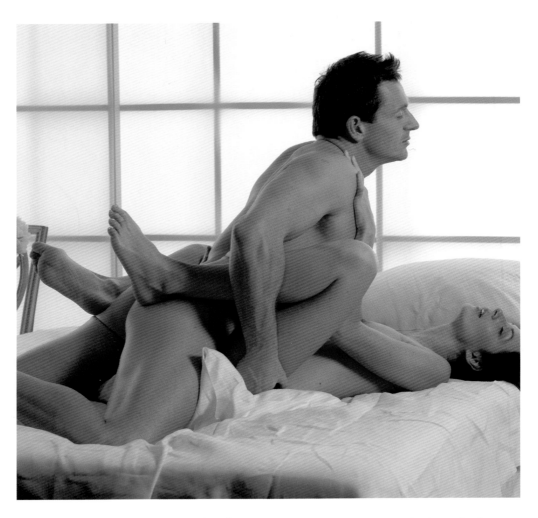

ABOVE | Man on top 1. Placing a pillow under the woman's bottom will increase contact between the clitoris and his pubic bone.

OPPOSITE | Man on top 3. Resting her feet on his shoulders makes penetration very deep. Both partners can still watch each other's faces.

man on top 1

The woman places a pillow under her bottom and bends her legs. The man can then kneel over her, holding her waist while he enters. The pillow helps to increase the contact between the clitoris and the man's pubic bone, so that it can be stimulated as the penis thrusts. Try different angles to get it perfect. This positions allows mostly for shallow penetration and you both need to be quite agile. The man can gently pull his partner's body towards him on each thrust. He can stroke her breasts and stomach and move off easily to stimulate her clitoris with his tongue. Since the woman is stretched right out in front of the man, he will be able to watch his penis thrusting in and out, which is visually very exciting.

PLUS POINTS This is good for a woman because her partner has more access to her breasts and clitoris.

MINUS POINTS This can be very tiring for a man, as he is holding himself and his partner up.

man on top 2

The woman wraps her legs around her partner's waist, with a pillow or two under her back if necessary. Her partner pulls her up so that he is holding her bottom. She can also stroke his back. The woman pulls the man inside her and can control the rhythm of the thrusts. Since this allows deeper penetration, her clitoris is more likely to be stimulated than if she were lying flat. The man enters his partner at a steep angle. If you can both manage it, lean forward for a kiss.

PLUS POINTS Because of the angle of penetration, a man who believes his penis is small will feel like a stud. The woman can stimulate herself at the same time, which both partners find a turn-on.

MINUS POINTS It can be tricky for the woman to get the rhythm right and for the man to let her.

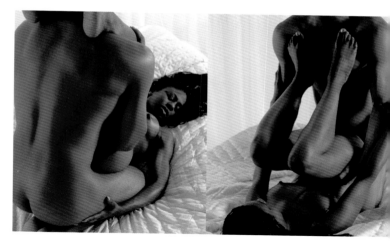

man on top 3

Here the woman pulls her knees up to her chest with one or both feet resting on her partner's shoulders. She can hold the man's hips for support and he can put his hands under her bottom. This is excellent for really deep penetration. If the woman then places her legs to one side, the side walls of her vagina will be massaged. She can also try pressing her hand on her belly to feel her partner's penis as it moves in and out. This is very arousing because you can watch each other's expressions and if the woman reaches down to masturbate herself, he will love watching this too. But some women will find the deepness of the thrusting too painful to tolerate for long.

PLUS POINTS Deep penetration makes this position extremely exciting for both partners – great for relatively quick sex.
He can watch his penis as it slides in and out and can also watch his partner masturbate herself, so it is visually a very stimulating position.

MINUS POINTS All men, but especially those with big penises, must avoid getting too carried away, as very deep thrusts can cause a woman considerable pain.

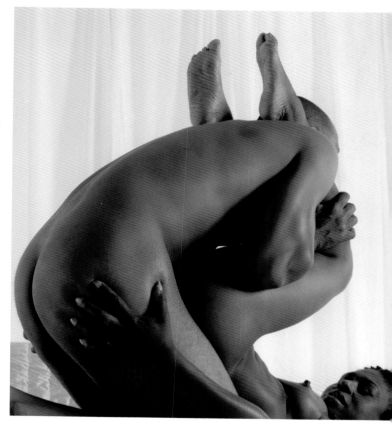

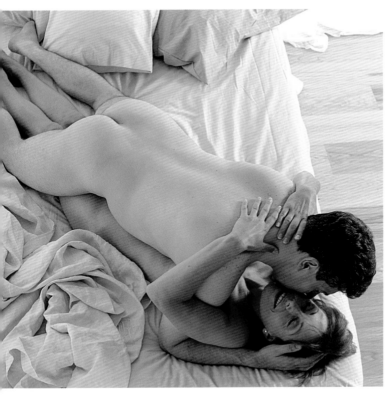

man on top 4

The man places his legs either side of the woman's and she squeezes her legs together, placing her hands around his head or neck.

This is a wonderful position for total body contact and slow sex with lots of kissing and caressing. If the woman keeps her thighs squeezed together after her partner has entered her, her vagina will be tighter and a stronger stimulation to her partner's penis. For the man there is only shallow penetration, so the penis can slip out if he's not careful. But it is also a very arousing and tantalizing position, so he has to be careful not to come too quickly.

PLUS POINTS As some concentration is essential to avoid the penis slipping out, sex is prolonged, slow and gentle, building inexorably to a spectacular climax.
It is ideal for women who worry about a slack vagina after childbirth as squeezing her thighs means that her partner's penis is also gently gripped – something he will find irresistible.

MINUS POINTS The eroticism of this position can be surprising, causing the man to come much more quickly than expected.
A small, light woman can feel crushed by her partner.

ABOVE | Man on top 4. It is precisely because this position is a little more difficult to maintain and the thrusts are shallow that the sensations are so powerful and intense.

RIGHT | Man on top 5. This position allows the woman to caress the head and face of her partner while he has access to her neck and breasts with his mouth.

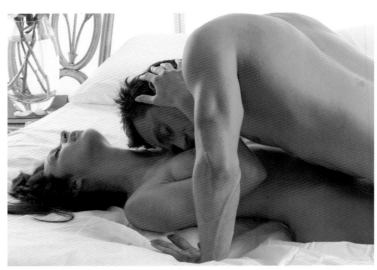

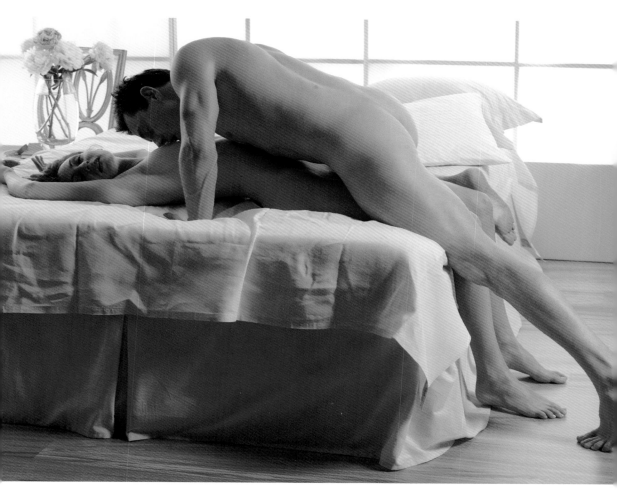

man on top 5

The woman dangles her legs over the edge of the bed, with the backs of her knees on the edge, and throws her arms back over her head. She may need cushions under her bottom on the bed in order to obtain a better angle for penetration. The man lies over her, supporting himself with his arms, with his feet on the floor. (A short man can put a couple of cushions under his feet.) The woman can suck her fingers and then masturbate herself – a great turn-on for both of you. This position is great for the man because he can see everything.

Although too far away to kiss, he can nuzzle and lick her nipples and both partners can watch each other's expressions as they come.

PLUS POINTS Watching his partner's arousal and abandonment to her passion is a turn-on for the man. He will have to be especially imaginative about ways to excite her, as his hands are occupied, taking his weight.

MINUS POINTS As the woman has limited control, she can feel dominated, but if she simply gives in to the moment, she will just feel wonderfully indulged.

ABOVE | Man on top 5. With her arms flung over her head the woman can abandon herself totally to the attentions of her lover.

woman on top

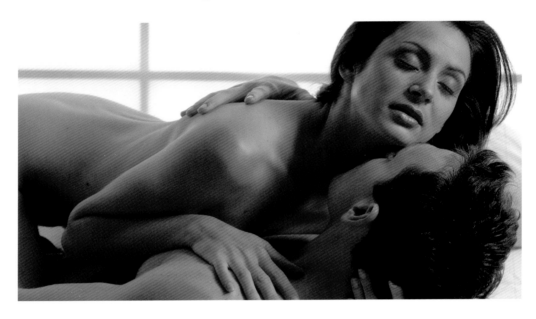

ABOVE | Being on top is an empowering position for women, which can be a real turn-on for him, especially if he is used to being the more dominant partner.

FAR RIGHT TOP | Woman on top 1. This position enables the woman to move freely, so stimulating whatever parts of her own body she likes at whatever pace best suits her, while simultaneously driving her partner into a frenzy of sheer sexual ecstasy.

THIS IS WHERE THE WOMAN dominates, and some of the most erotic positions are played out here. In these positions, the woman can regulate the depth of penetration of her partner's penis and decide on the rhythm of sex, and thus the stimulation needed to reach orgasm. The man can watch his penis thrusting in and out and admire his partner's breasts or bottom. For those men who tend to come quickly, your partner can slow the pace down and help you to control your orgasm.

basic woman on top

The woman climbs on to the man, facing him, with her legs pulled up slightly, so she has freedom of movement. Once he is aroused – and he probably will be already – she places his penis inside her before lying down on his chest. The man can caress his partner's bottom and help with the thrusting by pulling her up and down on to his penis. In this position there is plenty of intimate skin-on-skin contact.

PLUS POINTS There is no pressure for the man to "perform" and he can enjoy feeling especially loved. She has control of her own arousal, as well as his.

MINUS POINTS Some men dislike not being in control, although usually they can be persuaded.

woman on top 1

The woman straddles the man, facing him, but remains upright. Both partners have their hands free and can make good use of them. The woman can massage his chest, bend over to lick his nipples and upper body, rock back and forth, and go round and round with her hips. If she contracts her vaginal muscles around his penis, he will be in heaven as well. She can pause at the top of the penis as he comes out and touch the end of his member at the entrance to the vagina. She can touch her clitoris at the same time, if she can balance and her legs are strong enough. She can also lean back and grab his ankles for stability.

The man can caress his partner's breasts and body as she rises up and down. He can grab her around her hips and buttocks to help with the rhythm. And just watch her as she begins to come.

PLUS POINTS This position is both highly tactile and visually stimulating.

Penetration is very deep, so it is great for most men and for those women who particularly like that.

It's a fabulous way for a woman to indulge all her basic instincts and demonstrate her feelings for her lover.

MINUS POINTS It is quite a strain on the woman's thigh muscles and sense of balance.

Inhibited women or those who are sensitive about their bodies will probably not enjoy this position.

woman on top 2

In this position, the woman squats on top of her partner, facing him, and the man keeps his legs stretched out so that she doesn't fall off. The woman then guides his penis inside her. The man helps the thrusting movement, although he will not be able to do too much, by placing his hands under her bottom. It is up to the woman to set the pace and rhythm. This is a good position for deep penetration. However, the woman has complete control over the depth, so she can vary it as much as she likes.

To enhance the experience, the woman can pause at the top for a few seconds to give her man a tantalizing sense of anticipation. She can also pull both legs apart so that her partner can see his penis going in and out. He can fondle her breasts, caress her body and watch everything that is going on.

There are numerous variations for this position: she can pivot around slowly, kneel and sit on his groin with her legs crossed. Men must be careful, as it is more difficult for them to control their orgasm in this position. Maintaining a stiff erection is essential for maximum effect, as a floppy penis will slide out easily.

PLUS POINTS This is a very versatile position, so it is a good one for imaginative and creative lovers.

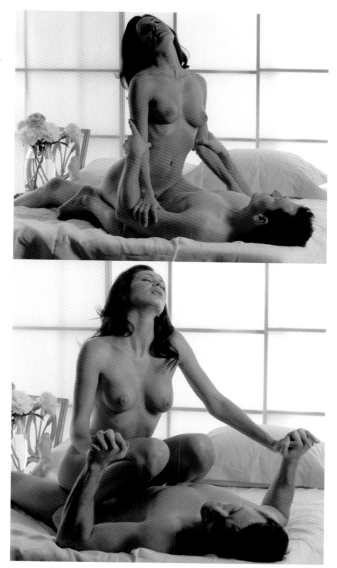

The woman is completely in control of all aspects of lovemaking – this is satisfying for her and hugely exciting for him.

MINUS POINTS She needs to be fit, as this position is quite tiring. It is also a strain on her knees.

ABOVE | Woman on top 2. When she is squatting on top, the man can support some of her weight by holding her hands, which will enable her to move more freely.

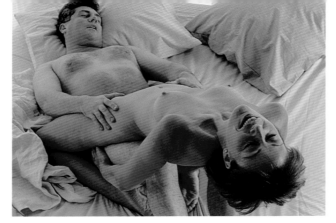

PLUS POINTS He can see his penis as it moves in and out and this is a real turn-on.

By leaning back and tensing her muscles, she is in a great position for his penis to stimulate her G spot.

MINUS POINTS She is unable to clearly watch her partner's arousal or see his face as he comes without changing her position to upright.

woman on top 4

The woman sits on top of the man, facing his feet with her bottom directly in line with his eyes, something most men relish. She can lean either forwards or slightly back. As well as watching her bottom bouncing up and down, the man can watch his penis thrusting in and out. For most men, this more than makes up for the fact that they can't see their partner's face and some women love to show off this normally concealed, even ignored part of their body.

If the woman leans back, she can stimulate her clitoris with one hand while resting on the other. However, she must take care to avoid hurting her partner's penis by sitting down roughly

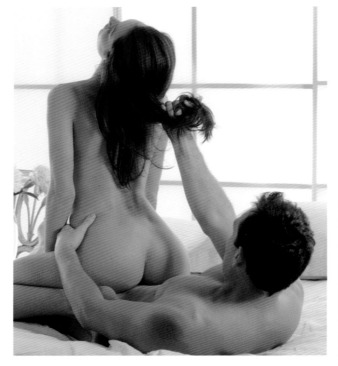

spice of life

The last thing sex should be is a series of mechanical steps that follow instructions – even from this book. Just because you start your lovemaking in one position doesn't mean that you have to stay there until you both come. You can move and change position entirely, from woman on top to man on top, for example, as the mood takes you. You might like to start in a gentle, relaxed way, such as woman on top 3, and then, as feelings intensify, switch to a position where deeper penetration is easier. Equally, you might choose to change from woman on top 4 to a position where there is more skin contact and you can see each other's faces. Follow your instincts and have fun, but keep your partner in the loop by telling them which position's next.

TOP | Woman on top 3. Lovely if you are in the mood for some slow rhythms.

ABOVE | Woman on top 4. Some women love having their hair gently pulled or teased during sex.

woman on top 3

The man lies on the bed and pulls his knees up and the woman sits on top, with her legs bent and feet flat on the bed, or out behind her, facing him. Once she has guided his penis inside her, she can then lean back to support herself on his knees. This is quite hard work for both people and it may take some time to get a rhythm going.

on top of it or bending it the wrong way. If she sits up slightly, he can contribute to the thrusting with his hips and she can be still. If she leans forwards, then the man can massage her back and buttocks and, if she likes it, place his finger around or into her anus. (Remember to have the lubrication handy before you begin.) There are many erotic nerves in this area which will enhance the feeling of intensity in her vagina.

In return, the woman can fondle his testicles, or, if she is very supple, bend right over and lick them. She will need to lean forward to obtain the right angle, but again, should be careful with the angle of the man's penis, as it is bending away from the body so it could cause discomfort.

PLUS POINTS Men usually find this different viewpoint of their partner during sex very exciting.
The woman can adapt her position to stimulate different parts of her own and her partner's body, constantly changing levels of arousal and pleasure.

MINUS POINTS Some women dislike not being able to see their partner's face.
This position can be inhibiting for a woman as she will be taking care not to injure her partner as she moves.

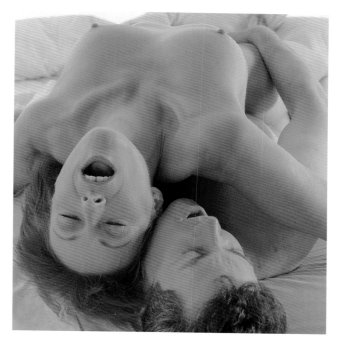

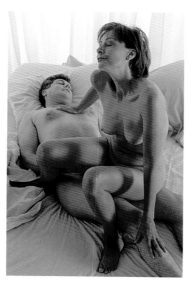

woman on top 5

Here the woman mounts the man's erect penis, facing him. She then pivots around, with his penis still inside her, until she is lying back on his chest. Her partner can then hold her by her bottom or hips to pull her back and forth. Pivoting can be tricky, as the penis can easily slip out, but once it is accomplished, this is a great position. The man can play with his partner's breasts in between thrusts and she can stimulate herself throughout.

PLUS POINTS This has great novelty value, as it is quite different from the usual woman on top positions.
There is lots of skin contact and the man can caress his partner's breasts and both can stimulate her clitoris.
With a little imagination, there are plenty of opportunities for exciting variations of this position.

MINUS POINTS The angle can make it difficult for the man to keep his penis in place.
Even a small woman can feel quite heavy in this position and some men find its restrictions a little suffocating.

ABOVE | Woman on top 5. This position would be perfect for couples who have a mirrored ceiling as they can watch themselves in action.

LEFT | Woman on top 5. Pivoting can be hard work, so the woman can pause on her way round. In a "side saddle" type position, the man can stimulate her breasts and either he or she can give clitoral stimulation.

rear entry

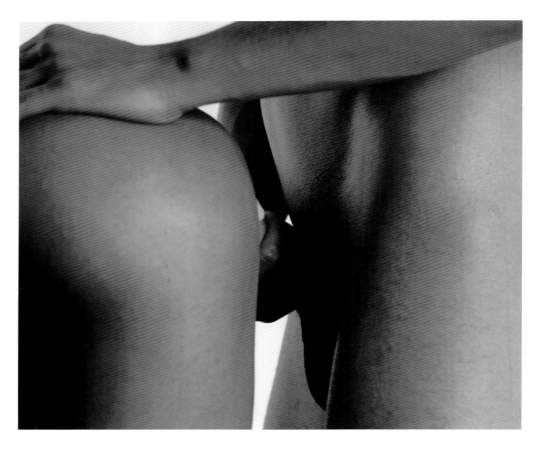

ABOVE | For a quickie, rear entry can be a tremendous thrill, but go gently as penetration can be deep.

ENTRY FROM BEHIND IS FANTASTIC for deep, penetrative sex. The penis is naturally angled to maximize impact for clitoral stimulation, although the woman may still need a little manual assistance, and the man's testicles rub and bounce against the vulva with each stroke, creating a most sensuous feeling for both partners.

Psychologically, some women find these positions difficult, as they have little control over the depth of penetration or the rhythm of the thrusts. A few find the position exceptionally unappealing, as it makes them feel almost like a depersonalized sex object. Rear entry positions can also be uncomfortable, with deep, heavy thrusting, as the penis goes in very deep and hits the cervix. Men should be careful and experiment to see what works without causing discomfort.

In spite of these provisos, these positions can be breathtakingly exciting for both partners, as, with limited visual stimulation, they concentrate physical sensation intensely. Consequently, the pitch of excitement increases very rapidly and orgasm tends to be an even more mind-blowing explosion than usual.

basic position

Sometimes known as "doggy" style, this can be extremely erotic. If you are both on the floor, make sure the carpet is soft, or kneel on cushions.

The woman kneels on the floor or bed on all fours with her arms straight or resting on her forearms. The man kneels behind her, holding her hips or waist. Then he enters her. Men who are shorter than their partners may need to kneel on cushions. Going up on one knee will help raise the level of the penis.

As the woman is being penetrated, she can touch her own clitoris or reach back and stroke the man's testicles. He will love this. He can lean over and fondle her breasts or stimulate her anus with firm finger pressure. (Many women enjoy the sensation of pressure just in front of the anus.). When doing this, he may be able to feel his penis through the wall between anus and vagina. You can use a small vibrator rather than a finger to do this if you prefer, but don't put the vibrator into the vagina until you've washed it.

Linger with the tip of the penis at the opening of the vagina, doing several smaller thrusts before going in hard and deep. If there is sufficient control to do this several times, she'll find this breathtaking and almost unbearably exciting. The natural curve of the vagina fits with the curve of the penis, so deep thrusting is possible.

This is a favourite position during pregnancy, as the "bump" doesn't get in the way. Take care not to cause discomfort with deep penetration, although sex in pregnancy is generally not dangerous.

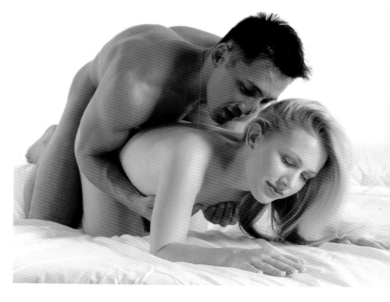

PLUS POINTS Many women love the slightly naughty feeling of being "taken" in this position.
This is great for an intense passionate romp, as both partners are aroused very quickly.
If he kneels up, the man can see his penis moving in and out and has a tantalizing view of his partner's body.

MINUS POINTS Penetration is so deep, it can cause discomfort to the woman.
The woman cannot see her partner's face.

ABOVE | The doggy position can suit your internal shape well, giving opportunities for using the hands as well as deep thrusting. Be sure to use extra-strong condoms here, as the strain may be more than they can normally stand up to.

LEFT | Most men find the sight of their partner's bottom an inspiration for imaginative sex and exciting positions.

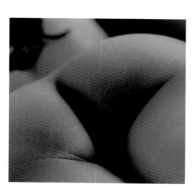

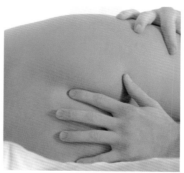

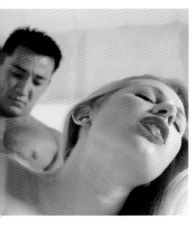

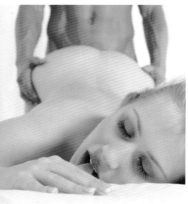

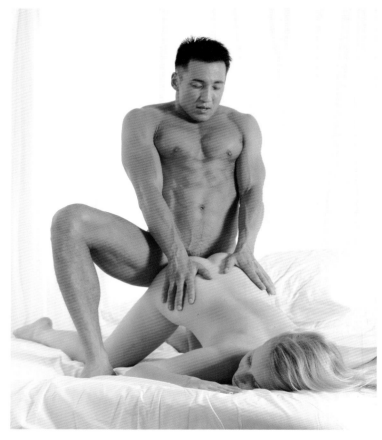

TOP AND ABOVE | Vocalize to let him know how you feel, as he cannot see your face.

ABOVE RIGHT | Rear entry 1. With one of the man's knees raised, penetration will be even deeper, so he should take it easy and be guided by his partner's verbal and physical responses.

OPPOSITE | Rear entry 2. Use pillows to raise yourself up enough to get the right angle.

rear entry 1

This is like the doggy position, but the woman, while keeping her bottom in the air, puts her head on the bed. The man is behind her on one knee, holding her shoulders or waist. This allows for even deeper penetration than the traditional doggy style. She can hook her legs over his, pulling him into her, and the couple can thrust simultaneously with a little practice.

PLUS POINTS This takes the weight off her arms so the woman finds it more relaxing.

MINUS POINTS It can cause headaches or a stiff neck if the woman is positioned awkwardly.

rear entry 2

Here, the woman lies down flat, legs spread out, and the man kneels behind her and then lies on top of her. She needs to raise her bottom high enough, perhaps with a pillow underneath her. Penetration will be shallow. However, this position is very comforting and close, with plenty of body contact and the opportunity for the man to kiss and nuzzle the woman's neck and lick her ear lobes.

PLUS POINTS He can whisper dirty things in her ear. Friction over her buttocks can be a real turn-on for her.

MINUS POINTS As penetration is shallow, there is a risk of the penis slipping out.

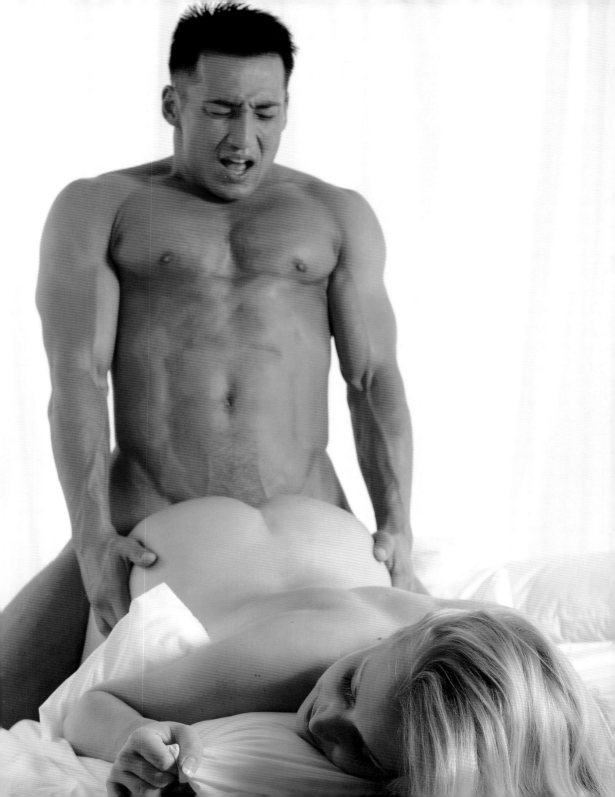

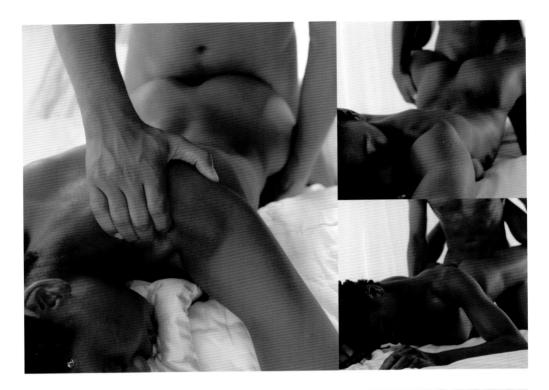

ABOVE LEFT | Rear entry 3. You may want to keep a firm grasp of the situation as this is quite a difficult position to perfect – but worth it.

ABOVE RIGHT | Rear entry 4. This is a variation on the wheelbarrow with the man kneeling so that most of the woman's weight is taken by the bed.

the thrust debate

Deep penetration can be equally enjoyable for men and women. It can stimulate the female G spot if the correct angle is achieved and men like the sensation of the tip of their penis coming into contact with their partner's cervix.

It's good psychologically too. It makes him feel like a well-endowed stud and it makes her feel that she is so irresistible that he can't control his surging desire for her.

However, shallow penetration can be equally gratifying for both parties. For the woman, the opening of the vagina is rich in nerve endings and for the man, shallow penetration provides constant stimulation of the frenulum and head of the penis, which can be squeezed and stimulated by the muscles at the vaginal opening. Many couples enjoy shallow penetration that involves rocking together back and forth: it is highly stimulating at the same time as being very relaxing, close and loving.

Partners soon find out what level of thrusting and penetration they prefer and consequently use positions that best suit them. Equally, they will choose a position for deep or shallow penetration depending on their particular mood or sense of sexual urgency. If deep penetration is your thing, plenty of lubrication heightens the experience, especially as many women don't secrete enough naturally.

rear entry 3

The woman kneels on the floor, leaning forward on to the bed, with her hands on or against the bed, and the man kneels behind her. (Put cushions down for this one, unless you want carpet burns.) This is quite an awkward position in which to enter the vagina, so experiment.

PLUS POINTS Good for a change of scene – sofa, armchair, footstool, coffee table and even the staircase are possibilities.

MINUS POINTS The man needs to be quite skilful to avoid a lot of fumbling.

rear entry 4

This is only for the fit and athletic. The man stands behind his partner and holds her straight legs while she bends forward and supports herself on her hands on the bed or the floor. You will both be more stable on the floor.

This position has a passing similarity to a wheelbarrow race on a children's sports day – with some very obvious differences. You don't have to run your partner around the room – unless you want to, of course – but you do need to have strong arms and she needs to be fairly light.

Once lifted up by the thighs, pull her on to your penis slowly while she supports herself. Neither of you will be able to do anything else with your hands. Unless you are an athlete, this will be a quick one, with vigorous thrusting. If you get into trouble, the woman can rest her legs on the bed or floor. You will have a wonderful view of your partner's bottom and back. There's not a lot the woman can do except enjoy. Lots of laughs are guaranteed.

PLUS POINTS This is great when you are in a really raunchy mood and want to feel like porn stars. Perfecting the technique is fairly tricky, but enormous fun for couples who love to laugh together.

MINUS POINTS This does have to be a quickie, as her arms will begin to hurt quite soon and the blood will rush to her head.

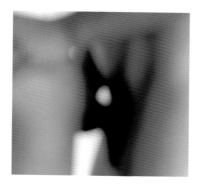

LEFT | Rear entry 3. The man may need some assistance to guide himself in.

BELOW | Rear entry 4. The wheelbarrow may be too strenuous to keep up for a long time. Have a rest and change of angle by both kneeling down, if you can manage it without collapsing in fits of giggles.

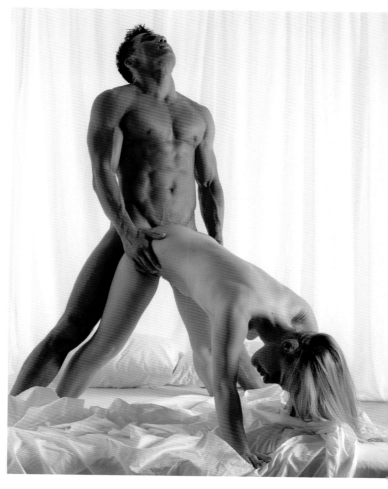

sitting positions

RIGHT | Sex in a sitting position is very loving and reassuring as there is plenty of skin contact and lots of opportunities for cuddling, kissing and caressing.

BELOW | Sitting position 1. Leaning back from each other allows greater freedom of movement and also provides exciting visual impact.

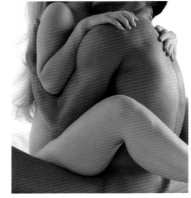

THIS SET OF POSITIONS is very intimate, allowing for lots of kissing and caressing. The movements are limited, but there is no need to rush so you can spend time perfecting them. They allows the woman to rock back and forth and thus to stimulate her clitoris. Why not try placing the chair in front of a mirror, so that you can watch yourselves? Some people find this very erotic.

basic sitting position

The man is sitting up with the woman on top – her legs wrapped around him. Initially, if the woman sits slightly away from the man, she can stroke his penis and he can stimulate her clitoris and caress her breasts. When he enters, they can rock their way to an orgasm.

PLUS POINTS This is very easy way to introduce an element of variety. Circular movements work well. It is a really intimate position, a little like giving each other an extra special hug.

MINUS POINTS With so much body contact, unless you're outdoors, you can become very sweaty on a hot day.

sitting position 1

The woman sits on the man's thighs, as he leans back. She puts her arms behind her, leaning back to support herself. Timing is of the essence here, as the woman raises her body up and down and her partner joins in with smaller thrusts. You can tease each other by looking, because you can't touch – unless you sit up slightly and take each other's hands. And you can both see the penis as it goes in and out.

PLUS POINTS Visual stimulation scores highly in this position for both partners. The hands-off effect is really tantalizing.

MINUS POINTS It can take some practice – not exactly a hardship – to get the timing synchronized.

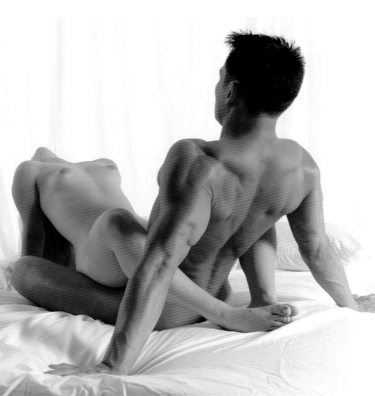

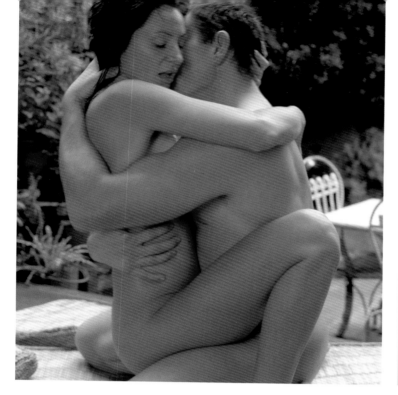

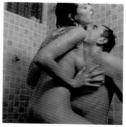

ABOVE | Sitting position 2. If you have a strong seat in the shower, use it.

LEFT | Sitting position 2. Enjoy sitting out in the garden on a balmy evening, as long as you're not overlooked.

BELOW | Sitting position 2. Chairs are great for this position. Rock back and forth, but be careful not to tip over.

sitting position 2

The woman is more in control in this one. If she places her feet flat, she can easily push herself up and down. Rotating the hips and making circular motions are excellent for clitoral stimulation. If you are on the floor raise yourself up with your legs and pause momentarily, then go down on to his tip and come up again before he has entered you.

The man can thrust upward at the same time, but it may take a while to get the timing right together. Since penetration will be quite shallow, experiment with the angles. He can also explore her upper body with his tongue. This is a lovely position for hugging, kissing and full body contact.

PLUS POINTS Great for women who like to be in charge. This is a good position for varying the location – from the garden to the office, on a chair or on the floor.

MINUS POINTS This position is slightly difficult for short women, but placing the feet on the rungs of the chair can solve the problem.

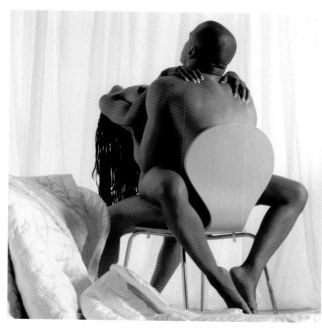

kneeling positions

BELOW | The man controls both rhythm and depth of penetration. The woman can create even greater pleasure by clenching the muscles of her buttocks and vagina to squeeze his penis – a delicious sensation for both partners.

THESE POSITIONS ALLOW the man to control thrusting in and out of his partner. While they are close and intimate because you are facing each other, they are physically harder for both partners and need determination and knowledge of each other's movements. You have to be reasonably agile for these positions, with good knees, so make sure you have plenty of pillows around.

basic kneeling position

The man kneels on the bed leaning over the woman, as she lies flat. He places his hands under her bottom to lift her on to him. Her legs are bent, with her feet flat on the bed and her back is arched. He has a full view of her body and, with plenty of eye contact, this is the perfect opportunity for talking dirty and discussing fantasies.

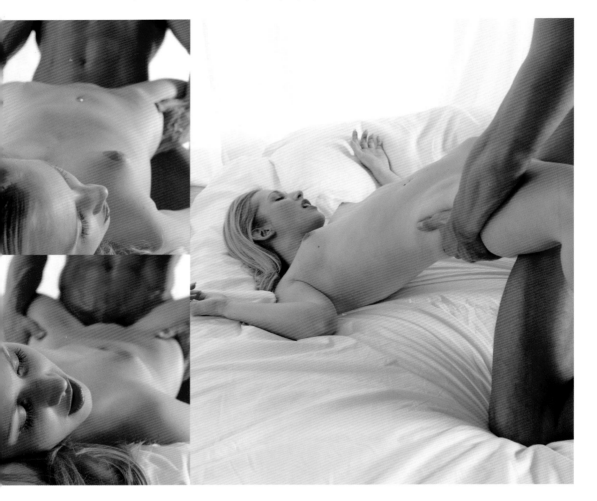

PLUS POINTS Penetration can be as deep or shallow as you like, as it is easy to vary depth and pace.

MINUS POINTS The man may find it difficult to support his partner's weight and penetrate her without shunting her across the bed.

kneeling position 1

The man sits on his heels on the bed. He lifts the woman on to him as she pushes herself up with one hand behind her on the bed, and the other holding on to his neck. He holds her buttocks with one hand and her back with the other, supporting her. This is quite a tiring and athletic pose, and would probably be best for quick sex. Again, there is plenty of opportunity for eye contact.

PLUS POINTS Deep penetration and clitoral stimulation mean both partners are rapidly aroused, so this is a great position for those times when you just can't wait. You can do this almost anywhere private, not just the bedroom – and a comfortable floor offers extra support.

MINUS POINTS He needs to be quite strong, but it helps if she takes some of her own weight on her hand.

kneeling position 2

The woman sits on a chair. The man kneels in front of her, holding her waist, and the woman's legs are wrapped around his waist. (There may be a problem with getting the heights right on this one, so choose a chair or footstool that is the right height and come forward slightly on the chair.)

This is a very sexy pose if you manage to do it right. The woman can lean backwards to facilitate entry, holding on to the man's neck. The man can put his hand on the chair to help steady his partner and can also reach his partner's breasts and clitoris to stimulate them.

PLUS POINTS This is a perfect position for making love quickly with your clothes on.
Penetration is deep – deeper if she places a leg over one of his shoulders.

MINUS POINTS Hard on his knees, but great for her.

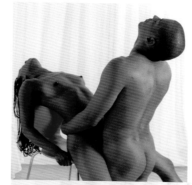

LEFT AND BELOW | Kneeling position 2. The woman's legs can wrap around his body, or stay firmly on the floor if the chair is not too stable.

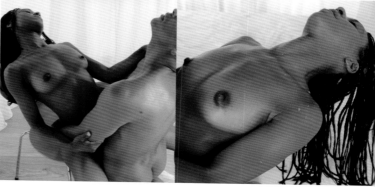

kneeling position 3

The man kneels back on his heels on the bed with the woman kneeling on top with her knees on either side of his. It may be easier if she raises one leg, placing her foot flat on the bed. She has her arms around his neck and his arms are around her waist. The man should thrust up and down. This is very intimate and erotic and you can stay in this position for a long time. This is a terrific position for fondling the woman's breasts, rubbing the man's back and stroking his neck, nibbling each other's ears and a long, delicious kiss.

PLUS POINTS Unlike most kneeling positions, this is a good position for prolonged sex, although it's also great for a quickie, as penetration is very deep.

MINUS POINTS Cramp in the leg muscles can bring proceedings to an abrupt halt.

mix and match

Kneeling positions are wonderfully adaptable and you can move very easily from one to another – a gentle, relaxed pose, such as kneeling position 3, to a more urgent and physically demanding one, such as kneeling position 1. Moving from most kneeling positions to rear entry or man on top are other options.

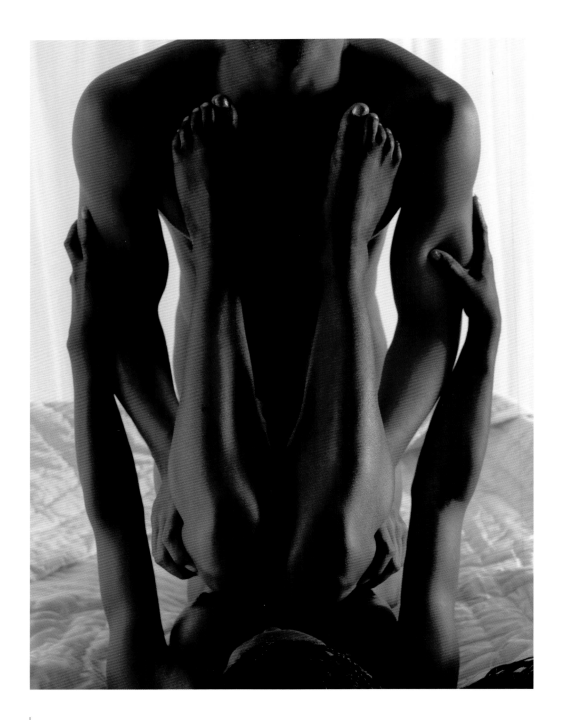

kneeling position 4

The man kneels back on his heels with the woman's legs wrapped around his neck or up on his chest. She lies back on some pillows. The man can lean forward and caress her breasts and nipples. If the woman has her legs wrapped around his neck, this is perfect for deep thrusting as they will be wide open and her partner has a great view of the penetration and can play with her clitoris. If her feet are resting on his chest, this will make her vagina feel tighter, as if gently gripping his penis.

PLUS POINTS If you are both quite fit and strong with well-toned muscles, this position is intensely thrilling. This is great for women who really relish feelings of passionate sexual abandonment.

MINUS POINTS This can strain the woman's back and demands muscular strength from the man.

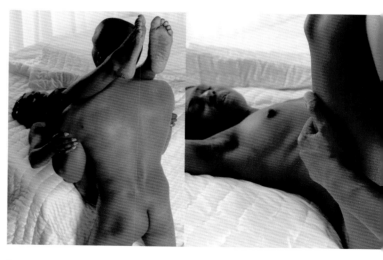

bed versus floor

Whatever the position, you don't have to limit your location to the bedroom, but kneeling positions are favourites for sex on the floor in other rooms. This is often for the purely practical reason that the floor offers greater resistance than the softer, springier bed, so you are more stable and less likely to topple over – a real risk with some of the more demanding and vigorous positions. The disadvantage is the same thing, the hardness of the surface. It's not always noticeable at the time, but afterwards you may find aching knees and, in several positions, a sore spine, a high price to pay. Even thick carpet provides only limited protection and can, in any case, cause painful friction burns. It takes only a few seconds to grab some pillows or cushions. It's even better if you fetch a quilt from the bedroom. Not only does this provide some comfortable padding, you can wrap yourselves in it afterwards for cosy, post-coital intimacy.

kneeling position 5

The man kneels on the floor, and the woman lies down on the bed or a couch or sofa. She puts her legs up against his chest, making sure she is right at the edge of the bed. The man holds the woman's buttocks and pulls them towards him as he gently enters her. It is essential that there is a carpet or quilt on the floor to protect the man's knees.

Here, the man has the opportunity for deep penetration and both partners can watch his penis thrusting in and out. He also has a great view of her breasts and can lean forward to massage and fondle them if he is agile. All the woman has to do is lie there, watch his face as he builds up to orgasm, and enjoy.

PLUS POINTS This is great for those who love the sensation of deep, powerful thrusting.
Sex in this position can be fast and urgent or prolonged and intimate, depending on your mood.
It is highly arousing visually.

MINUS POINTS This is not ideal for women who like to be in at least partial control of the action.
As with all positions where penetration is very deep, it is important that the man is sensitive to the possibility of causing his partner discomfort.

OPPOSITE | Kneeling position 4. Simply by moving her feet from his chest to behind his head creates all sorts of utterly delicious sensations.

ABOVE | Kneeling position 5. She wriggles right to the edge of the bed, but he must hold on tight, otherwise you may both end up in an untidy heap on the floor.

side by side

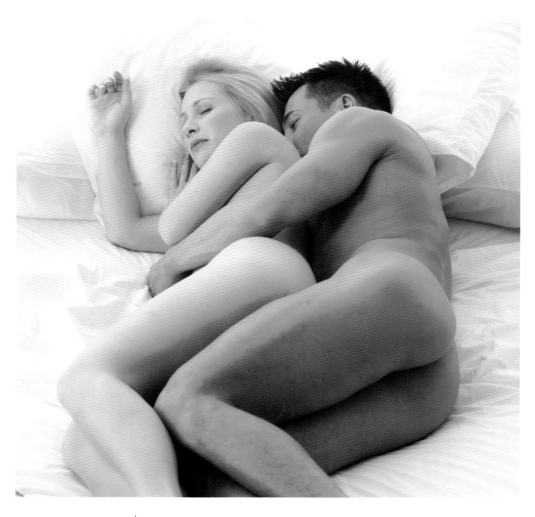

ABOVE | The basic side by side position is the most comforting, and so restful that it is easy to fall asleep afterwards without moving.

THIS IS CONSIDERED the least active of the sexual positions. It is perfect to do first thing in the morning when you just want some meditative and relaxing sex, on a lazy, hot afternoon or late at night when you're feeling romantic but sleepy. It is wonderfully cosy and very intimate, with lots of cuddling and caressing. It is good for tired people and those who aren't very agile. It is difficult for heavily pregnant women to find a comfortable sexual position that is not painful with deep thrusting, so this is a good one for them. It allows for hours of stop-and-go sex, and you can just fall asleep afterwards in exactly the same position, still connected if you are lucky.

basic side by side

Neither of you has to do a lot of work here, but there are infinite possibilities for touching, as your hands are free. The man snuggles up behind his partner as she draws up her knees towards her waist and he slots in behind her. This is pure skin-on-skin contact. He can kiss his partner's shoulders and neck and nibble her ears, while reaching around to cup her breasts. He can also reach down and stimulate her clitoris or alternatively, if there is some lubrication handy, place his finger around or into her anus.

The woman can reach back and massage his testicles or slowly masturbate him between sessions. She can also suck or nibble at his fingers. By lifting her leg over his, she can massage his thigh with the inner surface of hers – a surprisingly sensual sensation.

PLUS POINTS Good for a first-thing wake-up call as morning breath can be avoided.
This position still works if he has only a partial erection.
Great for whispering dirty things to each other.

MINUS POINTS This can be tricky for partners of very different height. The woman will need to bend her knees quite far and arch her back for the man to enter her. Not great for those who like to watch each other's faces.

side by side 1

From the basic side by side position, the man leans back. The woman places her leg over his and leans to a different angle. The man should grip the woman's hips when he enters her. This allows for deeper penetration than the basic position and involves a little more energy. It can feel slightly impersonal as you don't have much body contact apart from the genitals.

PLUS POINTS Women often find the sensation of being gripped firmly as penetration deepens very erotic. Men often find that feeling their partner's bottom pressed tightly against them is highly stimulating.

MINUS POINTS As you're further apart than the basic position, it is difficult to whisper in each other's ears.

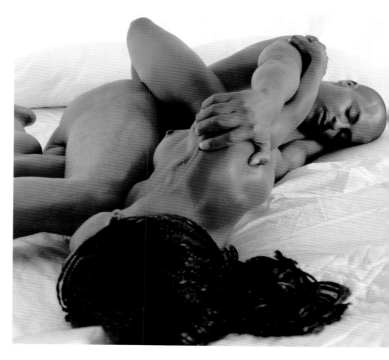

side by side 2

This is a great position for slow sex, but it requires agility and there is some choreography to learn. The woman lies in front of the man in spoons with his penis inside her. Slowly, both partners should lean away from each other with their legs stretched out straight, until their heads are at opposite ends of the bed. They then grab each other's hands or shoulders to prevent themselves coming apart. This position requires both verbal and non-verbal communication and co-ordination in slow movements.

PLUS POINTS Quite different from most other positions, this is good when you want some variety.
The man can watch and play with his partner's bottom, which is erotic for both him and her.

MINUS POINTS Not so great for the unsupple and unco-ordinated, but still worth trying if you share a sense of humour.

ABOVE | Side by side 2. This is also known as position X because of the shape.

BELOW | Side by side 1. Lean away from each other to vary the angles.

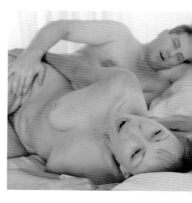

standing positions

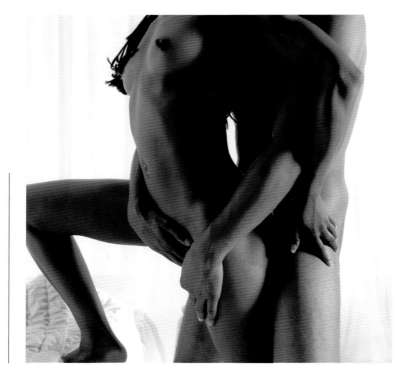

RIGHT | Standing position 3. Unfortunately, standing positions are often neglected in the bedroom in favour of more supine poses, but they may offer considerable scope for variation.

BELOW | Even in the basic standing position, it is easier for the man to enter his partner – and to stay there – if he lifts one of her thighs, supporting it with his hand.

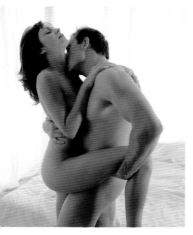

STANDING POSITIONS WORK better if you are both of a similar size, although you can always use the first one or two steps on the staircase to get the height correct. These positions engender very intimate embraces, because you have total body contact and can kiss and caress each other constantly. However, penetration is not very deep.

basic standing position

This is one you see regularly in movies, whether it's in the shower, up against a garden wall, or against a door. It's fantastic for passionate, spur-of-the-moment sex in a place you never expected it to happen. If you're in the shower, before you even start penetration, lather up your hands with soap and wash each other all over, leaving the pubic area until last, but then rinse thoroughly, as it may sting if used for lubrication. Then the man gently pins his partner up against the wall and enters her, grabbing her by the bottom. She can put her arms either up against the wall for balance or around his neck. He can suck her nipples and breasts and she can massage all down his spine.

PLUS POINTS Spontaneous sex is incredibly erotic, not least because it somehow seems a little naughty. There's plenty of scope for touching, caressing, nibbling, nuzzling, licking and every kind of body contact.

MINUS POINTS Falling over, especially if you are in a slippery shower, is always a risk.
Make sure the shower you are in is structurally stable.

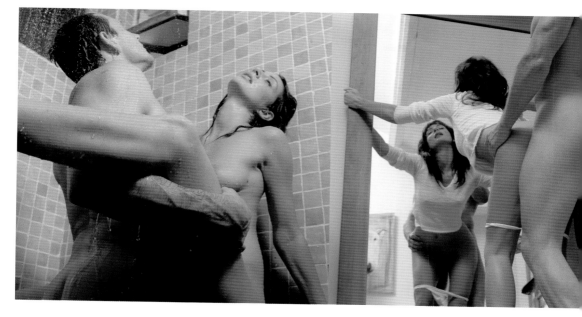

standing position 1

The woman stands with one leg over her partner's forearm or shoulder if she can manage it. A strong grip is needed to keep a balance, so it will be best if the woman has her back up against the wall. This position gives the woman deeper penetration than the previous one, with plenty of opportunity for kissing, licking and general nuzzling.

PLUS POINTS This is a great opportunity for any woman who practises yoga or even went to ballet classes as a child to surprise and delight her partner.

MINUS POINTS Only for the supple – otherwise pulled muscles and/or falling over may occur.

standing position 2

Stand in front of a mirror, so you both have a view of what's going on. The man enters his partner from behind, holding on to her hips. The thrusting will be shallow, so you both might have to lean slightly forward in order to keep the penis inside. The man can nuzzle into his partner's neck and there's plenty of skin contact.

PLUS POINTS An irresistible temptation to talk dirty as well as to watch yourselves.

MINUS POINTS It is quite difficult for the man to prevent his penis from slipping out, so there is not much scope for vigorous movement.

standing position 3

This is another rear entry position. Both stand by the bed (just in case you fall over) with the man holding his partner's thigh, so her leg is lifted and foot resting on the bed – her knee being bent will allow deeper penetration. He lowers himself slightly and enters her from the rear. With one hand free he will be able to offer some clitoral stimulation as well.

PLUS POINTS Because this is more stable than other upright positions the woman has more opportunity to match her partner's thrusts.
He has a hand free for extra caressing.

MINUS POINTS While he can caress her body, she will be unable to reach much of his.

ABOVE LEFT | Standing position 1. Only for the supple.

ABOVE RIGHT | Standing room only for position 2.

dangerous liaisons

Astonishingly, thousands of people each year are, apparently, admitted to A&E (the Emergency Room) with injuries sustained while attempting unusual sexual positions. When trying out exciting new positions with your partner, remember to keep within your limitations and although alcohol may remove inhibitions, it doesn't make you any more flexible, more supple or any younger.

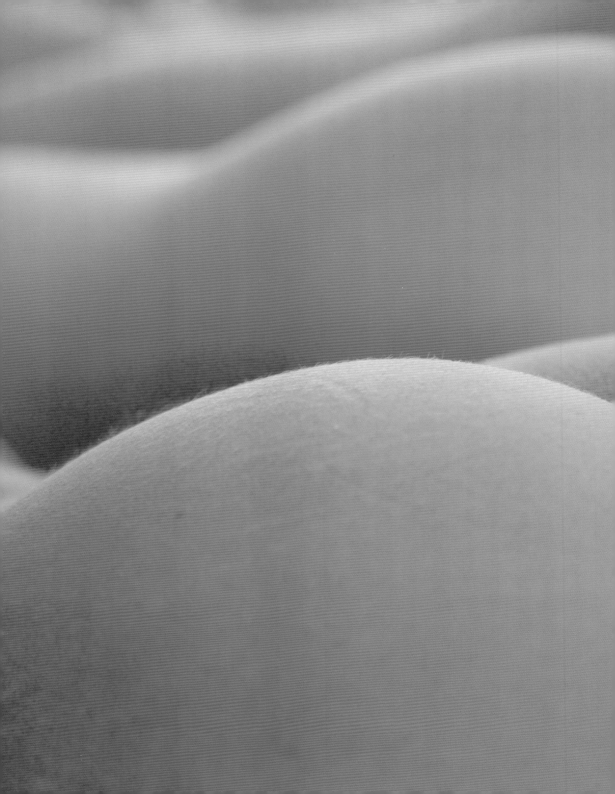

x-factors

There is more to a sensational sex life than vaginal sex, delicious and important though that is. Both oral and anal sex can bring some spice to a relationship, creating unique sensations of extreme pleasure – both when giving and when receiving.

please your partner

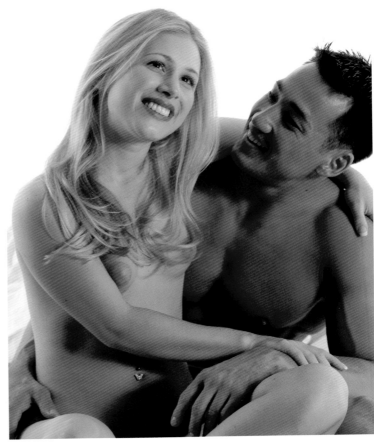

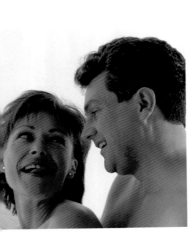

IN THE LAST FEW DECADES there has been a definite trend towards demystifying sex and dispensing with sexual taboos and many sexual barriers have been broken down by increased information and greater liberation. Masturbation is now considered normal practice, although some women are still only just beginning to feel comfortable with admitting to self-pleasure. It's much the same with anal sex and oral sex. Pleasing your partner with your mouth – or vice versa – is as natural as doing it any other way. In fact, with the added bonus of that most mobile organ, the tongue, the erotic potential might even be increased.

Sex is all about pleasure and intimacy. If you find pleasure from anal penetration or oral sex, then where's the problem? Equally, if you're not keen, there's no reason why you should feel obliged to include them in your sexual repertoire.

talking about it

Reading about positive aspects of what, in the immediate past, was regarded as a sexual taboo, might well create a desire in you to try it out for yourself. But even the most liberated people sometimes find it tricky to discuss their innermost sexual thoughts with their partner. How, then, do you go further still and raise adventurous topics such as fellatio, cunnilingus and anal penetration?

Perhaps you and your partner already have a great sex life, but you feel there is always time and space to try something new. Whatever your reasons, it may be hard to put them into words for fear that you may offend your lover by making him or her feel inadequate or threatened. You may also be concerned that they may regard you as a little perverted for bringing up the possibility of more risqué sexual options. The likelihood is that they won't feel anything except excitement at the prospect of jazzing things up.

So where to begin? A straightforward request is probably too blunt and might provoke a straightforward negative reply that closes off that prospect forever. Instead, be a little more subtle and sensitive. If you'd like to explore anal sex, for example, you could take his or her hand during foreplay and gently guide it to your anus. If he or she pulls back in fright or horror, then just smile and explain that you have never done it before and thought it might be fun to give it a try. Don't make a big deal of it and he or she probably won't either. In fact your partner will probably be keen to please you and as curious to try something new as you are, so why not mull it over together?

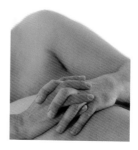

ABOVE AND BELOW | By discussing issues such as oral and anal sex beforehand, you are less likely to hurt each other's feelings and overstep each other's boundaries.

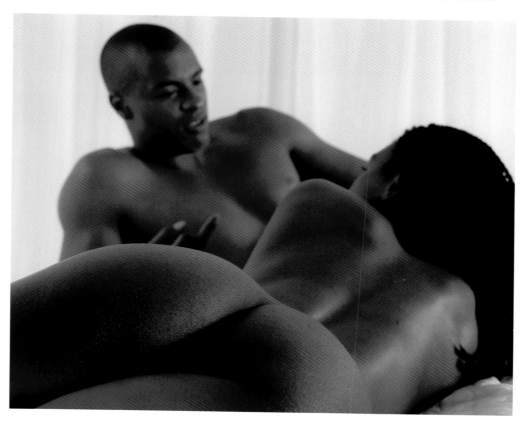

oral sex

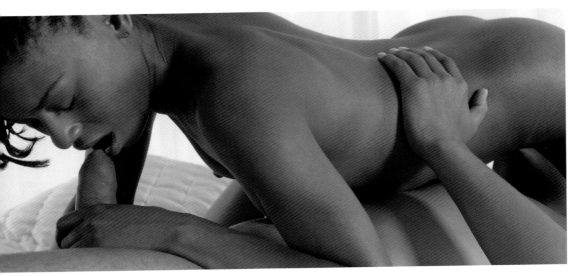

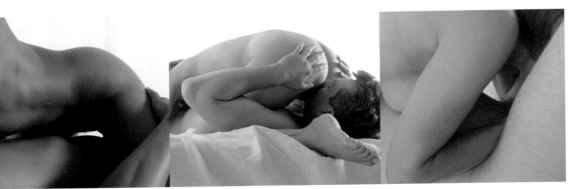

ABOVE | Whatever position you choose, the tongue is an extraordinarily flexible organ and can be made hard or soft. Try it on your hand to vary your technique and then practise on your partner.

THE ACT OF ORAL SEX is an extremely intimate and trusting one in which you invariably find yourself opening up to your partner and allowing them access to your most sensitive and private places. When you think about it subjectively, it is actually quite a bizarre ritual. Licking, sucking, tasting and pleasuring your partner is a very emotional experience that requires commitment, not only to your partner but also to the task in hand. All too

many people think of oral sex as a prelude to penetrative sex. In actual fact, it is really a quite separate act. The techniques used for explosive oral sex are extremely different from those of penetrative sex. By refining the art, you can get a greater understanding of your partner's sexual preferences. It is an exciting journey of exploration into your partner's hot spots – a journey that is equally, if not more, exciting for them.

For many people, the difference between being an average and an exceptional lover lies here. Skilful fellatio and cunnilingus – giving good head, providing a great blow-job or going down with the best of them – whatever you call it, is worthy of an award. There is nothing more sensual and pleasurable than lying back and being orally stimulated by a genital genius.

You must remember that tastes – literally and metaphorically – differ tremendously in this department. What may be a great oral sex technique on one individual may be totally inappropriate for another. In order to be a great oral aficionado, the secret is timing, listening and responding. Once again, it's all to do with communication. Take time to do oral sex, and do it sometimes without penetration in mind. Listen to your partner's moans, groans and body movements to work out what is working for them and what isn't. Respond according to what is working and *keep doing it.*

Make it apparent to your partner that you are enjoying yourself too. Oral sex is not something you just do to someone else; you are participating and sharing in the activity and relishing the intimacy, the effects you are having and, in fact, the entire experience. (If you're not, perhaps you shouldn't be doing it all.) Some people worry that the active partner in oral sex is not getting their "fair share". Sexual pleasure and orgasm are not like a bank balance – you don't have to keep in credit all the time.

soixante-neuf

The 69 is tricky. Many people find it hard to concentrate on stimulating as well as being simultaneously stimulated. It can be difficult for the man to hit the woman's spot in this position, as his chin is stimulating her clitoris. Similarly, it is the less sensitive top side of the penis that receives most stimulation in this position. Height differences can cause problems too, making one partner curl and the other stretch.

So why do it? Well apart from the fact that it is a real giggle, it can also be quite effective. The sight of each other's most private places up so

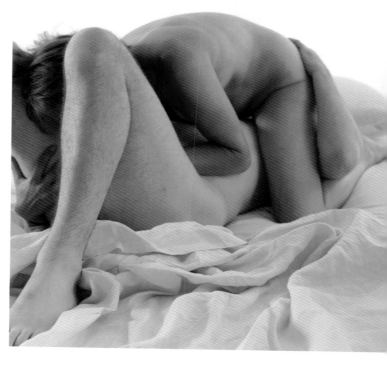

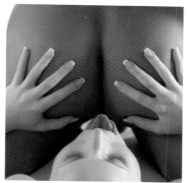

close can prove to be an astonishingly erotic experience. If the woman goes on top, she is more in control and her partner can stimulate her dangling breasts. The man can massage her buttocks – most men find their partners' bottoms arousing – or just concentrate on her genital area.

ABOVE | Soixante-neuf is an expression of ultimate togetherness and complete trust in each other.

LEFT | Rimming is the term used to describe licking around the anus. It is a highly pleasurable experience but as always the area must be scrupulously clean. If rimming a casual partner a dental dam of clear film (plastic wrap) is a good barrier method to prevent contracting sexually transmitted infections.

fellatio

PUTTING YOUR MOUTH around a man's penis requires trust on both sides – you assume that he's washed and that he won't choke you, and he assumes that no biting will be involved, something men commonly have nightmares about. The secret to giving good head is, without a doubt, enthusiasm, but most men agree that the mere idea of a blow-job is a massive turn-on. If you don't want to do it, then simply refrain – a half-hearted effort will disappoint him and make you resentful and there are lots of other delicious things to do. However, if you are willing, it's unfair for him to expect you to do so if he's not prepared to return the compliment himself every once in a while.

BELOW | Fellatio works from any direction. Straddle your partner's chest, for example. He won't be able to see what you are doing, but can enjoy the rear view.

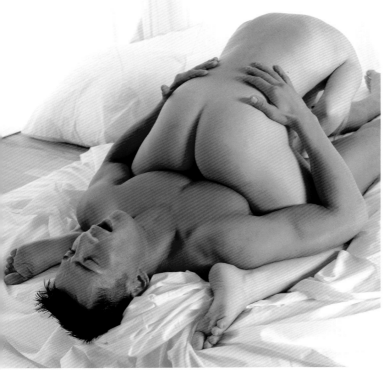

where to begin

The best blow-jobs are those given as a luxurious, time-consuming package. Rather than heading straight for the penis, it's often nice to incorporate an element of anticipation. Lie him flat on his back and begin either at his feet, working up, or at his chest, working down. The secret here is to ignore time and to immerse yourself in both his body and his needs. Sucking toes, licking nipples, massaging his inner thighs and flicking a tongue around his belly button are just some of the delights you can provide for him, but stay away from the genital area to begin with. He will read the road you are following, so as you start to home in towards his groin, he will be almost literally bursting with excitement. Once down there, you can tease him by licking around the outline of his penis on his belly, allowing your breath to pass over it or brushing your lips suggestively over the head of his penis before using direct stimulation.

technique

From this point there are a variety of techniques that you can use. Different men like to be stimulated in different ways, so why not try them all and see which ones he likes the most? You can discuss what his likes and dislikes are or simply read his body. If he's groaning and grinding, then you are on to a winner. If he is quieter or pulling away from you, try something else.

Position yourself so that you are comfortable. Most women like to be between their partner's legs, with him lying back. This positions the tongue so it can easily stimulate the front of the penis, the most sensitive area, and also allows your partner to look down and watch you in action, which will excite him even more.

Use a lot of saliva to lubricate the lower part of the shaft, which you can stimulate with your hands. Wrap your lips over your teeth. The merest hint of anything sharp near a man's penis will have him leaping away from you in fear.

Get your tongue working. Little flicks of the tongue around the head and over the frenulum are very stimulating. Roll your tongue both quickly and slowly around the head and, if you can, use the thin layer of skin that joins your tongue to your mouth to stimulate the frenulum.

The term "blow-job" is really a misnomer, as you don't actually need to blow. As you go up and down the penis, you can create an airtight seal with your lips. This means that as you move up the penis, a vacuum will naturally suck so you don't have to. Use quite a firm grip with your mouth and twist your head around at the same time for added stimulation. Use your tongue too, applying extra pressure or using a quick flicking action.

The head of the penis is often more sensitive in uncircumcised men. You can place the tip of your tongue underneath the foreskin and run circles around the head, or you can pull the foreskin back with your hands by wrapping them around the shaft, just above the base, and pulling down to the base. This exposure heightens sensitivity and will make it more exciting for him.

A good blow-job is a partnership of both the mouth and the hands. While your mouth concentrates mainly on the top end of his penis, your hands can be working on the lower shaft. The

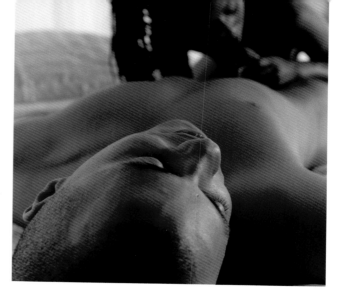

most successful technique is to synchronize your movements, allowing your hands to follow the pumping action of your mouth.

spicing it up

Experimentation with different tastes and textures can spice up a blow-job even more. Try sucking on a mint beforehand. The added ingredient of menthol in your saliva will provide a different sensation on your partner's penis. Sucking ice cubes or licking

ABOVE | Don't neglect his testicles and perineum while you are giving him a blow-job. It will enhance his experience if you gently stroke these areas with your free hand.

BELOW | Sitting or lying down, make sure you are both comfortable before you begin.

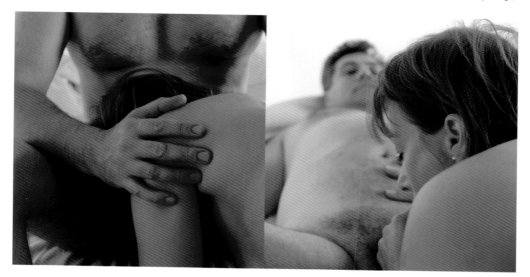

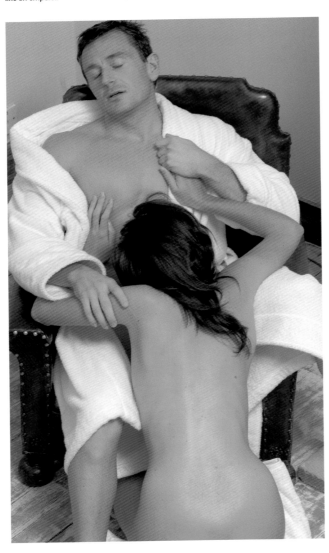

BELOW | In the chair – he sits in the armchair and she kneels on the floor in front of him. This is liable to make him feel like an emperor.

ice cream and then drinking hot drinks also adds variety in the form of hot and cold sensations, but beware of extremes. Your favourite spreads, such as chocolate or jam, can also make it a tastier experience for you and you can have lots of fun with the application.

Some men like to have their prostate or anus stimulated during oral sex and many of them say that orgasm is greatly heightened when the prostate is stimulated at the same time. Using a little lubrication, massage around the area for a while to relax him before gradually slipping in one finger. Once inside, very gently massage the area towards his belly button, taking care not to scratch with your fingernail. Licking around the anus, known as rimming, is also a source of pleasure for some men.

Another technique worth trying is called "flicking". Don't panic – despite the name it's actually a pleasurable experience for him if done properly. During a blow-job, slide the shaft out of your mouth and then flick his penis gently against your cheek or neck a few times; you get a breather and he gets a different sensation.

blow-job basics

edging This is a great move if your mouth needs a bit of a breather. Hold his penis in one hand and place your lips at the bottom end of the shaft on the top side. Use your lips as if you were kissing and create a light suction, then move your mouth and head steadily up and down the shaft, increasing and decreasing the pace. You can use your other free hand to caress the head or glans of his penis at the same time.

rolling This produces a wonderful sensation as it concentrates on the head of the penis, the most sensitive area. Place your mouth over the head of the penis so that it is completely in your mouth. Use your tongue to stroke all around the edges of the head in a circular motion, quickening and lessening the pace and changing direction every now and again. When your tongue passes over the frenulum at the front of the head (facing you) use the bit of skin that attaches your tongue to the bottom of your mouth to stimulate it. You can also

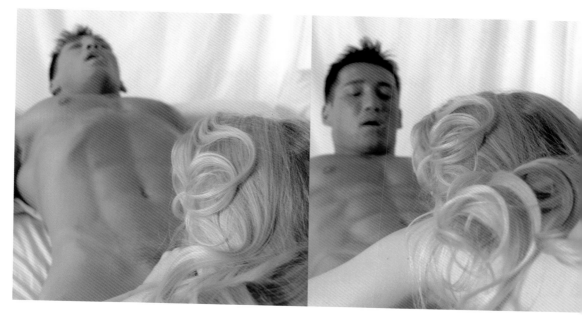

use your tongue to massage the tip, as if you were licking an ice cream.

balling Men's balls are very sensitive and you can give a lot of pleasure by playing with them. Just before a man comes, his balls contract and move up towards to the body to prepare for ejaculation: by gently gripping them at the top and pulling down (gently, gently) you can hold off his orgasm. Put both his balls in your mouth and sucking them and massaging them with your tongue can produce a wonderful sensation.

pumping Placing your mouth over his penis, form a tight vacuum with your lips, making sure that they cover your teeth to prevent scratching him. Then, using a slight sucking action, move your head up and down the shaft. Keeping your neck relaxed and taking a breath when you get to the top, and breathing out through your nose as you move down the shaft, will help you take more of him in your mouth and prevent you from gagging. Use either one or two hands to follow your mouth up and down the shaft, gripping it as you would a tennis racket. You can have quite a firm grip, the firmer the better.

humming As you are sucking him, try humming or moaning at the same time, as the vibrations from your voice box will penetrate through to his penis and make it more stimulating.

the swallow debate

The pros and cons of swallowing semen are individual to each woman. Some women don't like the idea of it, others wouldn't consider spitting and see swallowing as the ultimate finale. Men's preferences vary almost as much.

Knowing when a man is about to ejaculate can be quite tricky. Things to look for – apart from an obvious screaming announcement – are a tightening of the muscles and increased rate of breathing. His facial expression, if you can see it, is often a giveaway, too.

If you don't want to swallow, you can either withdraw and finish him off with your hand, or you can spit, but do it discreetly, or it will put you both off. Another alternative is to ask him to come on your breasts, which is known as a pearl necklace, or face. Semen is, after all, very good for the condition of your skin.

ABOVE | Decide before you begin giving him a blow-job whether you want to swallow or not. If you don't want to swallow, try not to be too obvious about it; excessive spitting and face-pulling is likely to spoil the whole experience for him.

cunnilingus

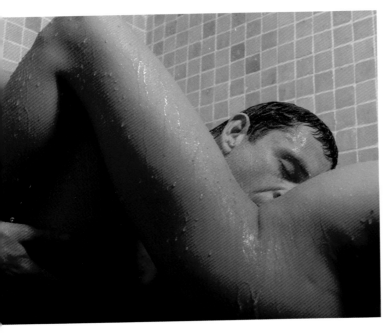

ABOVE AND OPPOSITE |
Whatever the position for cunnilingus, it must be comfortable for both partners. Then he can lavish time and attention on her, while she can abandon herself to pure sensation.

THE WHOLE ISSUE of oral stimulation for women – going down – is one that sends spasms of fear through many men. How a woman wishes to be stimulated is so individual that it takes a lot of time and communication to get it just right. It is difficult to gauge exactly how to stimulate the clitoris without some help from your partner and even then it can be tricky, as many women know how to stimulate themselves but often find it difficult to explain and teach. As your relationship progresses and you begin to read each other's bodies, cunnilingus gets better and easier; practice does, after all, make perfect.

where to begin

Performing cunnilingus, as with fellatio, is a luxuriously time-consuming act. Bear in mind that you may be doing it for a while and make sure that you are both comfortable. The best positions

are those in which both your bodies are pointing in the same direction, but as long as your tongue can reach her vagina, then any position will do.

Begin by kissing and sucking around the vulva, luxuriating in everything, excluding the clitoris. The clitoris is highly sensitive and needs plenty of forewarning before it is touched. Heading straight there can cause discomfort and, at times, even pain. Gently spread your partner's outer labia with your fingers and kiss and suck her inner labia in the same way that you would if you were kissing her passionately on the mouth. When you notice her starting to respond, glide your tongue between the folds of the inner labia. If her response is a sharp jerk or she pushes away from you, stay away from there for a while, concentrating, instead, on the outer edges and massaging her pubic mound with your hand.

Once your partner is sufficiently relaxed and turned on, you can expose the clitoral shaft which runs down from the top of the labia to the clitoral head, underneath the inner labia. You may find it helps to spread the labia with two hands to make the skin taut, exposing the shaft. This area of densely packed nerve endings is extremely sensitive and a soft tongue, hard tongue approach usually works best. Try to stimulate it first with your tongue relaxed and soft and if she begins grinding towards you, you can increase the pressure by tensing and firming your tongue muscles. Remember to keep your tongue well lubricated with saliva.

How you stimulate the clitoris is very individual to the woman. Some like a soft sucking or caressing action, while others prefer a harder and sharper flicking action, either up and down or sideways.

If the clitoris enlarges, then she likes what you are doing; if it shrinks, then stop. However, remember that just before orgasm, the clitoris often retracts and seemingly disappears, so it is important to read other signs from her as well.

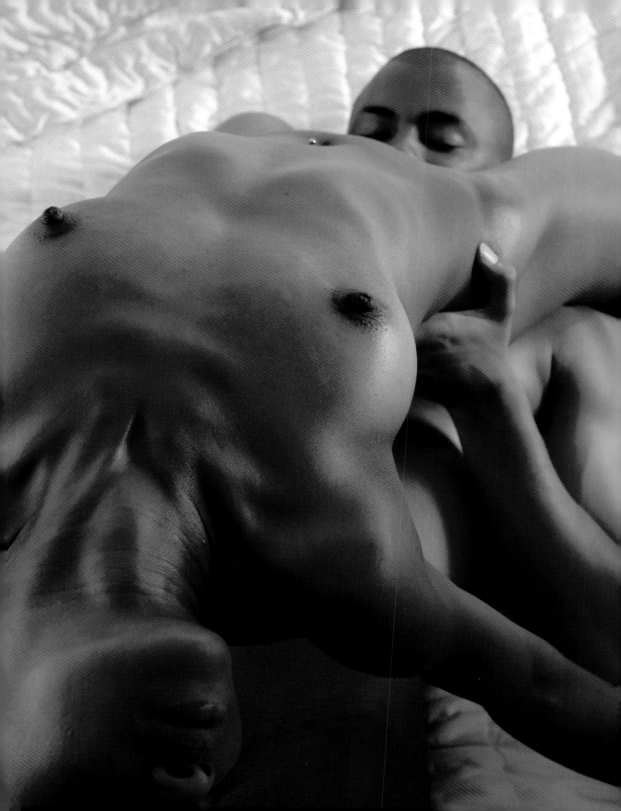

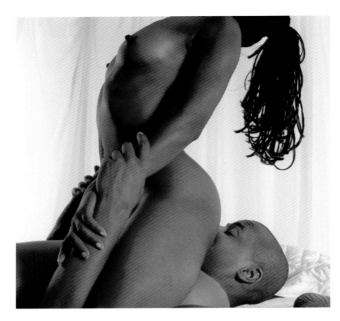

spicing it up

In the same way as fellatio, drinking hot and cold drinks before oral sex can lead to different sensations for your partner, but do be aware that the clitoral head is hypersensitive and may not necessarily respond well to extremes. Occasionally the head can become irritated, which will certainly cool down the proceedings.

Incorporating a vibrator can add to the experience; place it under your tongue, so the vibrations transmit through you.

To really extend playtime, bring her to the brink of orgasm and then stop for a good half a minute, do the same but stop for less time, and so on. Some women may not appreciate this, so it's best to discuss it first.

keep the rhythm going

Just before your partner is about to come, make sure you don't change a thing. Whatever you're doing is working, so just hold your ground and

ABOVE | For many men, cunnilingus with their partner sitting on their face is the realization of their dreams.

RIGHT | You need to be sensitive to your partner's responses. As she becomes increasingly aroused, you can put on the pressure and move your tongue more rapidly – but don't try to force the pace.

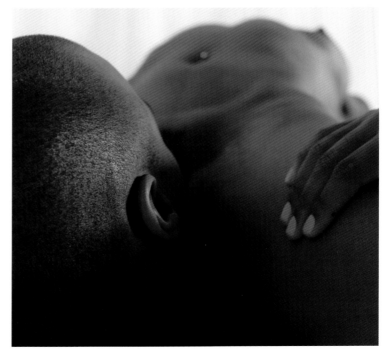

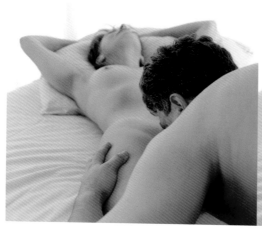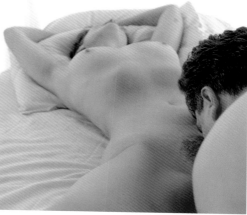

prepare for the tsunami. When she comes, don't necessarily stop unless she asks you to, but lighten the touch slightly and perhaps take the emphasis away from the clitoris. Continuing stimulation can increase the orgasm and some women even report multiple orgasms from good oral sex.

licking the clitoris

Imagine you're drawing small circles on and around her clitoris with your tongue. The smaller circles will concentrate on the tip and larger ones will deal with the base. Alternate the speed and direction of the circles, as some women respond better if the circles rotate in a specific direction.

Draw figures-of-eight over her clitoris with your tongue. This may be too much stimulation for some women but for others it will work wonders. Experiment with the speed and frequency.

Use your tongue to either flick the clitoris up and down with a short pause between each flick, or from left to right, aiming just underneath the base of the head. Vary the pressure of the flicks along with their frequency.

the bridge

Remember doing the bridge in the gym, when you raise your arched body up, supporting yourself only with your feet and hands? Well this is a variation for the more supple lover. He sits while

the woman positions herself face up with her knees hooked over his shoulders and her head between his knees or legs. From here she arches her back and uses her hands to support herself, raising her genitals closer to his face.

the edge

She lies down on the bed, on her front or back, with her bottom over the edge of the bed. He kneels on the floor between her legs and uses his hands on her bottom or pelvis to support her. She hooks her legs over his shoulders and he can raise her up or lower her down with his hands.

the triangle

She positions herself face down on the bed or floor with her bottom in the air and her legs straight and spread, similar to a triangle. He then sits so that the tops of her thighs are supported by his shoulders with his legs straight out on either side of her head.

face sitting

The man lies on his back while the woman crouches or kneels over his face, facing in either direction. This is great for women as they can control the pressure by either easing off or grinding down, but be careful not to suffocate him in the throes of passion.

ABOVE | There are no hard and fast rules for cunnilingus. Try to keep in tune with your partner so you can both get the most out of the experience.

anal sex

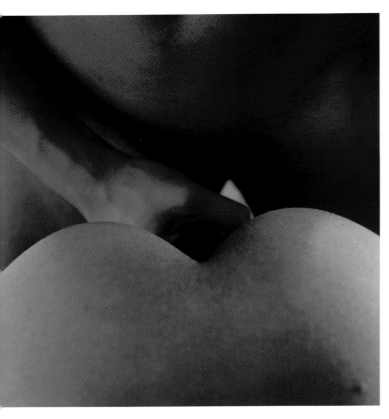

THOSE WHO PRACTISE anal sex insist that it can be one of the most stimulating experiences in the sexual repertoire. They claim that because the area concerned is jam-packed with sensitive nerve endings, when stimulated they produce a more intense and dramatic orgasm. Some people have tried it and found it a painful experience not worth repeating. Others see their anus as a one-way passage and find the mere thought of incorporating it in sex play plain disgusting and unnatural. The fact is that the anus is composed of two anal sphincters – rings of muscle – that are designed to control only outgoing matter. With training however, they can learn to facilitate a two-way traffic.

demystifying anal sex

Although no one should ever be forced to take part in any kind of sexual act that they are not comfortable with, it is worth mentioning that many people, both men and women, find anal sex a hugely enjoyable experience.

So why the taboo? There are several reasons, the most obvious of which is that, just like masturbation, people rarely admitted to the practice in the past. Secondly, when the AIDS virus became so prevalent in the western world in the 1980s, anal sex came to be seen as a gay practice that increased the risk of HIV and AIDS.

However, today people have a greater understanding of these viruses and so are less cautious about practising anal sex. Although it is true that unprotected anal sex can increase the risk of HIV and AIDS – the thin membrane in the rectum can easily be torn – with proper safety precautions (which should be used in all sexual adventures with new partners, be they anal or vaginal), the risk of contracting these viruses is minimal. The key word here is simply precautions. It is possible to buy harder-wearing condoms that are specifically designed for anal penetration or penetration where there is extra strain.

ABOVE | Absolute trust in your partner is the key to relaxation – essential for practising anal sex.

RIGHT | Couples who practise anal sex agree that it has added a new dimension of pleasure to their sex lives.

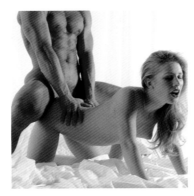

the gay factor

Anal sex is not an exclusively homosexual practice. In fact, only about half the gay population practises it. We already know that the male prostate gland is an area of great erotic potential that, when stimulated by a man or a woman, enhances sexual sensation and orgasm. The prostate gland, however, can only be accessed through the anus, so should it be ignored just because of inhibitions? If this is so, then we could be missing out on a whole array of potential sexual experiences purely because of the implied connotations.

In fact for men, practising anal sex on a woman is a tighter and more intense experience. For women, if it is done correctly and carefully, the vaginal and rectal walls can swell during arousal, stimulating the G spot and providing sensations that they could not get from vaginal penetration. Men receiving anal sex from a woman with the help of a strap-on, finger or vibrator can have their prostate stimulated at the same time as their penis.

the hygiene factor

This is another reason for the taboo. There's always the chance that a bit of faeces will still be in the rectum when it is penetrated, although most of the time it is stored in the colon until defecation. To combat this problem, you should empty your bowels before anal sex and not just when you need to go. If this is still not satisfactory, then you can buy an enema kit from the chemist and clear the system out in the bathroom beforehand. This may seem somewhat over the top, but performing anal sex does call for a little preparation.

getting down to it

The secret of successful and satisfying anal sex is trust and communication. Before you even think about doing it for the first time, you should be absolutely certain that your partner is someone you can trust. Discussing it beforehand is also important and if you can't do this, forget about it. Without these two essential ingredients you can only end up hurting, and possibly damaging yourself or your partner.

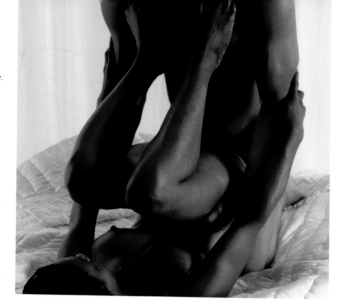

relax and do it

The difference between anal pain and pleasure is relaxation. When you are tense, your natural reaction is to clench your buttocks, so it's important that the environment and pre-anal play is relaxing and complementary. A massage, soft lighting, a warm bath and soothing music can all help in setting the right scene.

When practising anal sex for the first time, the key is to use plenty of lubrication and take it very slowly. Initially, you will probably find the sphincter tightens up, making entry seem impossible. Get your partner to use more lubrication and gently massage the area for a while before even contemplating putting anything up there. Stimulate each other's genitals at the same time, as nervousness can lead to loss of arousal. If this happens, it's best to stop and try again later.

For the first few times it is advisable just to insert a clean, manicured finger, slowly and gently. By doing this, the rectum learns to relax and not to "clam up" every time anything goes near it. Gentle massage with the inserted finger, bending slightly towards the coccyx (tailbone), following the natural curve of the rectum, can also help you to relax. It's a good idea if the receiver inserts his or her own finger up the anus to get a better understanding of how it all works.

ABOVE | Men enjoy the tighter feeling of anal penetration. For a woman, the stimulation of the G spot is exciting.

ABOVE | Gentle, lubricated massage is the way to start.

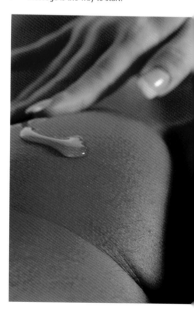

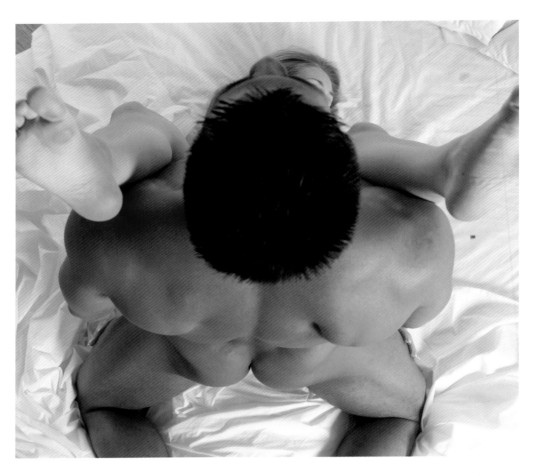

ABOVE | Once anal sex has become part of a couple's sensual repertoire, they can experiment with confidence to explore a whole range of different positions.

Entry is usually the most difficult part and must always be done slowly and with care. It's often better if the receiver lowers herself or himself on to the partner's well-lubricated penis or dildo with the partner applying constant pressure and a guiding hand. (Unlike the vagina, there is no natural lubrication in the anus.) Remember, though, that both entry *and* exit must be done slowly. A quick exit can cause a lot of pain and even damage. Remember, slow equals safe.

Once in, thrusting should be minimal to start with. Keep applying the lubrication and check frequently that your partner is all right. If there is any discomfort, stop for a while, with the penis or dildo still inside, and calm things down by stimulating the genitals or by giving a soothing massage. If the discomfort continues, it's best to stop altogether and try again another time. Remember that before entering the vagina after the anus, you must wash your penis to prevent any potential infection.

strap-on fun

Some men like their female partner to wear a strap-on anal dildo to stimulate their prostate. Others feel it has some stigma attached. Once tried, lots of straight couples enjoy the delights of anal sex and it becomes a regular part of their lives.

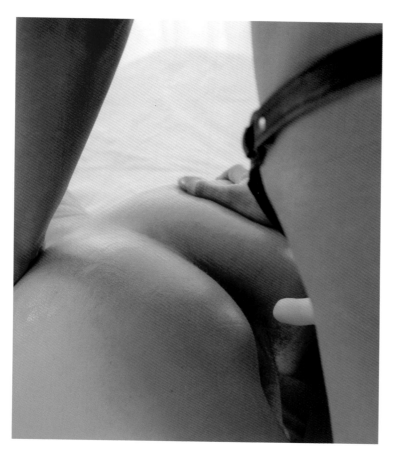

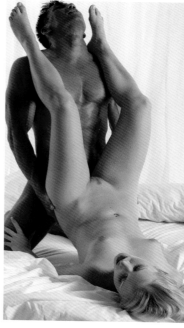

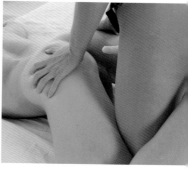

anal sex and the law

The term sodomy refers not only to anal sex but also to "lewd and lascivious behaviour". Many countries and US states use sodomy laws as a means of preventing homosexual behaviour regardless of whether penetrative sex is present or not. However, sodomy laws affect gays and straights alike.

In Massachusetts, for instance, sodomy is illegal. Anyone convicted faces a maximum sentence of 20 years plus another eight for "lewd and lascivious behaviour".

Countries that have sodomy laws include Jamaica, USA, Morocco, Saudi Arabia, India, Mauritius, Trinidad and Tobago, Malaysia, Tunisia and the Seychelles. Countries where sodomy is punishable by death include Afghanistan, Pakistan, Yemen, Iran, Saudi Arabia, Mauritania and Sudan.

In the UK there is no sodomy law at present, and in the Netherlands, full marriage rights are given to homosexual couples who enjoy a relatively free life.

ABOVE AND LEFT | Being penetrated by a woman may be disconcerting to begin with, but many find that seeing their partner with a strap-on is highly erotic.

TOP | There are as many positions for anal sex as there are for vaginal rear entry.

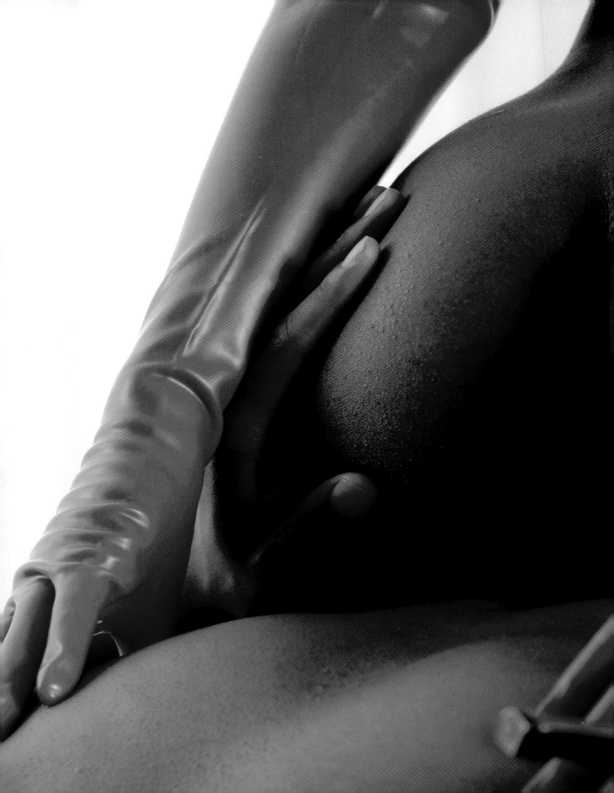

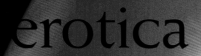

erotica

There comes a time in many couples' lives when sex can become rather routine and occasionally you might need a little stimulation from outside. Incorporating pornography, reading erotic literature together or shopping for sex toys can add that extra zing to your lovemaking, especially if you both have a good sense of humour.

the senses and sensuality

BELOW | What used to be called "sex aids" now come in all shapes and sizes. Artists and designers are turning their skills to making sex toys more approachable and more aesthetically pleasing.

THIS CHAPTER IS A JOURNEY through the more advanced and esoteric practices of sex. It covers sexual acts that push the boundaries out just that little further. You don't have to be a leather-masked, latex-wearing, whip-wielding dominatrix to appreciate this chapter. Erotica is more to do with stimulating the senses, all five of them, removing the emphasis from actual penetration and

technique. To that end, this chapter could be seen as the most sensual of them all – a delicious exploration of the darker side to sex.

Although sado-masochism (S&M), body manipulation and whipping are touched on in these pages, this chapter is more about the sensuality of using different media in your sex play. Wearing leather in bed can be very arousing,

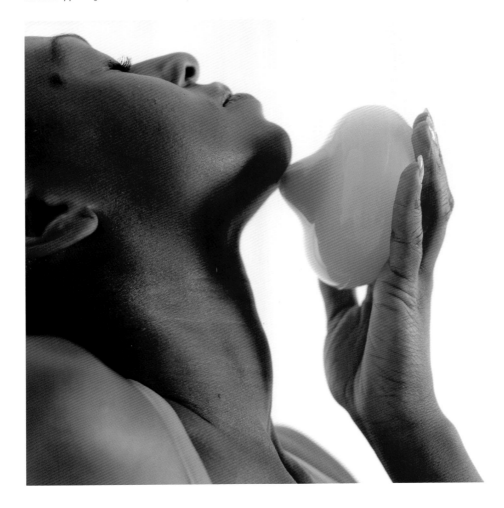

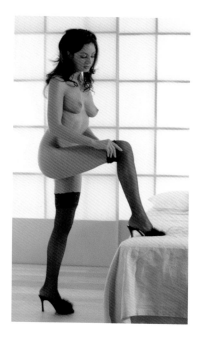

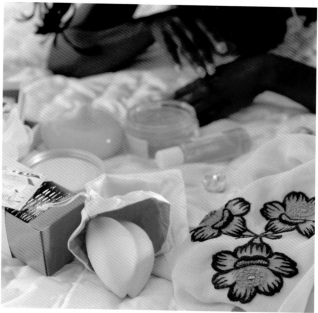

for example, purely because of its sexy connotations and the texture of it against your skin. It does not necessarily mean that you are about to embark on some sinister role play with your partner, involving nipple clamps, whips and chains. It could be quite the opposite.

sensuality

There are plenty of ways to introduce the sensual touch to your sex life. For instance, silk scarves, with their cool soft slippery texture, are sexy when used to tie up your partner. The emphasis is not so much on the tying up, but on the sensuousness of the material against your skin. This form of tying up allows you to luxuriate in your partner while he or she lies back and enjoys the sensations.

Try to incorporate much more sensuality into your sex play by concentrating on your five senses:

touch Be aware of the pressure you use when caressing your lover, use just your fingertips and then the pads of your fingers when stroking each other. Use different textures on your skin: feathers, silk, satin, velvet, rubber, a soft brush.

sound Choose music to go with your mood. Jazz is always mellow and helps you relax, or you may be a Beethoven or Mozart type of person who likes a good crescendo. Brazilian, Cuban and other World music is very sensual and can strongly influence the way you move and groove together.

sight Create your own magic space with lighting, candles or dimmers. Use fairy lights around a mirror or tea lights along a mantelpiece. Soft lighting is conducive to relaxation and the flickering flames can be hypnotic.

smell Rub musk or vanilla scented oil into your body, sprinkle rose petals on your bed, use scented candles, burn incense, or have your favourite flowers in full bloom.

taste The best taste is the taste of sex – that musty, musky, heavy, natural perfume that attracts us to one another. However, you might also enjoy some delicious tidbits to tempt each other with. Choose different flavours and sensations: the satin of melting chocolate, the juiciness of ripe mangoes, the saltiness of caviar, the softness of yogurt or cream, the coldness of ice cream.

ABOVE LEFT | Stockings and high heels may be a cliché, but they are still a turn-on.

ABOVE RIGHT | Sex accessories are abundant. There is a huge variety of places that will help you to stock up.

BELOW | Hold-ups or stockings, for some men it is a matter of fetish – for women one it is a question of comfort.

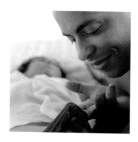

erotica and pornography

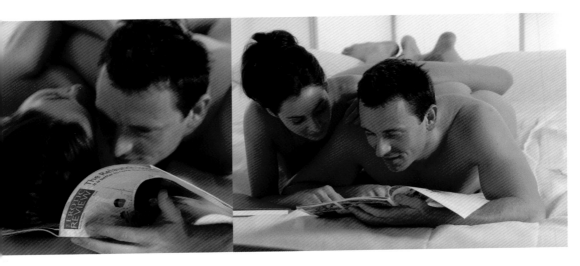

ABOVE AND ABOVE RIGHT |
Erotica is often more exciting than straightforward porn, but the range of sexy literature and magazines covers the entire spectrum. Reading it together – or to each other – can be a great turn-on.

I KNELT DOWN in front of him again. His cock, already thickly inflated, sprang up. I moved my hand over his balls, back up to their base near the anus. His cock stood up again, more violently. I held it in my other hand, squeezed it, began slowly pulling it up and down. The soapy water I was lathered with provided perfect lubrication. My hands were filled with a warm, living, magical substance. I felt it beating like the heart of a bird, I helped it ride to its deliverance. Up, down, always the same movement, always the same rhythm, and the moans above my head. And I was moaning too, with the water from the shower sticking to my dress like a tight silken glove, with the world stopped at the level of my eyes, of his belly, at the sound of the water tickling over us and of his cock sliding under my fingers, at the warm and tender and hard thing between my hands, at the smell of the soap, of the soaking flesh and of the sperm mounting under my palm.

Taken from *The Butcher* by Alina Reyes, this is a perfect example of contemporary erotica. Reading it is like drinking a glass of single malt whisky or fine wine – it makes you feel really good

all over. In addition, it stimulates the erogenous zone that straightforward pornography simply cannot reach – the brain.

Erotic literature can be a great aid to sex. It can provide the warm-up act before your lover comes on stage or can be part of the programme together in bed. The choice is vast, whether books, poetry, films or magazines. It gives you access to your fantasies and often provides brilliant material to act out in the reality and privacy of your bedroom.

Most people think of porn films and dirty magazines when they think of literature associated with sex. Getting away from the hard stuff, there is a wonderful variety of sensual and erotic films that are guaranteed to get you in the mood. You may be inspired by a raunchy sex scene in an elevator, or the idea of being blindfolded, lightly tied up and fed delicious morsels on the kitchen floor.

At the other end of the scale, the gritty porn film and dirty magazines can be appealing because of their explicitness and lack of subtlety. Many people watch porn and read dirty magazines as masturbation tools or as extra stimulation in sex play. Both men and women find it exciting to view something that appears so naughty. It helps to vent fantasies that are active in people's minds but which would perhaps never be brought into reality. To this end it is by no means wrong or subversive to use porn, providing of course that it is legal.

make your own movie

Many people think that porn movies are generally smutty, badly acted and could be done better, so why not give it a go yourself? All you need is a camcorder and a bit of imagination.

Start by sitting down with your partner and discussing the "theme" of your movie. Don't make a script as all the best porn movies rarely have a good script anyway, but just get a general idea of how events will run together. Some ideas could be: the doctor's visit; the prostitute visiting his or her client; an alien sent from outer space to learn more about human procreation; the electrician coming to fix the television.

Set the scene, get any props that you might want, and dress up appropriately for your roles. Position the camera so that you have a good view of the room and, most importantly, the bed. Finally hit record and begin.

Making your own porn film is not only hilarious fun, but also watching it afterwards together can be an extremely erotic experience. Seeing yourselves making love from a different angle gives you a whole new perspective. Alternatively, if you don't have a camcorder then you could create your own kinky photo shoot – just be careful about where you get the pictures developed.

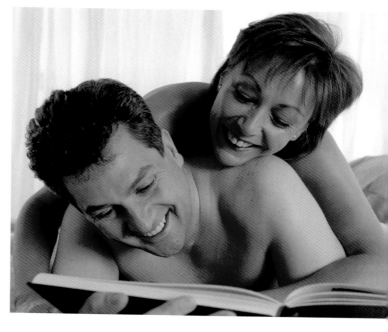

ABOVE | Sharing a pornographic book may end up as a joint exercise in humour or it might give you some interesting ideas.

erotic poetry

The choice of erotic poetry is vast, but sometimes the classics are the best, like DH. Lawrence's poem from *Women in Love*. Here is a taster of the first few lines, best sampled while resting under a ripe fig tree, accompanied by your partner, a good bottle of wine and the sun on your skin…

The proper way to eat a fig, in society,
Is to split it in four, holding it by the stump,
And open it, so that it is a glittering, rosy,
moist, honied, heavy-petalled four-
petalled flower.

Then you throw away the skin

Which is just like a four-sepalled calyx,
After you have taken off the blossom
with your lips.

But the vulgar way
Is just to put your mouth to the crack, and
take out the flesh in one bite.

Every fruit has its secret.
The fig is a very secretive fruit.
As you see it standing growing, you feel at
once it is symbolic:
And it seems male.
But when you come to know it better, you
agree with the Romans, it is female.

sex games

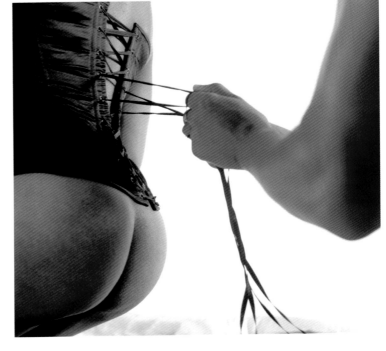

party games

dice games Get two dice. Write down one sexual position for each number on the first die. Then write down six places for the second die (the car, the broom closet, the stairs and so on). Roll the two dice together and obey dutifully.
truth or dare Take it in turns between either answering a personal question (truth) or performing some naughty act (dare) – great after a couple of glasses of wine.
spin the bottle This is a game for an adult party. Each of you should write a list of sexual forfeits. Spin an empty wine bottle, and the person it points at must undertake the next forfeit.

LET'S FACE IT, repeated sex with the same person can get rather, well, repetitive. A common complaint is, "Our sex lives have become boring. What can we do to spice things up?"

play time

Sex is meant to be fun. When you recognize that glint in your partner's eye, you will know that it's time to go and have a bit of adult play time. There are lots of games that you and your partner can share to enliven the average bedroom and not all of them have to involve his wearing your underwear. You can play naked scrabble, hide and seek in the garden, have dinner in the nude when the kids are away at camp – and cook it wearing nothing but an apron. The list is endless, and the main goal? To have a laugh and enjoy each other.

dressing up

Nurses, doctors, chambermaids and dominatrices: these are all well known in the repertoire of role-plays that many people enjoy. Less obvious scenarios include the bored housewife and the plumber, starring in a porn movie, a visit from a high-class call girl and even pretending to be complete strangers.

Dressing up and role-play are not just for drama students; you can re-create your bedroom as a dungeon of depravity, a hospital of hedonism or even Lara Croft's lair. It's an opportunity to put those fantasies into reality. You can buy outfits or make your own. Your boyfriend's a fire fighter? Wear his uniform; it's bound to keep him smiling the next day at work. Your girlfriend is a doctor? It's what white coats were made for.

board games

Dust off those board games you play only at Christmas. Although there are games that you can buy that involve an element of stripping or sex play, you can just as easily reinvent the rules of the old favourites. Instead of paying the fine when you have to "go directly to jail", change the cards for your own set, with whatever your desire dictates as the forfeits.

strangers

The following ideas allow you to act out your desires. Surprise your partner on your anniversary by secretly booking a hotel room. Tell him or her to meet you at a specific time in a restaurant nearby but make sure he or she understands that this is a blind date and that you have never met before.

Arrive at the restaurant and introduce yourself. Order wine and sumptuous food, and flirt in the manner that you did before you met one another. As the evening progresses, become more provocative. Tell him or her that you are wearing no underwear or that you have a partner but would be interested in playing away from home on this occasion. As the meal comes to a close, ask them if they would be up for a one-night stand of no-strings-attached unadulterated sex.

As you leave, do not tell them where you are going, but arrive at the hotel and accept the booking under pseudonyms such as Mr and Mrs Smith. Then, staying in character, play the ultimate sexual host or hostess, asking what they want you

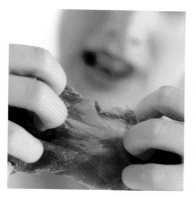

to do to them. If you can stay in character then this is guaranteed to release the naughty side to both your natures and result in some pretty hot and exciting sex.

midnight feast

Have some oysters and champagne hidden in the refrigerator, making sure your partner doesn't see them when he or she comes home. Have a normal evening, with a light meal, and then say that you want an early night because you have a headache. Make sure you set an alarm or stay awake while your partner sleeps so that at midnight you can quietly get up and set the scene in the bedroom with candles and soft music. Retrieve the champagne and oysters and bring them into the bedroom. Start the music and gently wake your partner. Eat and drink together and enjoy a night of passion. This is best done on a Friday or Saturday night so you can catch up on the sleep you will inevitably lose.

teaser

This is a great oral sex game to get you and your partner literally bursting with anticipation and sexual energy. Begin by lying him or her back on the bed and explain that they are not to move, and if they do then they will be punished. Massage their whole body from their chest, arms, legs and down to their toes, avoiding the genitals. Then start to kiss and caress the chest, sucking on his or her nipples and massaging with your hands. Work your way down slowly, paying attention to every crack and crevice of their body, and begin to work your way towards their genitals.

If they move, "punish" them by beginning all over again from the top. Give them oral pleasure, beginning lazily at first, every now and again stopping and moving to another part of the body. Make the breaks less and less frequent but every time they twitch or groan, begin from the chest again. This will build up so much sexual tension that they will soon learn and become stiff and still with anticipation. The final orgasm will be monumental and will have them eating out of the palm of your hand for days to come.

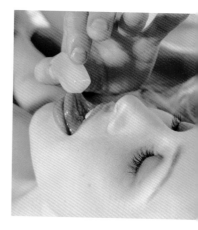

ABOVE | The sensation of an ice cube against your skin excites nerve endings in a way that hands and fingers can't.

BELOW | Removing your sight with a blindfold may heighten other senses.

BELOW LEFT | If you are sharing a croissant you must have made it as far as the morning after.

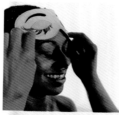

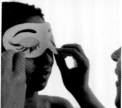

bondage, s&m and spanking

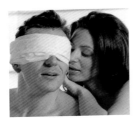

ABOVE | Tissue paper is a soft alternative with no hint of danger involved.

BELOW | When tying each other up, it is worth investing in some handcuffs or other restraints, such as this self-sticking bondage tape, to avoid ending up struggling with tight knots that simply won't come undone.

MENTION BONDAGE to most people and images of sinister black masks, chains, long whips and complicated harnesses spring to mind. Although there is definitely a culture of people who love all that, there is also a lighter side to the scene that a larger proportion of people indulge in.

Bondage can be described as any sexual act that involves the restraint, humiliation or even pain of a partner. In spite of the potential harm it can do, it is important to add that bondage is a consensual act, in which both parties agree exactly on what they are about to do to one another. Take away the word "consensual" and it becomes a criminal offence. It's a fine, but definite line.

light bondage

This can include a little light bottom spanking or having your arms and feet tied to the bedposts, bed head or even the banisters, using handcuffs (often covered in fake fur), stockings, ribbon, silk scarves or your work tie. To save yourselves

considerable embarrassment later, before you start, make sure you know exactly where you have put the key if you are using locking handcuffs. Whatever you use, it can be fairly tight, or looser just to simulate restraint.

The person who is being restricted is often referred to as the "bottom", and the person inflicting the restraint as the "top". There are some who enjoy both roles and they are known as "switches". For the top, the pleasure in bondage is found in feelings of power and control. For the bottom, it is more about submission and victimization. In light bondage, the thrill is mainly a psychological one coupled with the fact that, when restrained, you no longer have to worry about reciprocating pleasure. You can concentrate exclusively on your own sensations, without any feelings of guilt about my turn/your turn. Some women who have difficulty achieving orgasm with penetrative sex, find that a little light bondage resolves the problem.

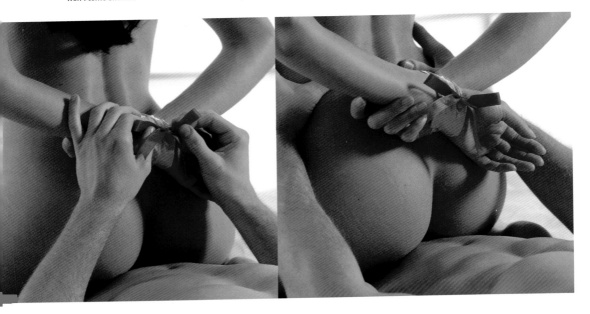

heavy bondage

This has a huge following and people who are into it form tight group connections. Orgasm takes second place to the infliction and receipt of pain. Many claim that when receiving extreme pain of this kind they are transported into a meditative state.

Bondage practitioners are very serious about their craft and it is not something that the experts take lightly. There are special codes, etiquette and release words that are used to prevent serious harm from being done. Anyone contemplating getting into heavy bondage must read about it first and learn how it all works. A lot of literature and advice is available.

sado-masochism

Like all forms of bondage, S&M is a game of role-playing in which the "sadist" inflicts the pain and the "masochist" receives it. It often involves whipping or body piercing, but extreme S&Ms have been known to brand the bottom with hot irons to enforce loyalty.

Research has shown that before climax the brain releases feel-good hormones called endorphins, which help the body to tolerate pain. After climax the top must stop, as the body becomes less tolerant of pain. S&Ms usually use a release word to prevent serious damage. "Stop" and "You're hurting me" are, apparently, no good, as the bottom will often shout these words when they don't actually want the top to stop or slow down and use them as part of the game. Instead, the word "red" often means stop and "yellow" means ease off a little.

submission and domination

SubDom, as it is known, is similar in practice to S&M. However, where practitioners of S&M concentrate on the infliction of pain, SubDom is more about relinquishing control. It is more of a mental game that involves a lot of trust and discussion for both parties to get satisfaction and enjoyment. The dominator will remove all control from the Sub (or bottom) in the form of slavery by commanding the bottom where to sit, when to speak and how to behave.

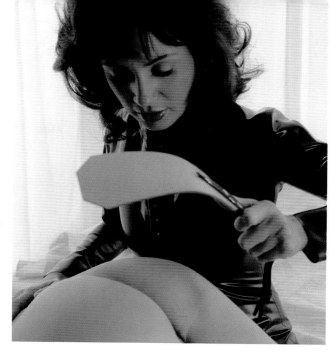

Most people either like to be a bit dominant or a bit submissive during sex, often switching roles depending on their mood. If you are playing the dominant role then you can command your partner where to lick you, what position to get into, how to touch you, where and for how long. Try switching roles so that you each get a chance to "play teacher" and each get a chance to be "dutiful student".

paddles and spanking

Spanking is used in bondage but also by "vanilla" sex practitioners, people who simply enjoy the odd thump on the rump.

Most people who spank each other for a bit of a laugh don't consider themselves as "real" bondage and discipline practitioners so don't really need to organize a release word as such before they begin. But remember to keep within each of your boundaries to prevent either of you from getting unintentionally hurt. In the heat of the moment you may forget your own strength. Begin slowly and gently with a light slap or two and then, if you want, increase the pressure in response to your partner. Keep it light-hearted and fun, and make sure you give as good as you get.

ABOVE | If you want something kinkier than a hand, go with a wide paddle, as this produces more of a dull thud than a whip's sting.

BELOW | A little light-hearted bondage can be fun. These pink accessories are soft and gentle on the skin.

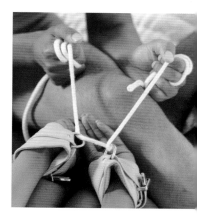

fun and fetish

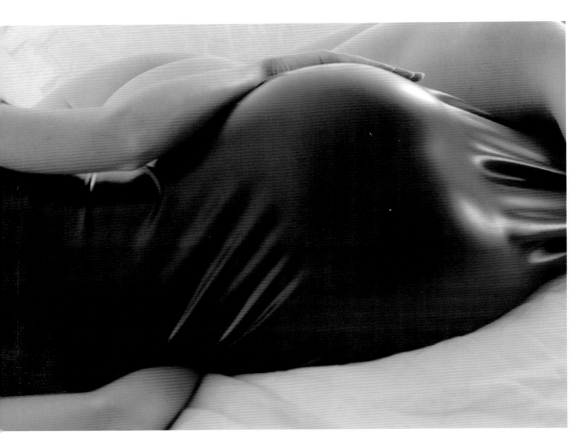

ABOVE | The feel of rubber and PVC against the skin can be a huge turn-on and some claim it makes them more sexually confident. Putting rubber and PVC garments on can be slightly less appealing – use plenty of talc to smooth your skin before you try.

OPPOSITE TOP LEFT | Piercing can be very erotic.

MOST PEOPLE LIKE TO PLAY around with fetishes – for example, getting their partner to keep her (or his) heels on while they make love. It's a titillating romp rather than a necessity. A stricter definition of a fetish, however, is a tangible object or an action that needs to be repeated over and over for sexual gratification. For example, we've already discussed talking dirty, which some people enjoy now and again. A talking dirty fetish, however, would mean that the person would not be sexually aroused unless the dirty talk is used in all sexual acts.

Fetishes are fine if both partners have the same one, but if they don't, then the relationship can break down and external guidance may be necessary. However, it's worth remembering that a person with a fetish usually loves his or her fetish immensely and is unwilling to part with it. It's usually better if the partner of someone with a fetish learns to accept the sexual foible, rather than trying to repress it. This assumes, of course, that the fetish is morally acceptable and legal. For example, an exhibitionist who gets sexual pleasure only or mainly from exposing his genitals

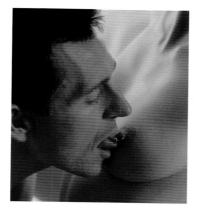

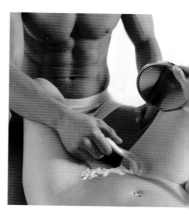

Cutting, piercing or branding may be permanent or temporary. Elaborate S&M piercing fetishes can involve piercing many needles shallowly through the skin with a variety of strings attached so that the strings can be pulled or weights hung from them. This is advanced S&M that is beyond the scope of this book. It requires trust and knowledge. There is a lot of literature on this type of sex play and anyone who wants to have a go at it needs to get informed advice.

watersports

Body fluid fetishes include a whole area of "dirty games" where body fluids are shared. This might be simply sharing sweat, saliva or other excretions, or sometimes involves urinating on your partner.

Some games involve exchanging blood, or body fluid bonding. Couples who try this have usually taken the precaution of being tested for disease before they begin – precautions should be taken so you are not putting yourself at risk.

ABOVE | Try the infamous Brazilian wax, or get your partner to shave you.

BELOW | Tantalize him with a pair of spiked heels and rubber accessories.

to strangers should not be allowed to continue this fetish and must face both the legal and moral consequences of his actions.

Common fetishes include leather, fur, latex, stilettos, handcuffs and feet (shrimping), but some go as far as exhaust pipes or mud wallowing. Cross-dressing is a popular fetish. Some women go so far as to wear a fake penis ("packing"). There are many theories about why people find cross-dressing stimulating. One idea is that men and women feel more relaxed when they are able to express the other gender side to their personality. Some men find transvestism erotic. In most cases these men are straight but merely find eroticism in wearing female clothing. Many of these men are afraid to share this fetish with their partner for fear of rejection and of being thought of as less of a man.

body modification

Tattooing and piercing are fairly common nowadays, with a huge number of people decorating their bodies in some way. Doing it for sexual gratification highlights the difference between high-street trend and sexual fetish.

Piercing, tattooing, cutting, branding and body sculpting through corsetry are all forms of body modification. For some, having an absolute stranger wield a long needle and clamp around their nether regions is just not a problem. It's seen as a means of enhancing sexual sensation and a way of getting more sensation from a localized area.

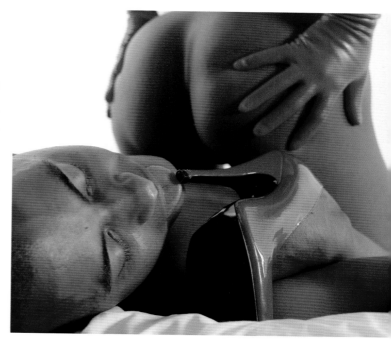

fantasy

VERY LITTLE HAS BEEN documented about male and female fantasy, probably because people guard their fantasies fiercely. Regardless of how liberated and open they may be or how close their friends are, people rarely discuss fantasy in the same way they may discuss, say, oral sex.

Nancy Friday was one of the first authors to bring women's erotic fantasies into the limelight in her bestseller *My Secret Garden* (1973). Until then, it was widely assumed that women did not have sexual fantasies, although most women must have known that they did. It has always

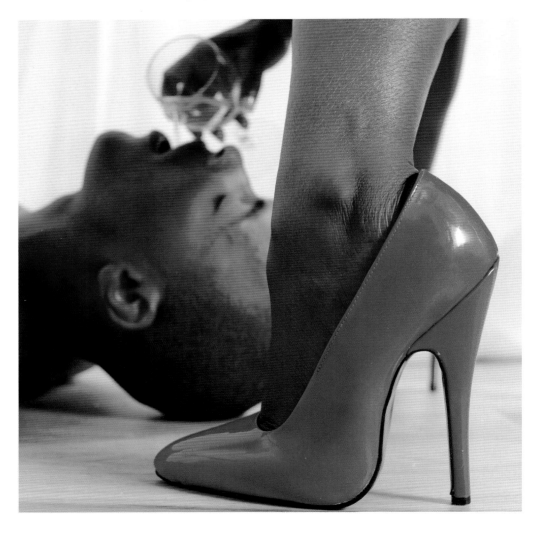

been accepted that men fantasize and whole industries have been built up to enable men to fulfil these with props and costumes.

Many people are embarrassed by the content of their fantasies. They may be extremely depraved and subversive; they may involve illegal acts that make most people angry or disturbed when they hear about them happening in real life. It is for this reason that many people become embarrassed and sometimes a bit disgusted by what they dream about during masturbation or lovemaking. Many people also worry that they fantasize about weird and wonderful scenarios while making love to their partner. This can lead to feelings of intense guilt and doubt. It is worth remembering that it is human instinct to be drawn precisely to those things that are forbidden.

Hardly surprisingly, men and women fantasize about different things. In general, men's fantasies tend to be impersonal, often involving several partners and complete strangers. Other common themes include watching others, especially two women, making love and watching their partner or another woman masturbate. Women's fantasies tend to be more about intimate, one-to-one relationships. Popular themes involve sex with a celebrity, sex with another woman and being dominated or dominating. Both men and women fantasize about having sex in public.

brain stimulation

Fantasy is one of the most important components in lovemaking. As humans we have very complex brains and mental capacities so it is often not enough merely to stimulate our genitals. We have to be in the correct mood and mind-set before we are relaxed enough to let our bodies go. Sometimes your fantasies are simple enough to enact: having sex in a smart hotel or on the kitchen table; being wooed in a romantic candlelit room. Others that involve a cast of thousands may be more difficult to arrange.

Many people fantasize about sex with a film or popstar. Try thinking about your fantasy figure while having sex with your partner. What they don't know won't hurt them. Just be sure not to scream

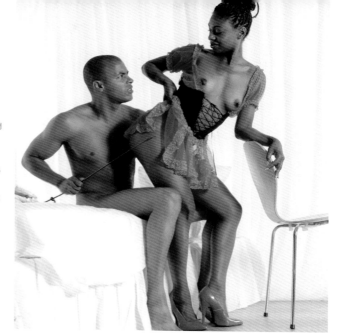

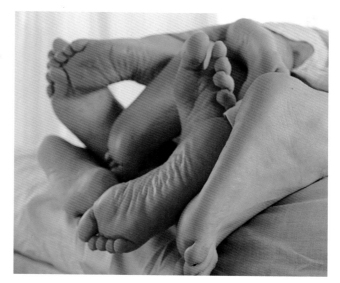

out the wrong name during a moment of heightened excitement. Keep your fantasies as a private store of erotic movies that you can switch on whenever you like. Remember that your brain is the biggest and most sensitive sex organ in your body and where the mind leads, the body will follow.

TOP AND ABOVE | It could be dressing up and role-playing, or having more than one partner in bed – whatever turns you on, as long as your accomplices are willing.

toys toys toys

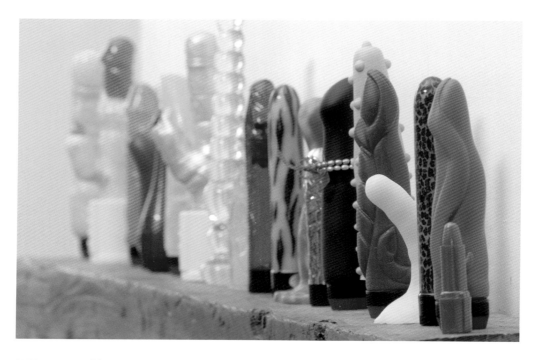

ABOVE AND OPPOSITE | There is a wide range of sex toys available and a new style of sex shop which caters for women and is less seedy than the stereotypical sex shop.

BELOW | A classic rabbit vibrator has a clitoral stimulator.

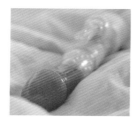

SEX TOYS ARE COMING out of the bedside drawer and going on the coffee table. Vibrators and other sex toys have become *de rigueur* as the face of sexual awareness has changed. There are so many toys to choose from, in all sorts of shapes, colours and sizes. Design and aesthetics are as important as function and nowadays sex toys are becoming desirable designer items.

And they're not just for women. There are as many gizmos and gadgets for men, from anal love balls to penis rings. We are becoming more open to the idea of incorporating toys into sex play. Sex toys have the advantage of spicing it up between the sheets, whether you are a man or a woman together or going solo.

The whole purpose of sex toys is fun, but you may need to be careful about how you introduce the idea to your partner. Many men feel that they are being criticized as inadequate lovers if their partner buys a vibrator. Equally, a woman might wonder about her partner's sexuality if he suddenly starts using anal love balls.

Sex toys are great incorporated into foreplay. They are exciting to use on each other and many can be used to arouse both men and women. A small, flexible vibrator with rubber nodules, for example, is just as great for stimulating the prostate as it is for hitting the G spot. Most vibrators are better for external stimulation than for penetration and feel fabulous on all kinds of erogenous zones, such as the insides of the thighs and the nipples, as well as the genitals.

Reassure your partner that you don't prefer the toys to them. It's just a different and fun variation. Sometimes you like oral sex, sometimes penetration and sometimes playing with toys.

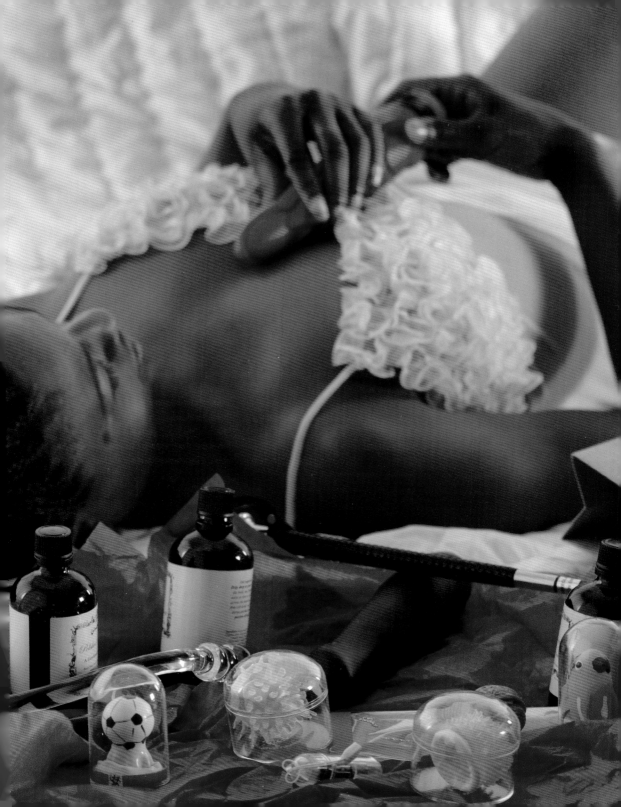

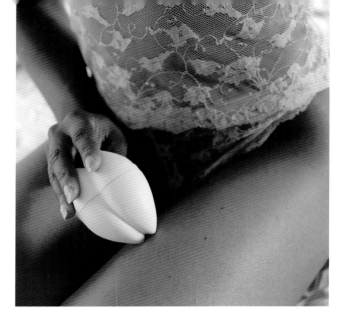

ABOVE | Designer toys are a far cry from the usual pink plastic fare. This vibrating "seed pod" is made from a soft, warm-to-the-touch elastomer material.

BELOW | These love balls are coated ball bearings which can be inserted into the vagina. Great for exercising your pelvic floor muscles, they come in a variety of weights and sizes.

bring on the toys

It's easy to confuse a vibrator with a dildo, so what is the difference? Well, the vibrator vibrates and the dildo doesn't. Vibrators are used more for genital massage and are not necessarily phallic in shape. Dildos are shaped like penises and are designed more for anal or vaginal penetrative use.

vibrators

Not just for women, many men use vibrators to stimulate their penises and report similar sensations to those of women. The advantage of the vibrator for women is that those who need constant clitoral stimulation to achieve orgasm can incorporate it into lovemaking or masturbation. Some women find the vibrator more effective than the hand, tongue or penis.

When using a vibrator, experiment with the different sensations it can produce. It may feel strange to begin with, but persevere. It can be used for massaging the clitoris, penis, testicles or anus, and not necessarily for penetration.

Vibrators can be made out of plastic or, more recently, soft elastomers, resins and silicon, and the most popular size is about 10cm/4in. The softer ones are better suited for penetration and are also quieter, as the softness absorbs the sound. The more rigid plastic variety may be better for more direct stimulation. As with any aspect of sex, it's important to keep it clean. Always wash and dry your vibrator after use. Remember to keep a supply of batteries handy, as there are few things worse than a pre-orgasmic power failure.

the rabbit

One of the most popular and most expensive vibrators, the rabbit first hit the big time after *Sex and the City*'s Charlotte fell in love with her rabbit. It has the standard vibrating shaft and the added bonus of the "ears", providing a clitoris tickler at the front. Some also have an anal probe at the back. It's guaranteed to make you hopping horny.

the mojo

Designed by Marc Newson in silicon, this nipple-shaped five-speed toy concentrates less on vaginal penetration and more on clitoral stimulation. It's good for hitting the spot, but some women miss the vaginal penetration aspect.

dildos

Like vibrators, dildos are made in a variety of different shapes, sizes, colours and textures, and are associated with penetration. They are usually phallic in shape, but this can vary from a lifelike penis (often complete with testicles) to a simple cylindrical structure. Dildos have a history that stretches back 30,000 years, so if you're feeling embarrassed about buying one, remember you are by no means the first.

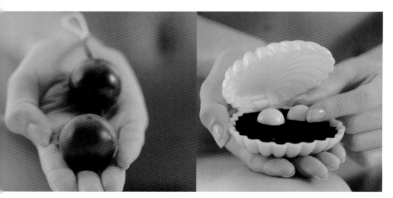

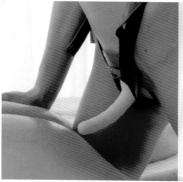
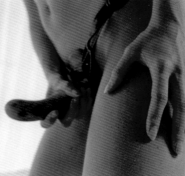

As well as being fun, dildos also have certain health benefits for women. Regular use of a dildo can help to strengthen the vaginal walls by exercising the muscles. They can also help to control the effects of vaginismus, a condition in which the vaginal muscles become tense and spasmodic, making penetration painful.

Dildos are often made from porous material that can accumulate infected semen or blood and vaginal discharge. If the dildo is shared, so is infection. If you want to share a dildo, protect it with a condom.

When buying a dildo intended for anal penetration, make sure that it has a flared end to prevent it disappearing up the rectum. You will thus prevent an embarrassing emergency trip to the local hospital. If you use a dildo for anal penetration, be sure to use a condom and dispose of it once you are finished, as the anus harbours many bacteria that could cause infection if the dildo is then used for vaginal penetration.

harnesses

Used in conjunction with dildos for strap-on sex, harnesses allow the wearer to ignore gender boundaries so that the woman can anally penetrate her partner or he can double penetrate her (vaginal and anal penetration at the same time). If he has erectile problems, he could also opt for the synthetic version to do the job. There is also an option that allows the woman wearing a dildo to have one inside her own body at the same

time. Strap-ons allow women to know what it is like to be the penetrator and the male to be the penetratee. Their use enables couples to role-play and has unlimited possibilities. They can be used by anyone – gay, straight, male or female.

love balls

These are two weighted balls of about 3cm/1¼in in diameter which are placed inside the vagina. The weights rock and jiggle together as you move around, so the balls move around. The advantage of them is that they help you with your pelvic floor exercises. They are also fairly discreet and can be worn anywhere. Some women love them, while others can't feel a thing.

lubrication

The production of love juice is not necessarily directly related to how aroused you are. In fact, it is hormone-controlled and its presence or absence can depend on a host of things from certain times in the menstrual cycle, effects of childbirth and hysterectomy to the drying effects of alcohol and marijuana. There is nothing worse than having to stop a steamy session because of drying up.

Some of the properties in commercial sexual lubricants kill sperm, so avoid it them if you are trying to have a baby. Lubrication is an essential component in anal play, as the anus and surrounding area produce no natural lubrication. Be sure to use water-based lubricants if you are using sex toys or condoms.

ABOVE | Strap-on sex toys can be made in any colour and shape to order, for anal sex or for woman-on-woman vaginal penetration.

BELOW | Vibrators come in all shapes and sizes – a ring must be one of the most discreet.

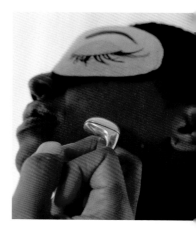

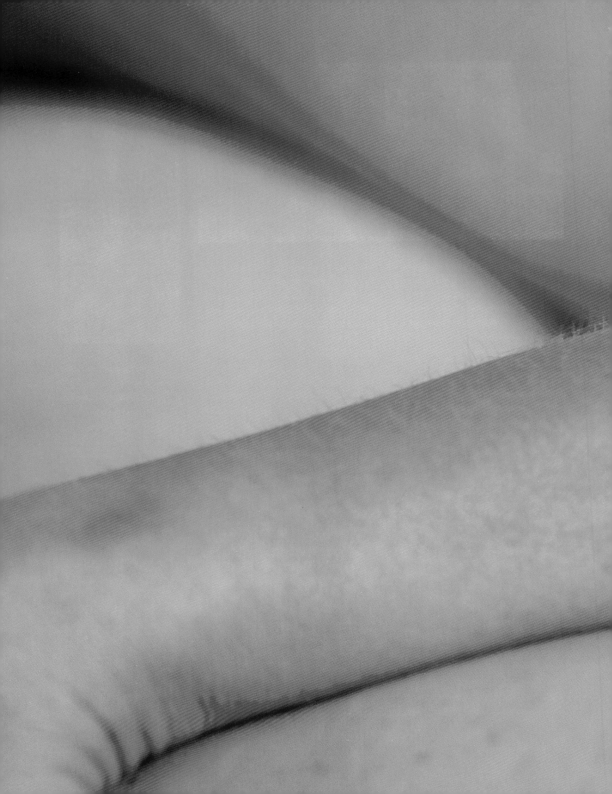

shaking it up

Many long-term relationships experience occasional periods of over-familiarity and predictability. Add some spice and fire to your relationship with some fun and exciting new ideas, allowing you to rediscover both your own and your partner's desire.

out of the bedroom

WHEN YOU HAVE BEEN TOGETHER for a long time, it can be difficult to keep the flames of passion burning brightly, especially if – whether out of habit or because you have children – the only place you have sex is your bedroom. As well as location, give a thought to timing and recall those days when you first met and couldn't keep your hands off each other. If you think about it, making love after a demanding day at work, cooking dinner and clearing up afterwards, then helping the kids with their homework, will almost certainly be less exciting and, frankly, more of a duty for both of you than rampant sex in the garden shed in the middle of an afternoon's weeding.

One of the most popular alternatives to the bedroom is the bathroom. As there is usually a lock on the door, even if the kids are at home, you are assured of some privacy. Sex in the shower or the bath is extremely sensual, as the hot water stimulates all your touch receptors, making your skin more sensitive. It is also very refreshing and revitalizing. Don't just go for the main event – relish the eroticism of lovingly soaping and rinsing every part of each other's bodies. Concentrating on giving your partner an invigorating body brush will not only produce its own rewards, but will also remind you why your lover's body is so special.

BELOW | The steamy atmosphere and sensuous effects of hot water on bare skin heighten the pleasure of making love in the shower.

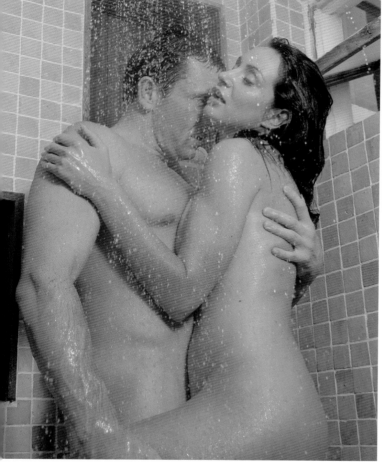

alternative venues

Chairs and sofas are also great places for making love and performing oral sex. Try sitting in your favourite chair in the front room with the curtains and windows open to add an extra notch of excitement and danger. Rocking chairs and recliners are fantastic, as the gentle motion gives a little extra movement to allow deeper penetration.

Cellars and attics are fun because of their secret atmosphere, although a little forethought about cushions and blankets might be a good idea. These places can become your own erotic dens and, if role-play is your thing, then there are unlimited scenarios, from dominatrix dungeons to caveman dwellings.

Stairs are fantastic settings for sex because the different levels allow you to experiment with positions that may otherwise not be possible. The vertical 69 is a challenge to the fittest. The woman sits on the second or third step while her partner kneels on a higher step, so her head is between his legs. Then – very carefully – he manoeuvres his

a change of scene

Try some of the following to spice up your sex life.

• Book into a motel for the afternoon – as Mr and Mrs Smith if you're not paying with a credit card.

• Hire a cabin cruiser for the weekend and enjoy the sensation of rocking on the water.

• Get away from it all with a tent or camper van (trailer) and make love under the stars.

• Splash out on a chauffeur-driven limousine, but make sure that it has privacy screens.

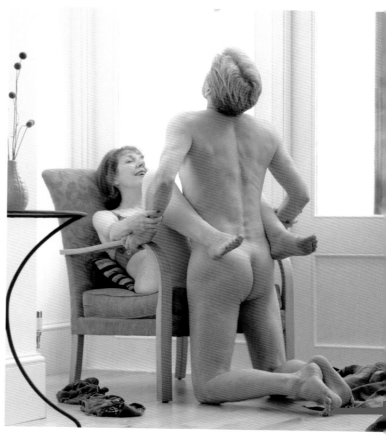

body so that he is head first down the stairs, supporting his weight with his hands on the floor at the bottom of the staircase, with his knees a few steps higher. Underneath him, the woman may need to move slightly or change the step she is on. Both partners' mouths are in contact with the other's genitals.

An easier position is for the man to kneel on the stairs, with the woman sitting one step above, facing him. She can then sit back and hold on to the banisters, while he grasps her by the hips. For additional spice, he can handcuff or tie her wrists to the banisters with a silk scarf and torment her with his hands, tongue and penis.

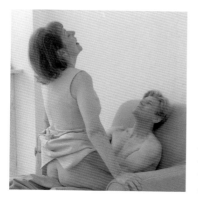

The kitchen, too, offers tasty possibilities. If the woman lies flat on the table and the man stands beside it, supporting her legs straight up in the air, the angle of penetration is intense. If she keeps her legs together, the tightness of her vagina will be immensely exciting for both partners. And, since you are already there, you can explore the possibilities of sensual and sexy foods – whether as an hors d'oeuvre or as a dessert.

There are couples who reckon that making love leaning against or with the woman sitting on an operating washing machine is one of life's truly erotic experiences. The vibration, especially if you time your "cycle" to the final spin, is said to be out of this world.

ABOVE AND LEFT | Chairs and sofas offer comfort as well as scope for some interesting and exciting positions. "Putting your feet up for half an hour" will never have the same meaning again.

the quickie

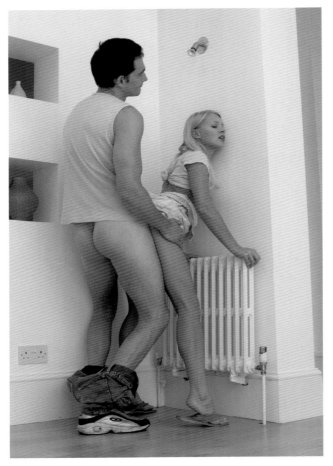

Quickie sex is a wonderfully erotic and lustful way of adding diversity to your love life. Although it cannot and should not replace the long sensual hours of foreplay and lovemaking that are essential in all loving and respectful relationships, it has a place, reaffirming each other's sexuality and reassuring your partner that you still find them the sexiest and most desirable person on the planet. Variety is not described as the spice of life without good reason.

mother of invention

Quick sex is often creative and inventive, two essential ingredients in lovemaking. Creeping up behind your partner while he or she clears the dishes in the kitchen in response to a completely overwhelming lustful urge is both delightful and flattering. There are no limits to when you can do it, whether sneaking off early from a party or a frantic session before you leave for work. It's up to you and your infectious desire.

The bedroom is usually the place where your loving, united encounters take place, so having a quick romp there may undermine the emotional importance of this room. The bathroom, on the other hand, is ideal. Steal in when your partner is having a shower and wordlessly show your intentions by kissing passionately under the hot jets.

ABOVE | Sometimes, the less glamorous the venue, the more exciting the sex.

RIGHT | Surprising your partner in the bathroom can have, well, surprising results.

RETAINING YOUR SENSE OF SPONTANEITY is one of the keys to a successful long-term relationship. It is all too easy to slip into a habitual pattern without noticing, especially when you have family responsibilities, a demanding job and a busy life. Seizing the moment and surprising each other with unplanned flurries of passion keeps excitement and desire alive, adding spice and maintaining the longevity of the relationship.

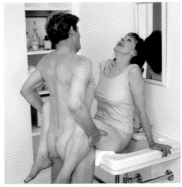

Sometimes the best places are those that seem to be totally unsexy and mundane, such as against a radiator in the front hall. It's almost guaranteed that you will both smile each time you pass that particular radiator in the future. Shamelessly grabbing your partner as soon as they walk through the front door for a passionate encounter on the hall floor is an unmistakable demonstration of your feelings – and who cares if dinner is half an hour late?

The living room is also a great place to have quick, spontaneous sex. While your partner is watching television, why not surprise her with a sexy striptease to distract her? Suddenly blast some music from the stereo as you rip your clothes off in front of her in time to the beat. It's bound to have her in stitches, and laughter is a wonderful aphrodisiac. Alternatively, while he is relaxing in his favourite chair, why not silently hitch up your skirt and sit on his lap, either facing him or facing away, gently moving and rotating your hips until he becomes aroused? It certainly beats making coffee during the advertisement breaks.

timing

If quickie sex is what you have in mind, you do need to choose your moment wisely or the whole idea could backfire. You must also be open and sensitive to your partner's response. Selecting the final five minutes of a nail-biting match on television to give him a blow-job or suggesting steamy bathroom sex when she is in the middle of shaving her legs would be inappropriate. Your partner will either end up "submitting" and feeling exploited and irritable or else push you away and you will feel rejected, unloved and unimportant. Neither of these is conducive to promoting harmony and closeness in your relationship. Quickie sex is, after all, just as much about mutual pleasure as is prolonged, sensual lovemaking – just different. Although being ambushed for a quickie is a great turn-on, sometimes your partner may simply not feel like it, and if they are still unwilling after a little gentle persuasion and encouragement, then it's probably best to postpone the idea until another, rather more suitable moment.

the sky's the limit

Quickie sex does add an element of surprise and keeps your relationship exciting, fun and light-hearted. Just breaking the pattern of day-to-day life can ratchet up the libido for days afterwards.

Nor does quickie sex have to be restricted to the home. If you're feeling reckless – and you really are going to be quick – what about the back seat of the car in a carwash? Try stopping a hotel freight elevator between floors – but watch out for surveillance cameras, there may be penalties for being found out. Airline security permitting, you could go for membership of the Mile High Club. The balcony of a holiday hotel can offer the frisson of exhibitionism without any of the danger, if only the top half of you can be seen. The list is as endless as your imagination – just make sure that you don't get caught *in flagrante*.

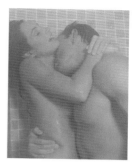

ABOVE AND BELOW | The occasional quickie helps keep the magic alive and can be a timely reminder of exactly how much you love and desire each other.

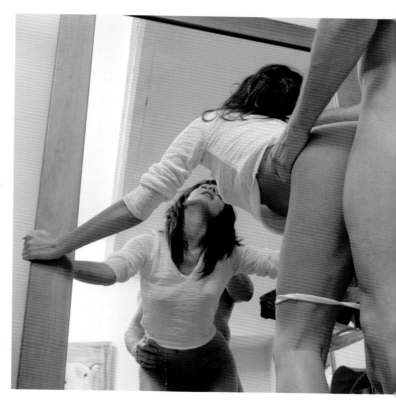

al fresco

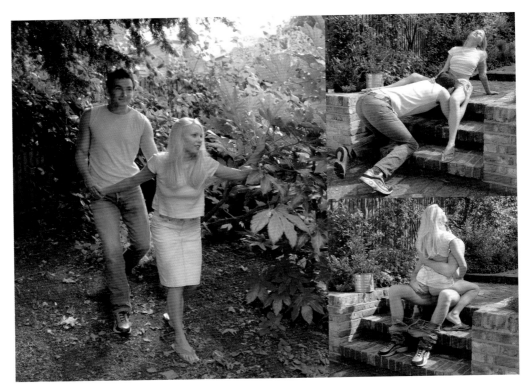

ABOVE | Fresh air and sunshine are natural aphrodisiacs. Whether you are walking in the woods or sitting in your own garden, why not follow your instincts and let nature take its course?

RELEASING YOUR SEXUAL ACTIVITIES from the confines of the four walls of your home and bringing them out into the open air can be a liberating experience. Enjoying each other in the outdoors puts you in touch with nature and makes the experience seem somehow more wholesome, purposeful and natural.

dangerous games

A word of caution here: having sex in public areas is illegal for reasons of public decency and it is vital not to cause offence. This is especially important to bear in mind if you are travelling abroad as some countries have harsh legal penalties. Equally, while some people find the risk – however slight – of being observed a positive turn-on, this can have precisely the opposite effect on others. As with all sexual activities, coercing an unwilling partner to have al fresco sex will sacrifice long-term fulfilment for short-term satisfaction.

There is something about the smell and feel of fresh air that ignites a basic passion in all of us. A long walk on a wintry day, with the wind literally taking the breath from your lungs, instils a sense of vitality, one of the most important ingredients of great sex. The proximity of lush vegetation, in the thick of a tall impressive wood or shaded by bushes and plants of nature's choosing, evokes fundamental animal desires and stirs our visceral energy. Even just strolling with your partner through a meadow, into a wood, along the beach or even to the local park is a wonderful prelude to get you both in the mood, whether you have sex outdoors or not.

basic instinct

The key to having great sex outside is to let nature be your guide and to go with whatever feels right. If the urge is suddenly to whip up your partner's skirt while you kneel before her and give her pleasure, it's doubtful she will complain. Open-air sex heightens the senses and intensifies feelings so that many people feel extra close and united. Being outdoors certainly gives an added dimension to the tried and tested positions that you enjoy in the privacy of your bedroom. Even the staid missionary position seems racy when you are outside. Sitting up, entwined in each other is also great, as you can do this with comparative ease. If you need to be quick, there is no need to remove all of your clothes, especially if the woman is wearing a flowing skirt.

The best place to have *al fresco* sex is in your own garden providing that it has suitably tall surrounding vegetation or a wall to prevent your being spotted by the neighbours. You can either spread out some blankets and pillows and,

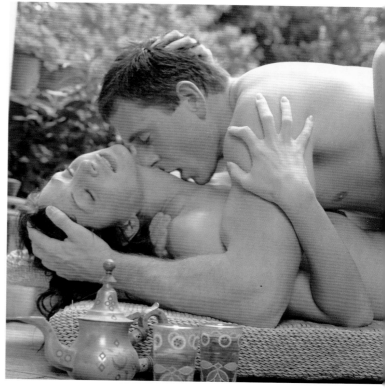

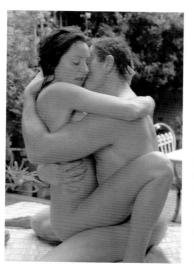

perhaps, some outdoor lights and candles if it is dark, or just go with the moment and get down and dirty in the mud. A garden hammock is a challenge worth taking on. It requires superb co-ordination, but can be done. A swinging garden seat provides a similar momentum with rather less risk of overturning.

Alternatively, if you live in the countryside, then research the area and work out where most people tend to walk and, more importantly, where they don't. Woods are always good, as there are many clearings and concealing bushes to choose from. Places that are harder to get to are usually better. A few things to consider are, how far away you are from a public footpath, where the nearest road is and whether there are any houses nearby. You don't want to end up making love in someone else's back garden.

ABOVE | A quiet cup of tea in the garden could turn into an intense and romantic lovemaking experience.

LEFT | Outdoor sex heightens the senses – touch most of all – and creates a powerful feeling of unity.

sharing sensuality

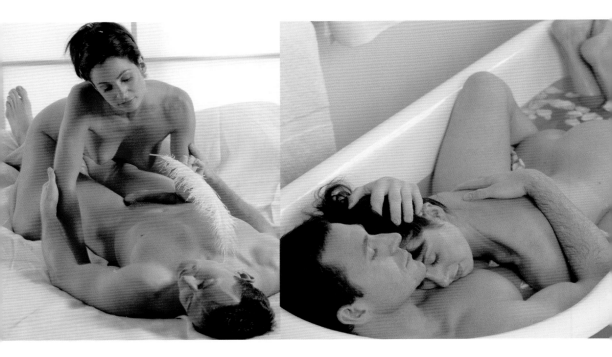

ABOVE | The light touch of a soft feather against bare skin is unbearably erotic.

ABOVE RIGHT | Get yourselves in the mood by sharing a warm, fragrant bath before an erotic session.

SHARING A WARM BATH is a perfect way to begin a massage and an evening of total indulgence and pampering. Many people associate water with relaxation and comfort and it is a wonderfully sensual stimulant. A warm, fragrant bath together is extremely erotic, as you luxuriate in the soft, silky textures of each other's bodies. The skin's responsiveness to touch is enhanced and the water's enveloping properties help you both to feel more united.

no touching

For added eroticism, give your partner a "hands free" massage. Tell your partner to close his or her eyes. The only rule is that you cannot touch one another with any part of your body. If you both have long hair, you can use it to caress one another. Make sure it is clean and smells nice.

Begin by putting your hair over your head and softly and slowly dragging it around your partner's body, starting from the head. You can add to the sensation by softly blowing on their skin at the same time. When you reach the most sensitive areas such as nipples, groin or armpits, allow your hair and breath to linger, gently circling and stroking to build anticipation.

Now try using a feather to caress your partner. Feathers are very sensuous, as the soft, light texture can be used in so many different ways. You can drag it slowly over the skin, following a path of your own choosing, or try a sharper, flicking motion, concentrating on specific areas. Whether you are male or female, being stroked by a feather is a delicious sensation. Make sure that your partner's eyes are tightly closed or that they are blindfolded before you start stroking them –

losing the use of one sense heightens all the others. Ask them to guess what it is you are using. If they guess correctly, reward them by spending extra long on their genital area. If they guess incorrectly, reprimand them by tickling their armpits or nose.

feathering

If you are stroking your man and he becomes aroused, ask him to lie on his back and place the feather between his hard penis and his stomach. Rub it up and down or forwards and backwards. Then get him to open his legs and, as you sit between them, run the feather up from his perineum, over his testicles and along the shaft before going back down again. Vary the sensation, so that on one stroke you keep the feather light, barely touching him, on another you use a firmer, circular motion, and on a third, you sweep it in quick sharp strokes, left and right, up and down.

Use your imagination to find other sensuous textures. Try the contrasting sensations of a bead necklace running over the skin, the softness of a leather glove, the barely there lightness of silk stockings or satin lingerie, the slight roughness of lace or the tactility of fake fur.

Another deliciously erotic sensation is the feel of ice against the skin. Run an ice cube over your lover's body and watch how their nipples harden as you gently circle the cube around them. Gently slide it around their genitals, holding it in your mouth at the same time, so they feel the heat from your breath and the chill from the ice. Be careful around the clitoris, as an ice cube may be too much for some women. Opt instead for running it over her inner labia for a more muffled chill.

Another way to excite the senses is to sprinkle the petals of your lover's favourite flower over their body so that they can luxuriate in the smell and the soft tickle of the velvety texture.

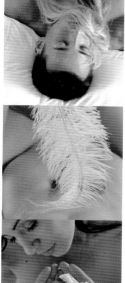

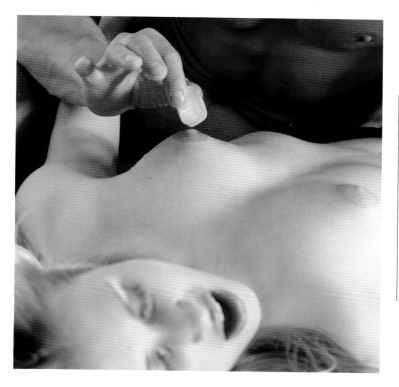

ABOVE TOP | If you have long, silky hair, brush it all over your lover's body for a unique "hands off" massage.

ABOVE CENTRE | Flick the feather over the aroused genitals for the full effect.

ABOVE BOTTOM | Showering your lover with fragrant petals is romantic and sensuous.

LEFT | An icy touch is a thrilling and tantalizing sensation.

erotic massage

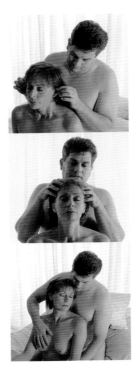

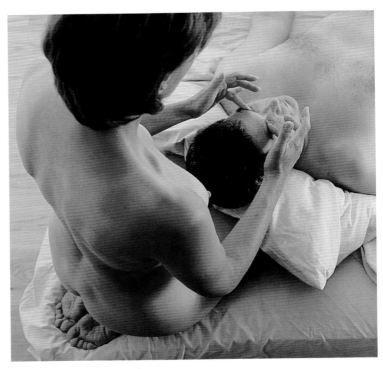

ABOVE TOP | The ears are a powerful erogenous zone – massaging them can be erotic.

ABOVE CENTRE | A head massage is superbly relaxing, helping to release all the day's stress and tension.

ABOVE BOTTOM | You can massage your partner's breasts by kneeling behind her.

ABOVE RIGHT | Massaging the delicate skin of the face feels strangely intimate.

A HEAD MASSAGE is one of the nicest gifts you can give your partner, especially if they have had a hard day, as it releases all tension.

Ask your partner to sit comfortably, while you sit or stand behind. Take off jewellery that might catch on their skin, then place your fingertips on the scalp. Run your open fingers softly through the hair. With quite a firm circular motion, rotate your fingers around the scalp, changing the size of the circles and gradually increasing the pressure. Concentrate on areas such as behind the ears, along the hairline and the base of the skull.

Now concentrate on the forehead, gliding your thumbs from the top of the nose in an arch to the sides of the head and back. Repeat, following the line of the eyebrow, and adapt it by using

small circular strokes with the balls of your thumbs. Next, sweep your thumbs gently down the sides of the nose and across the sinuses, then out towards the cheekbones before repeating.

Cup your hands into a loose fist and support the back of the ears with the side of your first finger, using your thumbs to make small circular motions all around the rims. Then move down to grasp the lobe between the tips of your thumb and index finger and gently pull it down, allowing it to slip through your fingers before repeating.

shoulders

A good place to start a full body massage is the shoulders and back, as these areas often contain the most knots and tight muscles. By easing the tension there, you pave the way for a totally relaxing and sensual full body massage – truly a great act of love.

Ask your partner to lie on their front. Put a small amount of massage oil on your hands and rub them together to warm it. Start at the top of the shoulders with both hands flat on the skin with the neck between them. Run your hands up the back of the neck, then down and along the tops of the shoulders in long sweeping strokes. Repeat with a firmer pressure using your thumbs. Begin to focus on specific areas, gradually increasing the pressure, pressing your thumbs into the muscular areas, using small circular strokes until you can feel the muscles loosening up. Punctuate the more intense circular strokes with the sweeping strokes to add variety and encourage relaxation.

Extend your massage down your partner's back. Place your hands flat on either side of the top of the spine and sweep down to the base. On the upward sweep, apply more pressure by using your body weight. Vary this stroke by sweeping your hands out to the sides using fanning strokes or a harder circular pressure with the heels of your hands. Avoid directly massaging the spine.

breasts

Massaging a woman's breasts is sensual and erotic for both parties. It is best done with the woman lying on her back. You may find it easier to straddle your partner, but do not sit on her. Begin by placing your hands palms down under each breast with your thumbs out to form an "L" shape and the breast cupped in the crook of the "L". Using quite firm pressure, circle your hands upwards and inwards and as they rotate inwards, bring the thumb and index finger together so that they end up lightly pinching the nipples before beginning again. If you want, you can concentrate on one breast, using a similar technique but this time with one hand following the other to complete the circle.

Another technique is to use your fingers and thumbs to pinch the nipple area gently before slowly fanning out your fingers across the breast. Use a light pressure around the nipple and increase the pressure as your fingers span out.

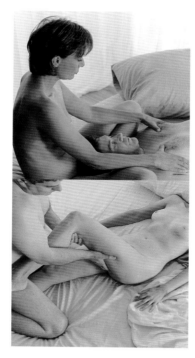

thighs

It is easier to massage the thighs with your partner lying on their back, as they can bend their knees. Cup one hand on the underside of the thigh and the other on the top, just above the knee. Increase the pressure in the tips of your thumbs and fingers as you glide your hands up the length of the thigh and down again. The inner thigh is very sensitive, so vary your strokes from feather-light to harder fanning, using the heel of your hand to give pressure in a constant sweeping motion.

buttocks

Sit at your prone partner's side and softly knead the buttocks with both hands, gradually increasing the pressure. Next, hold your hands above one buttock, keeping them taut, flat, straight and parallel, and use a sharp chopping motion to strike it. Use alternate hands and move up and down the length of the buttock. Then repeat on the other buttock before going back to kneading.

LEFT | Men also enjoy having their chests massaged, using a similar technique to breast massage. As the pectorals are less sensitive, you can use a firmer pressure. Use the balls of your fingers to do small circles on the whole area, but especially the sides and the groove of the armpit.

BELOW LEFT | You can tease your partner when massaging their thighs by lightly brushing your hands "accidentally" over their genitals on the upward stroke, gradually increasing the frequency and pressure of these "accidents".

BELOW | Breasts and buttocks are usually the fleshiest part of the body but need different treatments. The soft vibrations from your hands will also run down to their genitals and fuel their excitement.

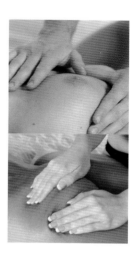

trying something new

BELOW | Nothing ventured, nothing gained. If sex is becoming more like a routine chore than a frenzy of ecstasy, you have the solution almost literally in your own hands. Try something that you have wondered about, but never done before, whether it is rimming, or using a vibrator. Suggest something you enjoyed with a previous partner, but have never done with your current one – you don't have to mention where the idea came from. Think back to the things you used to do together, but now no longer seem to have time for. Stretch your imagination and push the boundaries a little.

TRULY GREAT SEX is usually that which is totally uninhibited, where no holds are barred and where each partner feels completely at ease with their loved one. For many couples, perhaps the majority, this is not the case, even though they may have known their partner for many years, watched their body shape change and feel comfortable and safe in their presence. As time goes on, it gets harder to change, and couples reach a sexual stalemate where they have met their limits. In order to progress, a new level of intimacy must be achieved.

masturbating together

Most people view masturbation as an uninhibited self-pleasuring practice that they have done for many years in private. The idea of masturbating in front of someone else, regardless of how much you may love and trust them, can be daunting.

A good place to begin is to lie between your partner's legs, so they can embrace you, but you do not have the sensation of being watched. Get used to the idea of touching yourself in front of them without worrying about whether you orgasm or not, just to let them see how you like to

touch yourself. Once you are fully comfortable doing this, you can both try masturbating at the same time in front of each other and work on trying to orgasm simultaneously. It is worth noting that watching their partner masturbate is one of the top five male fantasies.

pushing the boundaries

It is precisely because couples feel safe and comfortable together that sex can actually become boring. For some couples, simply letting go of a few inhibitions – and almost everyone has some – can be enough to restore the magic. Try positions and activities that you haven't previously explored, even a little light S&M or anal stimulation.

Don't confront your partner as if this as a challenge or grit your teeth and systematically work through the entire Kama Sutra. However, if you would like to try, say, rimming – licking and kissing the anus – you could both test the water by gently licking and sucking each other's genitals, while stroking and massaging the anal area with your hands. Mirror each other, so that one copies the other. If one chooses to lead, then he or she massages their partner's anus in the way they would like him or her to massage them. The other partner can reciprocate by following this lead – or not, if they don't like it. This is a great way of communicating to each other how you like to be touched in new and sensitive areas.

crossing the line

Trying different positions may not be enough for some highly adventurous couples who feel that they need a more extreme stimulus to enliven a dull sex life and want to push the limits still further. A good place to start is the Internet, as there are plenty of websites catering for all manner of sexual tastes from swingers' clubs to voyeurism. This will give you the opportunity to discover the options, discuss them and form an opinion about whether you both really want to try something

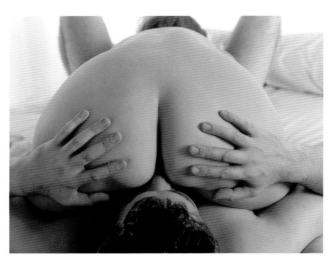

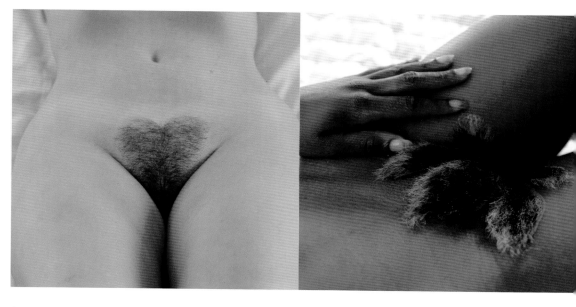

that, perhaps up till now, has just been a fantasy. A trip to a sex shop together would be another way to explore other possibilities, such as bondage and restraint fetishes.

It is important to discuss any activity that might be described as beyond the usual boundaries, especially if it involves other people. The reality of seeing your lover giving pleasure to a third party may be very different from the idea of it and could harm or even ruin a long-term relationship. If you both agree – and it must be both – to proceed with some more off-beat sexual thrills, set some limits about what is and isn't allowed and do some more research to make sure that you will be as safe as possible. If one of you is keen, but the other lukewarm or totally unenthusiastic, keep the idea at fantasy level and watch some blue movies or read porn magazines or raunchy books that will indulge this aspect of your libido.

a bit of fun

Never forget that laughter is a great aphrodisiac and that one reason couples reach a sexual stalemate is that life – and sex – has become boringly predictable and serious.

You might choose to give your partner a surprise the next time he or she sees you naked. There is a whole variety of things that you can do to your pubic hair that will guarantee that they will be equally amused and aroused. Many women wax or shave their pubic hair to keep it trim and tidy, but a variation on this is to shave it into fun patterns or even dye it for the total makeover. The amount of hair you have will determine how much you can do, but as it is pretty much already in a heart shape, it doesn't require too much skill or artistic flair to trim it and sculpt it into that shape, perfect for a Valentine's Day treat. Other shapes could be a star or a cross, or even a chessboard. A beard trimmer is an excellent tool for all genital artists, as it is often thinner and more precise than your average razor.

A merkin is basically a pubic wig or hairpiece, held in place with a special glue. They have been used throughout history for a variety of reasons, including health problems and "public decency", but today people use them for titillating fun. They vary in shape and colour, from fig leaves and flowers to national flags, and are guaranteed to raise more than a smile.

ABOVE LEFT | Heart-shaped pubic hair – the perfect private joke.

ABOVE | A fig-leaf merkin for playing Adam and Eve – watch out for the snake.

BELOW | Masturbating with your partner is deeply intimate.

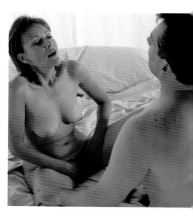

mind games

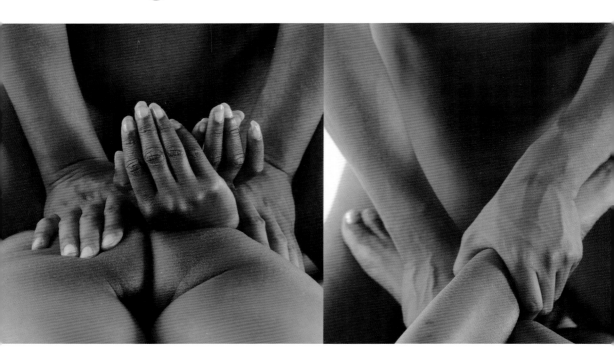

ABOVE | The woman can lie on her front while the man straddles her waist facing her bottom, restraining her hands together behind her back. He can then command her to wrap her restrained hands around his penis as he thrusts in and out of them.

ABOVE RIGHT | Hold your partner's legs bent and they won't be able to escape.

IN LONG-TERM RELATIONSHIPS, fantasies can play an important role in keeping the flames of passion burning. The difficulty often lies in sharing your fantasies with your partner, as many people are afraid of being judged. Most sexual fantasies range from the weird to the subversive and often people fantasize about things during the throes of passion that make them feel uncomfortable when they think of them out of the sexual context, but being unruly is a very human desire. An uninhibited and passionate session of being "naughty" with your partner is an expression of your innermost desires and an act of physical and emotional trust that can enhance a long-term relationship.

Your fantasies are personal and private and it is not necessary to divulge them, but there may be elements of them that you could bring up and explore with your partner. For example, a woman who fantasizes about having sex with two men at the same time could ask her partner to use a dildo or vibrator and double-penetrate her during sex.

restraint

Other common fantasies that couples can explore to spice up a long-term relationship involve restraint. These can range from holding hands or legs down while you stimulate each other, to being physically tied up. One advantage of restraining each other is that it helps you to communicate without actually having to speak. By holding your partner down you are telling them that you don't want them to worry about pleasing you, for now you are going to concentrate on them. All they need do is lie back and enjoy. It is fun to alternate playing the dominant role, in which you take charge of proceedings, with the submissive role, which takes the pressure off having to please and allows you to relinquish control to your partner's loving hands and kisses.

The great thing about restraint sex games is that they include a frisson of anxiety – which is immensely arousing – but do not have to include pain or fear. Forget the whip-cracking dominatrix and leather mask image of "heavy bondage" (unless that really is your thing) and concentrate on teasing and tantalizing. Loosely tie your partner's wrists and ankles to the bed with silk scarves, stockings or ties so that they are spread-eagled, or invest in a pair of furry handcuffs. Then slowly wreak havoc on their nervous system, by stimulating every inch of their body with your hands, tongue, genitals, a vibrator, a feather – whatever you like – repeatedly drawing back at the last possible moment. Remember, you are in control.

The idea of restraint can be intimidating, as however much you trust and love your partner the feeling and idea of helplessness is not always a pleasant one. To overcome this fear it is sensible to start with a few simple restraint positions such as holding down your partner's hands while covering their body with kisses, or tying your partner to the bed while you perform oral sex on them. Once you are aware of each other's boundaries and how far to take restraint, there are a number of different things that you can do.

Restraint can also be used within role-playing. Whatever your role-play fantasies are, whether it's doctors and nurses or parlour-maid and master, holding each other down or tying each other up can add to the element of excitement.

swinging

Previously known as wife-swapping in the 1950s, swinging has boomed into a lucrative alternative to straight sex. There are now swingers' clubs, swinging festivals and swingers' holidays available for like-minded couples who can go and fulfil their fantasies and desires in a relatively safe environment with other people who share their preferences. Swinging often culminates in group sex, as many swingers find the thrill lies in watching each other making love to different

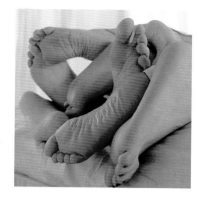

people. There are strict codes of practice and most partners have limits within their relationship as well. For example, usually if one partner does not want to have sex with a certain couple, then they choose not to as a couple, regardless of what the other partner may feel. It is almost always a joint decision. Swingers are usually very open people who are not interested in doing anything against anyone's will. Any couple interested in swinging should consider visiting one of the organized events to talk to other swingers and get more information before they decide whether or not they want to get involved.

see and be seen

Voyeurism and exhibitionism are other sexual activities that give some people a thrill. It is important to point out that watching someone else without his or her knowledge is both illegal and immoral. There is a current trend for car-park parties where people park their car, and allow others to watch them, and sometimes join in, having sex. This is aimed at voyeurs and exhibitionists as it is considered acceptable for other partygoers to wander around the car park, looking through windows and watching what is going on in each car. There are voyeur websites and some sex clubs have voyeuristic viewing rooms.

Obviously, there is an element of risk involved here, and by taking part you are laying yourself open to abuse. Not everyone who takes part in such activities will be as conscientious as you are.

LEFT | Sex in a group is not to everyone's taste, but for some people it can be a great fantasy.

BELOW TOP | Some positions require keeping a firm grip.

BELOW BOTTOM | Try different positions incorporating restraint. For example, he could lie on his back while she gets on top of him and forces him to surrender with her knees.

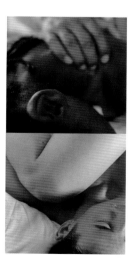

multiple orgasms

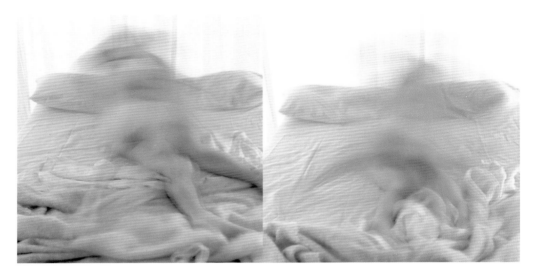

ABOVE AND BELOW | Genital geography can make orgasm during penetrative sex elusive for some women. CAT can solve this and is actually fun for both partners.

MANY WOMEN HAVE INFREQUENT ORGASMS or no orgasms at all and, over the years, this can take its toll on a relationship. This doesn't necessarily mean that they are not having good sex, but the dynamics of a woman's arousal are quite complex and it doesn't help that the design and position of the clitoris make stimulation somewhat hit or miss. The Coital Alignment Technique (CAT) and the Extended Sexual Orgasm technique (ESO) are two methods that have been designed to overcome some of these difficulties.

coital alignment technique

CAT is a position that has been adapted from the missionary position to greatly increase the likelihood of a woman reaching orgasm during penetrative sex. It is ideal for women who have difficulties achieving orgasm during penetration, although it helps only if these difficulties are technical ones and not psychological.

The clitoris of most women is approximately 2–3cm/¾–1¼in away from the vaginal opening, so clitoral stimulation during penetration is often

sporadic, indirect or totally absent. The difference with CAT is that the man penetrates his partner from a more acute angle, so that his thrusting penis stimulates her clitoris.

Start in the normal missionary position with the man on top, between his partner's spread legs, which she gently bends from the knees. As he enters her, he should lift himself forwards, further up her body, so that his thrusts make contact with her clitoris, keeping his upper body relaxed by leaning either to the left or right to rest part of his weight on the bed. The woman can wrap her legs around her partner's legs, keeping her pelvis stretched so that her ankles lie around the vicinity of his calves.

Another option is for the woman to keep her legs closed while her partner places his legs on the outside of hers. Try both ways to see which one suits you better. The latter may be more beneficial to women with a very sensitive clitoris which does not respond well to direct contact. From here, the couple should begin a light rocking motion back and forth, keeping in rhythm with

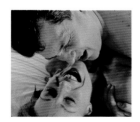

each other. He should grind and rotate or make figures-of-eight with his pelvis from time to time, as many women respond well to the stimulation of a circular motion around their clitoris.

extended sexual orgasm

ESO was developed by psychiatrist Alan Brauer and psychotherapist Donna Brauer and is designed to help women to extend their orgasms to up to 30 minutes in duration. The woman should begin by training both her mind and body, cleansing herself of any negative barriers or fears she may have about sex by focusing on the enjoyment of sex with her partner. What this means is that she should begin with a couple of weeks of daily pelvic floor muscle workouts and a regular masturbation programme concentrating on learning precisely the types of stimulation she finds the most effective.

ESO is done with the woman lying on her back and her partner between her legs, either kneeling or sitting. As he could be there for anything up to half an hour, he should choose a comfortable position. The man begins by applying lubrication to her entire genital area, massaging everywhere except the clitoris. When the woman begins to move her body to the rhythm of the massage, he should begin slow, rhythmic clitoral stimulation, while she flexes her PC muscles and takes deep breaths. When the first set of orgasmic contractions commences, he should shift stimulation from the clitoris to the vaginal walls, by inserting a couple of fingers, but keeping the rhythm steady and slow. Once she achieves her first orgasm, he should wait for it to subside slightly, but not so long that the contractions stop. He must then continue massaging the vaginal walls slowly and rhythmically and if she feels the contractions subsiding, move back to the clitoris, maintaining the momentum. This should trigger further contractions and so he should move back to the vaginal wall massage, continuing this back and forth movement until the contractions become continuous. Finally, he stimulates both areas at the same time, resulting in wave after wave of continual orgasms.

go again, and again…

For some women it is possible to have more than one orgasm. Some claim that the second or third is less intense, whereas others claim that intensity builds with each one. The techniques for achieving multiple orgasms in women are similar to those described in ESO, where stimulation after the first orgasm continues. Many women find that their clitorises are hypersensitive to touch after orgasm, so instead of stimulating the clitoris directly, her partner should stimulate the surrounding areas until feelings of arousal return.

For men, the multiple orgasm is more difficult to achieve, as many enter a refractory period after ejaculation, which usually means a light snooze. It is believed that men who can separate orgasm and ejaculation are able to experience multiple orgasmic sensations. This is one of the tenets of Tantric and Taoist sex.

In order to achieve this separation, men need to develop strong PC muscles with Kegel exercises. When the man gets to the point of orgasm, he should stop all stimulation and contract his PC muscles, then relax all the muscles of the pelvis and bottom area. He should then resume stimulation and repeat the whole process, before finally squeezing the PC muscles tightly at the point of orgasm. The man should then experience the pleasurable sensations of orgasm without releasing any semen. Anyone with a prostate problem should consult a doctor before trying this.

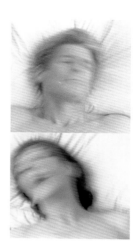

ABOVE AND BELOW |
Practising what is known as semen retention, by contracting the PC muscle, enables a man not only to prolong lovemaking and so stimulate his partner to orgasm, but also to have multiple orgasms himself.

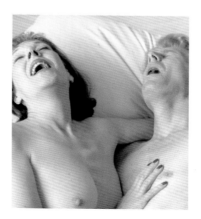

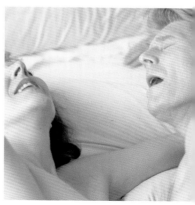

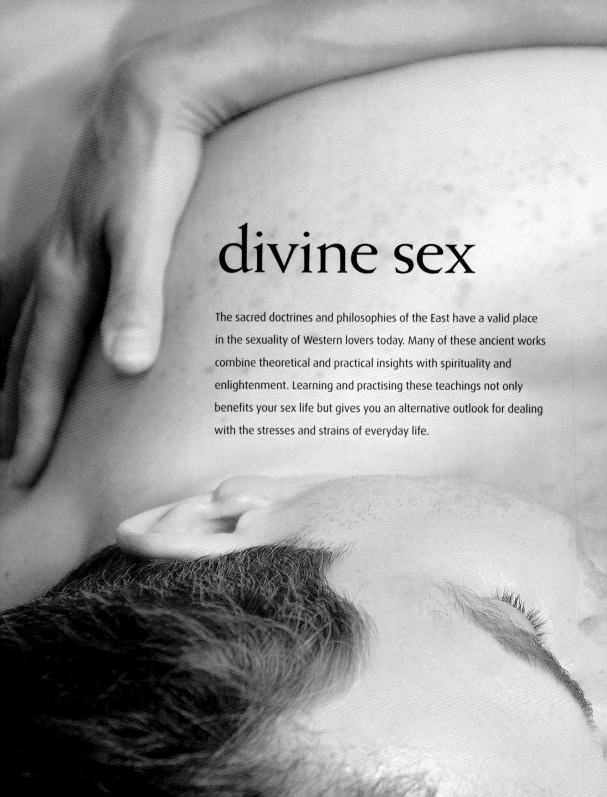

divine sex

The sacred doctrines and philosophies of the East have a valid place in the sexuality of Western lovers today. Many of these ancient works combine theoretical and practical insights with spirituality and enlightenment. Learning and practising these teachings not only benefits your sex life but gives you an alternative outlook for dealing with the stresses and strains of everyday life.

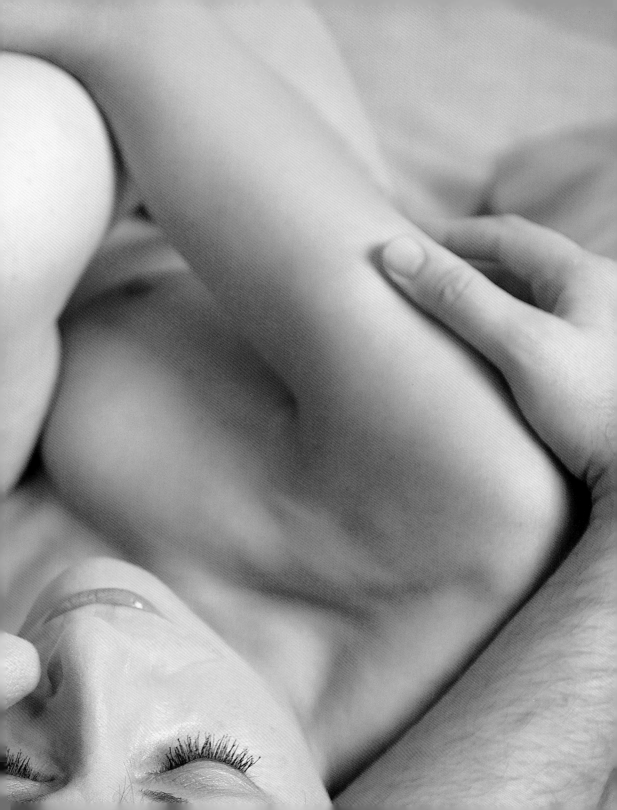

sex and philosophy

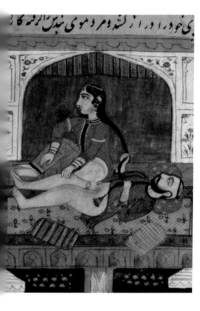

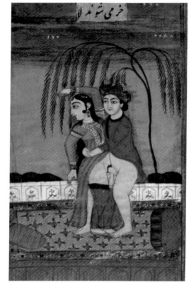

ABOVE | An 18th-century image from the Kama Sutra shows the woman on top while the man pulls her hair.

ABOVE RIGHT | Standing positions were most exalted.

SOME OF THE MOST FAMOUS ancient sex manuals originated in India many hundreds of years ago. The first, the Kama Sutra, is a collection of ancient Hindu writings on sex – known as Vedas – which were themselves based on an earlier oral tradition. It was followed by the Ananga Ranga and later by Tantric philosophy, both of which have used the Kama Sutra in their teachings as a sexual blueprint, adapting the positions and practices.

The Kama Sutra was put together by a student of religion and the divine, Mallanga Vatsayana, sometime between the 1st and 4th centuries AD. In its fearless and uninhibited approach to sexual passion it is more enlightening than the theories of many modern-day erotologists. Due to its explicit content and vivid descriptions of positions and potions intended to enhance lovemaking, it has often been misunderstood in the West as pornographic. In fact, it was intended as a guide to love, detailing courting practices, ways of treating marriage partners and consorts and more.

Over a thousand years after the Kama Sutra, Kalyana Malla's Ananga Ranga appeared. Although Malla used many of the Kama Sutra's sexual positions, embraces and other techniques, the Ananga Ranga had a different aim and content to the Kama Sutra. Whereas the Kama Sutra was associated with love and union, the Ananga Ranga was more orientated towards preventing the separation of husbands and wives and enhancing marriage longevity. Following up on this aim, Kalyana Malla describes the different types of men and women and catalogues their various seats of passion, characteristics and temperaments.

The origins of Tantra are harder to define. The oldest Tantric text seems to be the Buddhist Tantras that date back to around AD 600, but there are Tantric elements in the Vedas. More than a practice or step-by-step guide, Tantra is a philosophy, concerned with spirituality and divine energy, blending sacred sexuality, Eastern philosophy and the teachings of the Kama Sutra. It involves the use of meditation and yoga to master the ultimate goal of dissipating the ego and creating union with the divine energy that is within each of us.

Over the last three thousand years, Eastern cultures have worshipped and respected the power and life force of human sexual nature and recognized the importance of teaching this to the next generation. In the West, our social sexual development has been very different. Although contemporary Western society is more liberal and open than in the past, the arts of seduction, sensuality and wanton abandon have been underdeveloped by comparison with the East. By looking towards the East, we can borrow wisdom and teachings from a long history of enlightened sexual revolutionaries.

kama sutra

Although little is known of the compiler of the Kama Sutra, Mallanga Vatsayana, it is claimed that he was a student Brahmin, involved in the contemplation of the divine. He was probably based in the city of Pataliputra during a period of economic growth and social liberalism.

The Kama Sutra focuses around the three major concepts of Hinduism: *dharma* (the gaining of religious merit or righteousness and responsibility), *artha* (achieving goals, including personal wealth) and *kama* (love and the other sensual pleasures). The theory was that when one had attained these three goals, combining the moral, material and erotic, then one could aspire to acheiving *moksha*, or spiritual liberation.

The Kama Sutra is therefore not solely sexually focused and only a small portion of the text concentrates on the act of sex. In India it became a guide to human relations and interactions. It advises on other aspects of male-female relations such as courtship and marriage, the duties of wife and husband, enhancing beauty and attractiveness, and it provides a variety of recipes and incantations to help with sexual problems and difficulties.

Vatsayana's tone in the Kama Sutra is remarkably unprejudiced and liberal considering the time in which it was written. The emphasis is suggestive as opposed to dictatorial, frequently reminding couples that they should do whatever they feel is right for them at the time. It is a lover's guide, not a lover's law.

The West got wind of the Kama Sutra in the Victorian era, when women were not expected to enjoy sex and men did not therefore require any specific sexual skill or talent to please them. Its Victorian translators, F.F. Arbuthnot and Sir Richard Burton, published the book in English in 1883 for private circulation. It was not until 1963 that the first edition became available to the general public, a hiatus that greatly added to the mystique surrounding the Kama Sutra.

The Kama Sutra is in many ways a direct portal to the period and culture in which it was written. Although much of it is outdated, there are many underlying elements in the Kama Sutra that the Western world can still learn from. The most important of these is the sense of belonging to a civilized society that takes the pleasures of the mind and body extremely seriously.

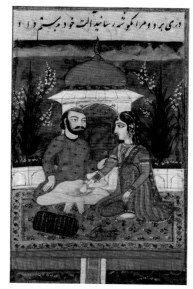

LEFT | In this 18th-century illustration, the woman is manipulating the lingham, or penis, of her partner.

BELOW | Illustrations of the Kama Sutra are often set in beautiful palaces, here complete with flowers, hand-woven rug and hookah.

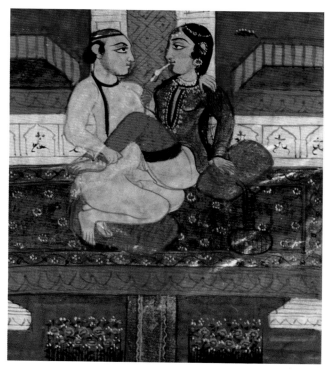

a modern kama sutra

THE KAMA SUTRA isn't just a list of exotic positions for sex. It describes in great detail the delicacy of foreplay and the importance of both parties being satisfied sexually, and also that they should share time together as a couple after congress.

the work of the man

In the Kama Sutra, the "work of the man" denotes any action that the man must do in order to give pleasure to the woman. Vatsayana suggests that when a man and a woman first come together, they begin by sitting on the bed talking about non-sexual topics and encourage each other to drink wine. While the woman is lying on the man's bed, engrossed by his captivating conversation, the man should loosen her undergarments and "overwhelm her" with kisses if she starts to protest.

When he becomes erect it is suggested that he should begin gently touching her with his hands. If she is shy or it is the first time they have had sex together, he should begin by placing his hands between her thighs. He should also caress her breasts, neck and armpits with his hands.

modern interpretation

The contemporary message of the concept of "the work of the man" is about the importance of foreplay. Take time to seduce each other in bed with words and actions and some good wine. The woman does not have to be passive; both should luxuriate in the sensuality of each other's body before actually having intercourse.

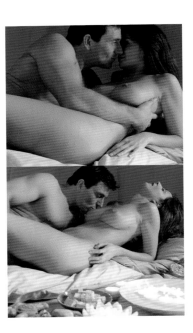

satisfying a woman

During sex, the man should concentrate on pressing the parts of the woman's body "on which she turns her eyes". Signs that a woman is enjoying herself are that she will turn (roll or close) her eyes, will become less shy and will press herself towards him to keep their sex organs as closely united as possible. When the woman shakes her hands, prevents the man from getting up, bites or kicks him, or continues writhing after he has orgasmed, it signifies that she is aroused and requires more satisfaction.

modern interpretation

It is interesting that Indian culture was so aware of the sexual needs of women at a time when the Western world seemed completely oblivious of them. Male reading of the body movements of women during intercourse allows you both to remain at the same tempo. If the man comes before his partner and ignores her need for sexual fulfilment he will invariably leave her frustrated.

sanskrit

The Kama Sutra was written in Sanskrit, the ancient and sacred language of India, in which Hindu literature from the Vedas downwards was composed.

Yoni is the Sanskrit word for the female genitalia, or vulva. The yoni is an object of veneration among Hindus as it is seen as a holy symbol of the goddess Shakti.

Lingham is the Sanskrit word for the phallus, which is worshipped among Hindus as a symbol of the god Shiva.

ABOVE RIGHT | The Kama Sutra was enlightened in its belief in foreplay and recommends that the man should begin by rubbing the woman's yoni with his fingers until aroused.

RIGHT | The woman can clutch the man, pulling him into her body, and demonstrating her physical pleasure.

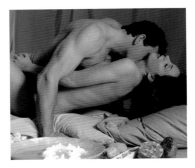

the end of congress

After sex, the two lovers must show modesty by not looking at each other and by going separately to the bathroom. They should eat betel leaves and the man should anoint the woman's body with sandalwood. He then must embrace her with his left arm and hold a cup in his right, from which he should encourage her to drink.

Together they should eat sweetmeats, soup, mango juice or lemon juice mixed with sugar, anything that is sweet and pure. The couple should then sit outside on a balcony and enjoy the moonlight, with her lying in his lap as they talk. As they gaze at the night sky he should show her the different constellations of stars and planets.

modern interpretation

Don't panic, most women today do not consider an astronomy lesson an essential post-coital activity, although if you do know a bit about stars and planets it can be romantic to share it. Following the above advice is actually a perfect way of spending time together after you have had sex. Enjoy these moments – share a drink, massage one another, feed each other with confectionery, fruit or have a light meal, before cuddling up together for a chat. Stargazing is optional.

the elephant woman

A Hastini, or elephant woman, is a woman with a large vagina. According to Vatsayana, if a man is unable to satisfy a Hastini, various forms of congress are recommended where the woman presses her thighs together, thus increasing the sensations for both parties.

An alternative is to use an apadravyas, an instrument put around or on the penis to make it longer or thicker. Apadravyas should be made of gold, silver, copper, iron, ivory, buffalo horn, various kinds of wood, tin or lead and should be cool and well fitted.

modern interpretation

Although it is not terribly polite to refer to women with large vaginas as elephant women, it is a fact of nature that with age and after childbirth, the vagina may lose some of its tightness. Pelvic floor and Kegel exercises do help to keep the vagina tight but for some women, it is just the way they are. Luckily for contemporary lovers, men no longer need to strap a buffalo horn to their genitals in order to satisfy a woman who has lost her grip. Today there is a wide range of gadgets that will satisfy all shapes and sizes and incorporating them into your sex lives can be great fun.

BELOW LEFT | At the end of congress, sharing some jasmine or mint tea with some sweet food is a marvellous way to bask in the afterglow of sex.

BELOW | Turkish delight is a modern equivalent to Vatsayana's "sweetmeats".

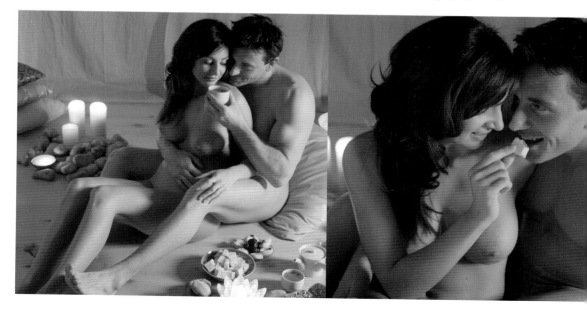

ananga ranga

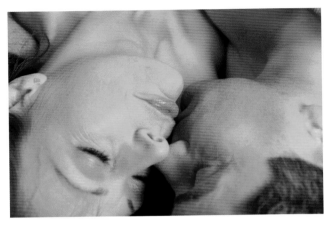

ABOVE AND BELOW |
Closeness continues to be important in a long-term relationship. The Ananga Ranga sought to increase intimacy and rid marriages of any stagnation.

INDIAN LOVE SAGE KALYANA MALLA wrote the Ananga Ranga during the 16th century. It was aimed at keeping husbands and wives from separating when their relationship went wrong. Like the Kama Sutra, the book was translated into English in the late 1800s, but it was not made extensively available until the 1960s as it was considered too racy.

The Ananga Ranga aimed to define more clearly the distinction between monotony and monogamy, releasing one from the other, and relieving the tedium of marriage. Malla believed that the chief reason that husbands go off with other women, and wives with other men, is that sex becomes boring and mundane: "the monotony which follows possession". He wrote a long treatise of erotic work, which incorporated the much older Kama Sutra, describing a multitude of ways of kissing, embracing and sexual positions.

"Fully understanding the way in which such quarrels arise, I have in this book shown how the husband, by varying the enjoyment of his wife, may live with her as with thirty-two different women, ever varying the enjoyment of her, and rendering satiety impossible." The Ananga Ranga seeks to help couples to renew their desire for sex,

which in turn helps them to re-establish strong bonds, both of friendship and love. Although sex is clearly important to all loving relationships, Malla removes the emphasis from sex and argues instead that this should be the end result of all the teachings and techniques that can be introduced to the relationship via the Ananga Ranga. It defines the different types of men and women and their needs, what kind of sex they enjoy and how to hold each other physically, mentally and emotionally.

The contemporary significance of the Ananga Ranga lies in its insistence upon the importance of maintaining passion in long-term relationships and its practical suggestions for rejuvenating stagnant patterns. Despite its antiquity, the concepts and practices set out in the Ananga Ranga are relatively new to the West. By combining the elements of Eastern magic and mystery with what we already know, we can begin to understand how and why problems have arisen in our relationships and begin to take positive steps towards healing wounds and strengthening bonds.

thirty-two lovers

The Ananga Ranga differs from the Kama Sutra in its recognition that the ability to maintain erotic interest in an exclusive monogamous relationship is not simple.

The book defines the difference between intimacy and familiarity and encourages sexual partners to break down the patterns of laziness that are bred from familiarity and to reinvent and renew the possibilities of sustained eroticism that can be derived from true intimacy. It teaches couples to use their minds and imaginations to achieve a more sophisticated level of eroticism and aims to teach lovers to experience their partner as if they were thirty-two different lovers.

embracing techniques

THE ANANGA RANGA'S CHAPTER on the "treating of external enjoyments" concentrates on the importance of various preliminaries that should precede sex and internal enjoyment. These include the various types of kissing and embracing, biting, scratching and hair pulling. These acts, according to Malla, "affect the senses and divert the mind from coyness and coldness." Foreplay is an essential part of all sexual encounters, as it helps to relax and acquaint the partners with each other's bodies and erogenous zones, allowing both to reach the same levels of excitement before penetration.

Malla recommends these techniques for embracing in relationships where cuddling has ceased to be spontaneous. Touching is one of the mutually satisfying ways for men and women to show their affection for each other – not just when they are going to have sex, but at other times as well. The types of pressure to be used are described as pressing, touching, piercing and rubbing. Once tried, these techniques might arouse interest in further contact, or can just be enjoyed in their own right.

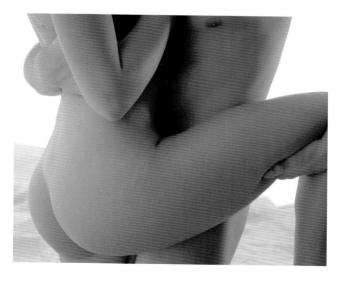

vrikshadhirudha

This is often referred to as the embrace that simulates climbing a tree. The woman places one foot on the man's foot and raises her other leg, resting her foot upon his thigh. She puts her arms around his back and holds him tightly.

modern interpretation

With the woman's legs parted in this fashion, and the man's hands relatively free, this embrace gives the man good access to the woman's breasts and genitals for light stroking and caressing, while she showers him with passionate kisses.

tila-tandula

The man and woman stand in front of each other and hold each other closely around the waist. Then, being careful to remain still, he should allow his penis to come into contact with her vagina, with only the veil of her skirt between the two. They should remain like this for a time.

modern interpretation

This embrace is best achieved if the woman is wearing loose clothing made of soft fabric, as the sensation of the material against both the man's and the woman's private parts will add to the experience. It may be hard to remain like this for a long time, as the sensation of each other's genitals in such close proximity is arousing, and can be too much for some.

urupaguha

The man and woman stand in front of each other and he places her closed legs between his own, so that his inside thigh touches her outside thigh. As with all the embraces, the couple should also experiment with kissing at the same time.

modern interpretation

This is an especially good embrace if the man is taller than the woman. The squeezing of her thighs provides gentle stimulation of her clitoris and his genitals are pressed against her.

ABOVE | Climbing a tree – it is as if the woman is trying to reach up for a kiss.

BELOW | Embracing doesn't have to be done by the book – if you are lucky it will happen spontaneously.

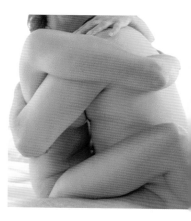

kissing techniques

THE ANANGA RANGA described osculations, or kissing, as particular styles to be studied and which were to be practised with the embracing techniques. "There are seven places highly proper for osculation, in fact, where all the world kisses." These are the lower lip, both the eyes, both cheeks, the head, the mouth, the breasts and lastly, the shoulders. Of course there is no reason why you should stop there.

nlita kissing

When the woman is angry, the man should forcibly cover her lips with his own and continue until her anger has subsided.

modern interpretation

This type of kissing can be a fantastic means of ending an argument in which there is simply nothing more that can be said. Couples who have been together for a long time often find themselves arguing over petty annoyances.

These arguments are usually cyclical in content and it can be hard to walk away or end the quarrel. A kiss such as this requires no words. It says, "Let's forget this, we are arguing over trivia and I love you."

sphrita kissing

The woman leans in to kiss her partner, who kisses her lower lip while she jerks her mouth away without returning the kiss.

modern interpretation

This is a playful, teasing kiss. When you move in to kiss your partner, allow him or her a taste of your lower lip before withdrawing and not allowing the kiss to continue. This is a great one to do in a quiet corner in the company of others. It tells your partner that you are feeling playful and frisky, but that he or she will have to wait until you decide when play will commence. It guarantees anticipation and excitement in your partner and is a seductive means of communicating without words.

BELOW | Nlita kissing – a great way of putting a stop to petty squabbles.

BELOW RIGHT | The teasing sphrita kiss can be initiated by either partner.

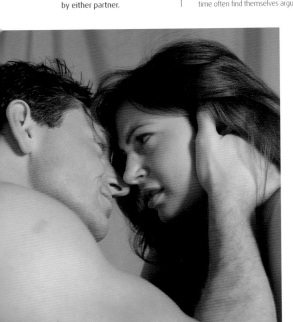
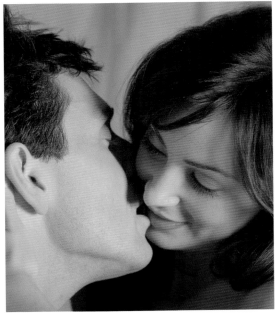

ghatika kissing

The man covers his partner's eyes with his hands and closes his own eyes before thrusting his tongue into his partner's mouth, moving it to and fro using a slow, pleasant motion that suggests another form of enjoyment.

modern interpretation

By removing one sense, in this case sight, the partners' bodies become more attuned to other sensations. In this case, sex is simulated with the mouth, building anticipation about how each will pleasure the other genitally. It is a provocative yet romantic method of kissing, ideal as a precursory invitation to a night of sensational sexual activity.

uttaroshtha

The man gently bites and nibbles his partner's lower lip while the woman reciprocates on his upper lip, then they swap over, both exciting themselves to the height of passion.

modern interpretation

This is like foreplay for kissing. With each other's mouths, the partners tease the nerve endings, so that by the time they begin a more passionate kiss, including tongues, all the sensory organs in the area will be in overdrive, and aroused beyond words.

pratibodha

When one partner is sleeping the other should fix their lips over their sleeping partner's lips, and gradually increase the pressure until sleep turns into desire.

modern interpretation

This kiss ignites passion first thing in the morning, and there is, after all, no better way to begin the day. Begin by gently kissing your partner, gradually increasing the pressure, sucking on his or her lips until they wake up.

tiryak kissing

The man places his hand beneath the woman's chin, and raises it, until he has made her face look up to the sky; then he takes her lower lip between his teeth, gently biting and chewing it.

modern interpretation

It would feel wonderful for a woman to surrender to this gently forceful kiss from a man.

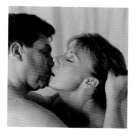

ABOVE | Here, playfully nibbling the lip is combined with pulling the hair.

BELOW LEFT | Ghatika kissing – this is a very suggestive way to arouse your partner's desire for more.

BELOW | Uttaroshtha kissing – he bites her lip, and she bites his; just be sure not to bite too hard...

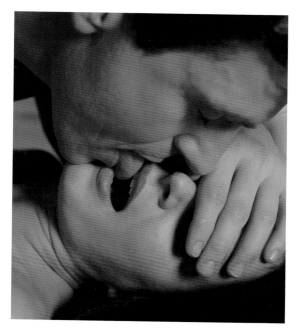

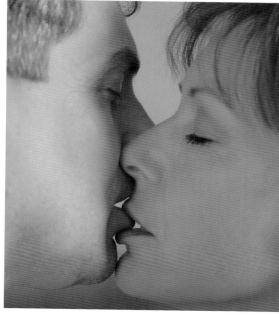

scratching, biting and hair pulling

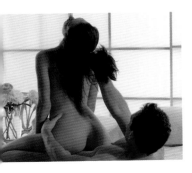

ABOVE | The ancient texts were witness to the effect that a woman's hair can have on a man.

BELOW | Light scratching can be extremely erotic if both partners are willing.

SCRATCHING AND BITING are, both the Ananga Ranga and the Kama Sutra suggest, to be tried only when love becomes intense. Description is given of the preferred, clean state of nails and teeth, and the willingness of both parties, before commencing.

scratching

The Ananga Ranga defines specific times when this type of sex play is advisable. Some examples include: when one partner is about to go away for a long period of time, or when both are "excited with desire of congress." It appears to have been done as a form of remembrance, so that when they are separated there will be a mark on the body to remind them of each other.

churit-nakhadana – gentle scratches

This involves the light scratching of the nails around the cheek, lower lip and breasts. The scratching should be light enough that it leaves no marks.

modern interpretation

The scratching described here is so light that it is more of a caress. The soft use of nails, however, indicates greater passion and energy than a more delicate touch.

the peacock's foot

For this specialist imprint the thumb is placed on the nipple and four fingers are spread adjacent to this on the breast. The nails are dug in to leave an indentation similar to that of a peacock footprint.

modern interpretation

Most women love to have their breasts caressed and squeezed during lovemaking. The preferred pressure and sensation is individual to each woman, with some having very sensitive breasts, especially around menstruation. Before digging your nails into your partner's breasts it is advisable to find out how much stimulation she prefers.

anvartha-nakhadana – to remember

Marks or scratches three deep are made by the first three fingers on the woman's back, breasts or genitals. It is most commonly done as a token of remembrance before the man leaves to go abroad.

modern interpretation

Many men and women really enjoy scratching if it is done correctly, as it is a form of sensual massage and can be very relaxing. Remember to be gentle and do not do anything that may cause pain. As with all these techniques, keep your nails smooth, clean and reasonably short.

biting

The Ananga Ranga suggests that biting should be done in similar places to scratching but lovers should avoid the eyes, upper lip and tongue. It also suggests that the pressure should be increased until the recipient protests, after which enough has been done. Neither party will be in particular favour if they bite the other too hard; soft nibbling is more advisable. Take cues from each other, rising to a passionate moment with appropriate strength, and a lighter touch when called for.

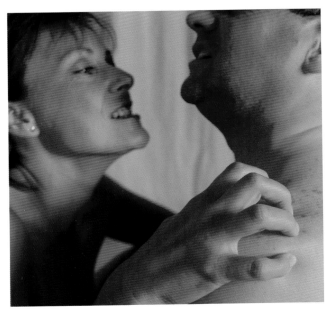

uchun-dashana – biting

This is the generic term to describe biting any part of the woman's lips or cheeks.

modern interpretation

Gently nibbling around each other's faces can be very sensual. Be careful around the bony areas like the cheeks, as they bruise easily. The lips should be handled with care too, as they are only protected by a thin layer of skin.

bindhu-dashana – teeth marks

This is the mark left by the man's two front teeth on the woman's lower lip.

modern interpretation

The lower lip is very supple and elastic and gentle sucking and nibbling on it is very pleasurable. In the days when the Ananga Ranga was written it was probably pretty acceptable for women to bear the marks of their husband's desire. Any imprint of passion today is reminiscent of the adolescent love bite, and not particularly desirable, so facial markings should be avoided.

kolacharcha – on departing

These are the deep, lasting marks left on the woman's body in the heat of passion and the grief of departure when her husband is going away.

modern interpretation

The fleshier parts of the body such as the thighs and buttocks can withstand more pain than the more sensitive areas around the face. They also have the added advantage of being hidden by clothing. Biting each other is a common outlet of sexual energy when in the throes of orgasm and many people, male and female, claim that they have been surprised at the depth of a bite afterwards. Many people enjoy sharp pain at the height of passion to enhance the powerful shudders of pleasure that they experience during orgasm.

hair pulling

Softly pulling the hair of a woman, states the Ananga Ranga, is a good method of kindling a lasting desire.

samahastakakeshagrahana – stroking

The man strokes his partner's hair between the palms of his hands, at the same time kissing her with passion.

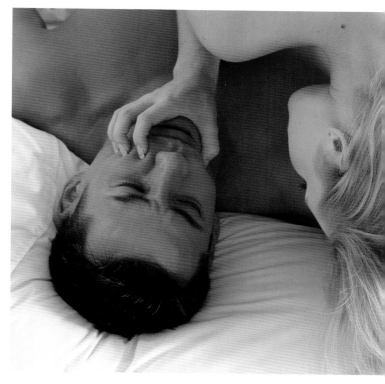

modern interpretation

Gentle pulling and playing with a woman's hair is very erotic and sensual. When pulling hair, make sure you get a good handful, as pulling at a small number of hairs can be very painful. Why not take this a stage further and gently pull tufts of each other's pubic hair – sure to bring each other to a state of excitement.

kamavatansakeshagrahana – pulling

This is done during sexual intercourse, when each partner grabs the other's hair above the ears as they kiss passionately.

modern interpretation

This type of hair pulling is ideal in the throes of passion when the body's touch sensors are dulled by the other erotic sensations that are flowing around. Stroking and massaging this area, including the temples, can be very seductive, especially if you whisper in each other's ears at the same time.

ABOVE | Churit-nakhadana – light scratching around the face – shouldn't leave a mark.

BELOW | He grabs her hair in kamavatansakeshagrahana.

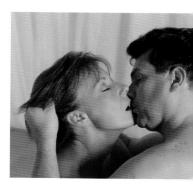

ananga ranga positions

MANY OF THE SEXUAL POSITIONS in the Ananga Ranga were adapted by Malla from the original work of Vatsayana's Kama Sutra. However, Malla's text was written in a very different social climate, where extramarital sex was frowned upon, so the emphasis is on variety with one partner.

the crab embrace

The man and woman lie on their sides facing each other. The man enters the woman and lies between her legs. One of her legs passes over his body (at about the level of his navel) while the other remains beneath his legs.

modern interpretation

The position provides deep penetration and increased friction. The man's movement is limited although the woman has more freedom. This position may be good when one partner is tired but both are still passionate.

kama's wheel

The man sits with his legs outstretched. The woman lowers herself on to his penis, facing him. She also extends her legs. He then stretches his arms out along either side of her body to support her. This forms the wheel-like figure for which this position is named.

modern interpretation

It is said that this position combines sex and meditation to create a higher level of awareness. It is meant to help the partners to obtain a balance of mind that is clear, calm and happy.

the ascending position

The man lies on his back while the woman sits cross-legged upon his thighs. The woman grasps his penis and inserts it into her, moving her waist backward and forward as they make love.

BELOW TOP | Kama's wheel – this is a great transitional position. Try it after ascending or before the placid embrace.

BELOW BOTTOM | The ascending position – this posture can give added satisfaction to the woman.

BELOW RIGHT | The crab embrace, lying side by side, enables plenty of physical contact along the body.

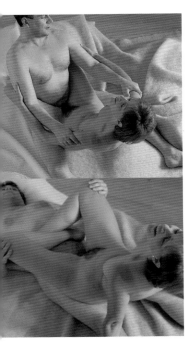

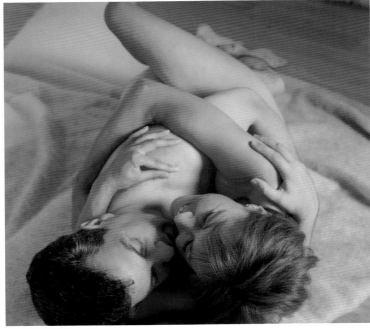

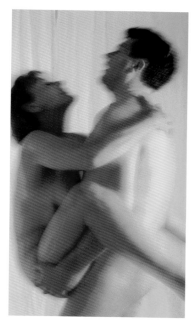

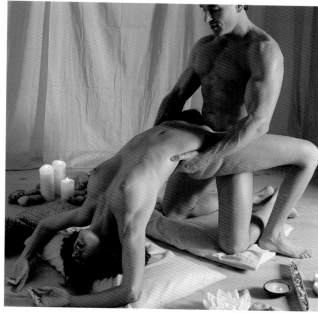

modern interpretation

The woman on top can control the movements and depth of penetration. By moving herself forward and back, her clitoris also receives stimulation from the gentle rubbing action against her partner's body. This is recommended for women who have not found satisfaction in other positions.

suspended congress

Both partners stand opposite one another. The man passes two arms under his partner's knees, supporting her by gripping her inner elbow or her bottom. He then raises her waist high and penetrates her while she clasps her hands around his neck.

modern interpretation

This one could be tricky, as its success depends on many factors such as the strength of the man, the weight of the woman, and the height of them both. It may be easier if the woman gets on a chair first, so that the man does not have to lift her from the ground and risk back injury. It may also help to be near a wall or rail to maintain balance. Good luck!

placid embrace

The man kneels and raises his partner to him by grasping her around the waist so that her head falls towards the floor. She in turn wraps her legs about his middle and lets her head fall freely.

modern interpretation

This position allows the woman to retain some control – by extending and flexing the grip of her legs she can draw her partner closer. Hanging with the head upside-down can also contribute a feeling of ecstasy and otherworldliness. Try this after kama's wheel.

ABOVE LEFT | Suspended congress – this one isn't for you if you have a bad back.

ABOVE | The placid embrace allows the woman to let herself go completely.

BELOW | You may have tried the crab embrace before without realizing it.

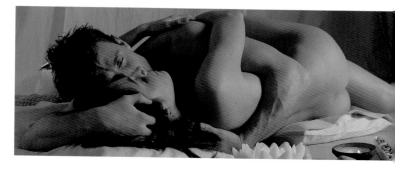

the art of tantric sex

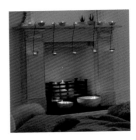

TANTRA FOCUSES on honouring and respecting your partner as the other half of yourself. Although Tantrists believe that sex is a divine gift that should be celebrated, Tantra is not a religion but a tradition, which can be practised by people of any faith or by non-religious people.

The word Tantra is derived from the Indian Sanskrit meaning, "liberation through expression". Based on early Hindu and Buddhist teachings, or tantras, Tantra unites elements of meditation, yoga and worship to provide practitioners with a more wholesome and intense sexual experience.

Tantra has many dimensions that can take years of study to fully appreciate. This does not mean, however, that people interested in Tantric sex must immerse themselves in study. Instead, it is perfectly valid to take some elements of Tantra and incorporate them into existing sex lives.

In Tantric sex the vagina becomes a sacred space (yoni) and the penis (or lingham) is a "wand of light". Kundalini denotes the life force and sexual energy that flows between sexual partners as they make love. Breathing and visualization exercises help to harmonize this energy. Tantric sex takes the emphasis away from the physicality

of the orgasm and concentrates more on spirituality, intimacy and connection. Men are often taught to suppress their orgasm, a Tantric skill known as maithuna, in order to devote their attention to the woman's sexual pleasure. If this all sounds rather pointless from the male perspective, it is worth remembering that once it is mastered, men reap the rewards, keeping sexually active for anything up to an hour with the promise of increased orgasm when it comes. It can also increase the chance of multiple orgasms for their partner and enable the man to "virtually experience" their lover's orgasm as well as their own.

tantra western style

Tantra cannot cure a failing relationship but it's a good prescription for a loving respectful relationship that has become a bit dull. Most people would prefer to tackle the problem of bedroom boredom rather than bailing out of a relationship. According to Tantra, boredom sets in when people make love with only their genitals, not their hearts and minds.

A couple should begin Tantric lovemaking with an idea of what they want and, more importantly, the genuine desire to give their partner what he or

ABOVE | Create a harmonious environment to share.

BELOW | Place your hand on your lover's heart so you can merge together.

BELOW RIGHT | Meditate with your partner, concentrating on each chakra in turn.

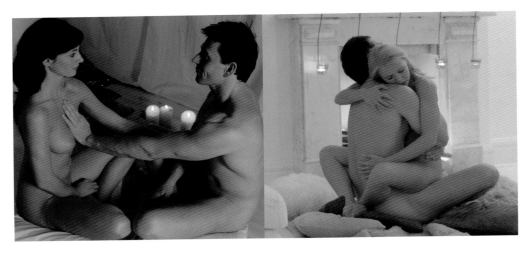

she wants. Tantric sex has no time limit: it can last minutes or hours, and it gives you and your partner the freedom and opportunity to explore each other's bodies and pleasure zones.

Much of Tantric lovemaking involves ritualistic foreplay that excites all the senses. Massage and the use of aromatherapy oils stimulate the senses of smell and touch. By caressing each other slowly and languidly the scene is set for a relaxed session of lovemaking, allowing time to explore each other's bodies and become more comfortable with each other's nudity.

meditation and breathing

Meditation in Tantra is an important principle, as it allows couples to move away from frantic passion, and emphasize tranquillity and harmony.

Dedicate an area for meditation and Tantric lovemaking and set aside a specific portion of uninterrupted time for you to either meditate alone, or with your partner. Make sure that the area is calm and warm, close the curtains, remove distractions, use aromatherapy fragrances such as cedarwood or frankincense, and light some scented candles to add to the atmosphere.

Begin by sitting on the floor with your legs crossed, back straight and hands resting in your lap. Ensure that you are comfortable before closing your eyes and focusing on your breathing. Breathe in through your nose and out through your mouth and become conscious of the soft rise and fall of your diaphragm with each breath. Try to concentrate on your breathing, and every time your mind wanders gently bring it back to your breath. With practice, meditation will create peace and tranquillity and leave you feeling refreshed and calm. Your meditation sessions will become longer, provided you remember to keep patient and relaxed.

tantra to share

Sit in front of each other and look each other in the eye as you place your hands on each other's hearts. As you breathe out, imagine that you are breathing the energy from your heart into your partner's heart. As you breathe in, imagine you are inhaling their energy into your heart. The physical

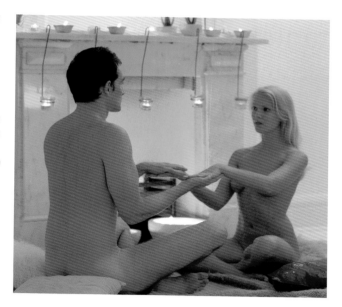

connection allows a circuit of energy to pass between you, so that energy flows from your heart, through your body to your partner's heart, and vice versa. Once you feel comfortable, begin alternating your breathing pattern with your partner's so that as they breathe in, you breathe out and so on. This should cause the energy to circulate evenly and harmoniously between you.

Sit before each other again, but this time merge your energy by placing your palms together, creating an electrical circuit. You can continue with the same breathing techniques or try chakra meditation, in which you concentrate on each chakra, breathing energy into each for two or three minutes. Begin at the base chakra and move up towards the crown, opening up each energy centre as you go. This may take some practice as each of you may require a different amount of time on each chakra, but be patient and before long both your sets of chakras will become harmonized with each other.

Don't be afraid to laugh! The point of this is not to reinvent you as Tantric gurus but to bring you closer together. Collapsing in giggles will not detach you from the spirit of what you are trying to achieve.

ABOVE | Create a circuit of energy between you – merge together for 15 minutes, allowing your breathing to synchronize naturally.

BELOW | A calming and private space in which to meditate will enable you to concentrate and not be distracted by external elements.

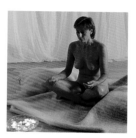

tantra lying down

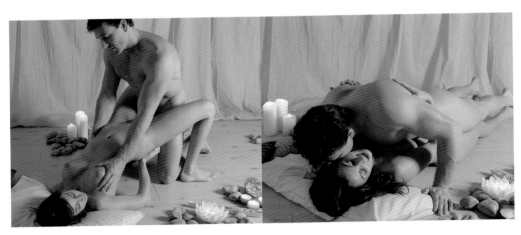

ABOVE | The flower in bloom, blossoming.

ABOVE RIGHT | The jewel case.

BELOW | Aphrodite's delight requires supple legs.

BELOW RIGHT | Dear to Cupid.

TANTRIC UNION IS A SEXUAL BOND that transcends the purely physical. Partners can forget their daily cares or status and concentrate though discipline on their being one with another person, thus achieving a higher state of ecstasy.

The positions of Tantra are based on those of the Kama Sutra. Here are a few examples translated into a more contemporary style, beginning with the supine, or lying down positions.

flower in bloom

The woman lies back, with bent knees, and spreads her legs wide, digging her heels in as close to her hips as she can. Then, placing her hands under her buttocks, she cups and lifts them with her palms, offering her yoni as a "flower in bloom". The man then enters her from between her thighs, and gently caresses her breasts. This may require some stamina and flexibility.

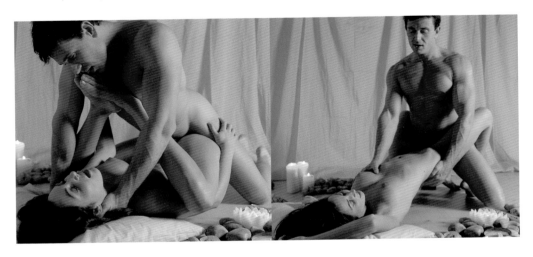

aphrodite's delight

This also requires quite a bit of flexibility from the woman. She lies back and the man clasps her feet, raising them to her breasts so that her legs form a rough circle. He then enters her, keeping her legs in place with the weight of his body, and clasps her around the neck as they make love.

dear to cupid

The woman lies back with her knees bent and the man kneels before her. He hooks her legs around his thighs and gently fondles and caresses her breasts as they make love.

the jewel case

This position is recommended for men with smaller penises. The man lies on top of the woman with his legs on top of hers, so that their legs caress each other from thighs to toes. This can either be done with the woman below the man, or side by side, in which case she should always lie to the left.

love's noose

The woman lies back as the man enters her. With her thighs pressed tightly together he encircles the woman's legs with his own. He should then squeeze and grip her thighs – very good for added clitoral stimulation.

the bud

The woman lies back and draws her legs up, clasping her knees to her breasts. This exposes her yoni (vagina) "like an opening bud" to her partner.

the mare's trick

The woman sits astride the man facing either way, and during penetration, rhythmically squeezes his penis, "milking it" with her PC muscle.

splitting the bamboo

The woman lies on her back and raises one leg over her partner's shoulder as he enters her. After a time she lowers that leg and raises the other.

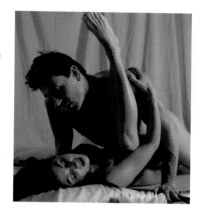

vadavaka

The art of vadavaka, or milking the man's penis, is a difficult one to be mistress of without significant practice. It can be tried in any sexual position, although some, like the mare's trick, will be easier than others where the woman is not in control.

Squeeze the PC (puboccygeus) muscle as if trying to halt the flow of urine. Pulsating in this way will heighten the pleasure of both parties. The grip may be improved by catching the glans of the lingham, or penis, behind the pubic bone, with the added advantage that it will be pushed up against the G spot here too.

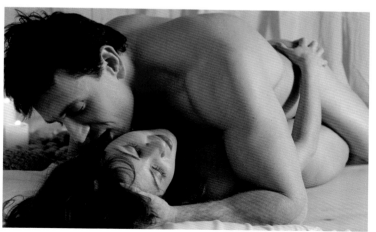

ABOVE LEFT | Splitting the bamboo – this may not be comfortable for the woman for a long time, so vary the posture or move to another.

LEFT | Love's noose – this is an advanced version of the jewel case and you may find you can move between these postures quite easily.

sitting tantra

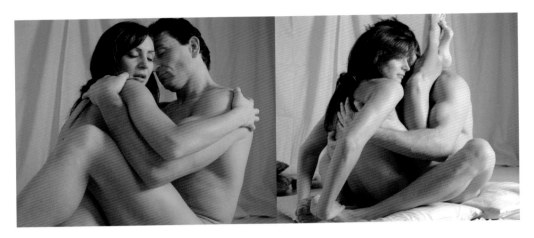

ABOVE | Feet yoke – this will be fun, once you have worked out how to do it.

ABOVE RIGHT | The lotus – it may be hard for the woman to keep her feet linked, but it isn't essential.

MANY OF THE SITTING POSITIONS are intended for long-drawn-out sex, where the couple becomes truly intertwined in mind as well as body.

the feet yoke

For this position you must both have reasonably flexible knees in order to achieve deeper penetration. The woman sits erect with one leg bent and the knee pulled in to her body, and the other leg straight out in front of her. The man does the same with opposing legs and penetrates her. If you cannot get close enough, then slip each straight leg beneath your partner's bent one, and gently pull one another closer together.

the circle

The woman sits with her left leg extended and encircles the man's waist with her right leg, laying the ankle across her left thigh. He mirrors this so that they are both entwined in a circle as they make love.

the peacock

This requires extreme female mobility! The woman sits and raises one foot to point vertically over her head, steadying it with her hand. In this position she offers up her yoni to her partner for lovemaking.

the lotus

The man and woman sit in front of each other, with his legs wrapped around the woman's waist. He then grips her ankles and locks them around the back of his neck like the link of a chain. She grips his toes or feet to steady herself as they make love.

awakening the chakras

The theory of chakras is that they are energy centres within the body that control our physical and psychological wellbeing. Kundalini energy is activated by the root chakra and allows spiritual energy to flow to the crown chakra, helping the body to achieve an ecstatic plane of consciousness.

There are seven chakras in the body. The first three, related to basic survival, are: root, associated with sexuality, pleasure and pain; belly, the central core of balance relating to sexual drive and reproduction, and solar plexus, concerned with power, intellect, will and ego. The four higher chakras relate to the mind, intellect and spirituality. The heart chakra is between the nipples, and being near the heart is associated with love, empathy and joy; the fifth, throat chakra, is associated with purity and expression; the sixth chakra, between the eyes, is often known as the third eye and is associated with intuition, compassion and intellect; the seventh chakra is the crown chakra, found at the top of the head. It is associated with cosmic consciousness, bliss and unity.

the swing

She sits in his lap, and the man and woman hold each other's arms and take it in turns to lean backwards, until a swinging or seesaw-like rhythm is achieved. This position restricts thrusting, so is good for when the man is tired, and also for allowing both the man and woman to have an equal role in lovemaking.

striking

The woman sits astride the man, and as they make love, he strikes her chest. Suggesting that the couple hit each other may seem odd to a modern audience. In the Kama Sutra, intercourse is likened to a quarrel "on account of the contrarieties of love and its tendency to dispute." Here the striking is almost a formalized kind of role-playing, where each partner strikes the other as if in anger, increasing the blows until orgasm.

Four different types of striking are described: striking with the back of the hand; striking with fingers contracted; striking with the fist; and striking with the palm of the hand. Different sounds should be made by the recipient of the blows, such as cooing or hissing, and they should then strike back in return. Even Vatsayana was scornful of the fashion for using implements to abuse each other, calling this "painful, barbarous and base, and quite unworthy of imitation." Striking was considered another form of "external enjoyment" to be used in the throes of passion, according to the strength and the proclivities of the parties involved. Obviously, this should not be undertaken without the informed consent of one's partner.

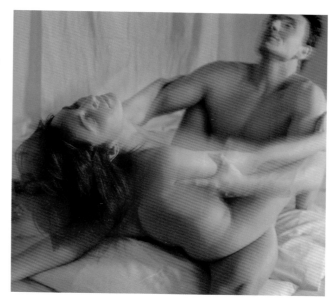

yab-yum

Yab-yum is the quintessential form of sexual union in Tantric lovemaking. It translates as "mother and father union", aligning all the energy centres (chakras) within the body, allowing kundalini energy to rise and a more spiritual level to be reached. The woman should sit on her partner's lap, facing him. Her legs should be wrapped around his waist and arms wrapped around each other. The idea is that the couple stay still and visualize, in the mind's eye, the energy rising from the root chakra to the crown, despite the temptation, of course, to move and thrust.

ABOVE | The swing can be fun once you get into the rhythm.

BELOW LEFT | Striking should be a passionate, rather than a painful, experience.

BELOW CENTRE | Yab-yum is one of the most loving poses allowing maximum contact.

BELOW | The temptation to be active can be strong.

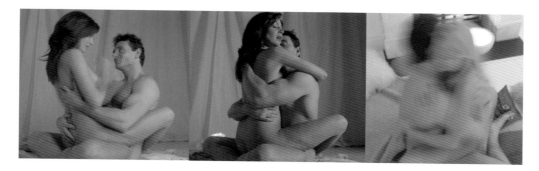

standing and rear tantra

STANDING POSITIONS were considered, by Brahmins like Vatsayana, to be a high form of congress, and they are depicted in numerous works of art. Rear entry postions were also enjoyed, taking their inspiration from the animal kingdom.

BELOW LEFT | The tripod – this is a position that could be done anywhere, but try next to the bed the first time, in case you lose your balance.

BELOW RIGHT | The ass – if the woman is not flexible enough to reach the floor, she could rest her hands on a chair.

please her yoni

It is the man's duty to please his partner and here are some suggested techniques.

manthana – churning
Grind your penis in circles once inside her, avoiding thrusting.

piditaka – pressing
Press your penis hard towards her womb and hold before withdrawing and repeating.

varahaghata – the boar's blow
Provide continuous pressure on one side of her vagina during penetration.

vrishaghata – the bull's blow
Thrust wildly in every direction while you penetrate her.

chatakavilasa – sparrow sport
Quiver your penis while it is inside her.

suspended

This posture requires quite a bit of strength from the man. He begins by standing with his back to a wall, but not leaning against it. The woman sits in his cradled arms with her thighs gripping his waist, feet flat against the wall and arms wrapped around his neck. As they make love she pushes back and forth against the wall.

the tripod

This requires a good sense of balance. He holds one of her knees firmly in his hand and stands, without support. As they make love she can caress and explore his body with her hands.

the dog

This is similar to the doggy position, in which the woman goes on all fours and the man enters her from behind. In Tantra, however, the woman should turn her head and gaze into her partner's eyes as they make love.

the ass

The woman stands with her legs slightly apart and bends forward, gripping her thighs with her hands, or with hands on the floor. The man then enters her from behind. Height differences can be combated by the width that she spreads her legs. For shorter men, she should spread her legs wider.

the stride

This is another one for the more adventurous and agile couple. The woman stands on her palms and feet so her body forms a triangle. From behind he lifts one of her feet to his shoulder, driving his lingham into her yoni with vigorous strokes.

the elephant

This is similar to spoons, in which the woman lies on her side facing away from the man. She offers her buttocks to him and he penetrates from behind, using his hands to gently caress the other parts of her body.

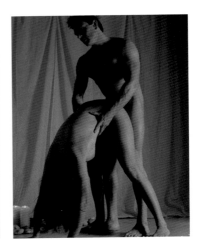

oral tantra

KNOWN AS "MOUTH CONGRESS" in the Kama Sutra, oral sex was considered a base activity practised by wanton women and eunuchs. These days it is a healthy part of most loving relationships, although some lovers are not sure how to go about it.

fellatio

There are different techniques described by Vatsayana for performing fellatio on a man. You don't have to put the whole thing in your mouth – the head is the most sensitive part.

nimitta – touching

Holding his penis with one hand, the woman shapes her mouth into an "O" and places it on the tip of her partner's penis. She moves her head in tiny circles, maintaining a light touch.

parshvatoddashta – biting to the sides

Holding the head of the penis in her hand, the woman clamps her lips lightly above the shaft, first on one side and then the other, being careful to keep her teeth hidden so as not to cause any pain.

antaha-samdansha – the inner pincers

The woman takes the whole of the head of the penis into her mouth. She then presses the shaft firmly between her lips and holds it for a few seconds before pulling away.

parimrshtaka – striking at the tip

The woman begins by flicking her tongue all over his penis, using a hard pointed tongue. Then she concentrates on the sensitive tip of the glans, striking it continually to evoke a heightened sexual sensation.

sangara – swallowed whole

This is done when the man is close to orgasm. The woman takes the whole of the penis into her mouth and sucks, working her tongue and lips until the man comes.

cunnilingus

Oral sex performed on a woman doesn't get much of a write-up in the ancient texts – it was considered just another form of kissing.

jihva-bhramanaka – the circling tongue

The man uses his nose to spread the woman's vaginal lips and then gently probes her yoni with his tongue. Then, with his nose, lips and chin, he moves in gentle circles all around her vaginal area.

chushita – sucked

The man fastens his lips to the woman's vaginal lips and nibbles at her before sucking on her clitoris. He uses varying degrees of pressure as he sucks on her clitoris until he finds one that she is comfortable with and, more importantly, one that gives her pleasure.

uchchushita – sucked up

The man cups and lifts his partner's buttocks, and uses his tongue to gently massage her navel, working down to her genitals. Once between her legs he should use his tongue to gently lap up her love juices.

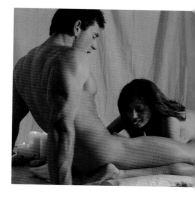

ABOVE | Striking at the tip – you don't have to put the whole penis in your mouth. The head is the most sensitive part, so concentrate here.

BELOW | Sucked up – hopefully, the tantalizing sensations will be almost unbearable by the time he reaches his destination.

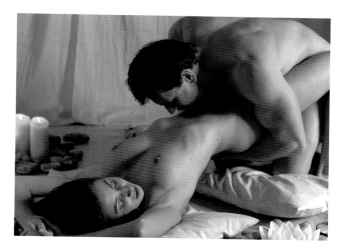

suppressing orgasm

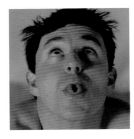

ABOVE | Controlling your breathing may help you orgasm without ejaculation.

RIGHT | Suppressing your orgasms may enable you to find an ecstatic plateau.

BELOW | Saluting one another acknowledges the other's body as the bridge to the spiritual world.

ACHIEVING ORGASM is often seen as the *sine qua non* of modern sex. Without that emphasis, lovemaking can become more relaxed and less goal-orientated. So sex without orgasm can be an activity in itself. Each partner tries not to reach orgasm for as long as possible.

The Tantric skill of maithuna is a technique for controlling response, designed to help intensify orgasm and also to help men to delay their orgasm to keep in harmony with their partner's sexual tempo. The technique is designed to help the flow of sexual energy and to ensure men feel energized after sex as opposed to exhausted.

● When you feel like you are about to come, breathe deeply. Many people hold their breath, as if forcing the orgasm to come out. By keeping the breathing regular the orgasm will become more intense as you flow with and not against it.

● Keep the tip of your tongue on the roof of your mouth or roll it into a "straw" to breathe through. This can help to circulate the energy and help men to withhold their orgasm.

● When you begin to orgasm, imagine the energy is flowing away from your genitals and up your spine. Do not contort yourself to try and help this physically. This is purely a visualization to

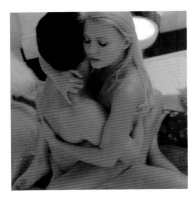

prolong orgasm. The more control a man has over his own sexual responses, the more he will be able to offer his partner.

saluting one another

At the culmination of your time together, you should sit before each other and salute each other, saying words such as, "You are a god/goddess." This acknowledges the other's body and gives praise for awakening each other's senses, and thanks for helping each other in the unity of spiritual Tantric lovemaking.

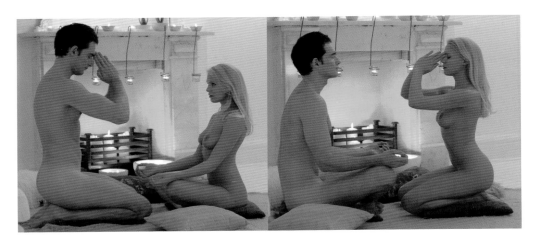

tantric energy orgasms

ENERGY ORGASMS CLEANSE THE BODY of repression, emotional pain and sexual blocks and barricades. It is a Tantric masturbation technique that requires deep concentration, visualization and lots of practice. Energy orgasms can vary in strength – extra time put into building energy generally leads to a more powerful orgasm. It is for men and women, and is said to be very different from an ordinary orgasm and may or may not feel sexual.

move like a butterfly

Begin by lying on a flat hard surface and bend your knees up. Start to take a few deeper breaths, empty your mind and release the tension in your mind and body. As you inhale, arch your lower back to rock your pelvis, and as you exhale, squeeze your PC (puboccygeus) muscle. (These are the muscles that stop the flow of urine when you pee.) By squeezing these muscles you are stimulating the G spot and clitoris or penis and testicles, and at the same time you are helping to pump energy throughout your body. Let your breathing and contractions be erotic and as you repeat the circular breathing technique, fan your legs open as you inhale and close as you exhale, like butterfly wings, to help to keep the energy flowing and maintain your rhythm.

Your energy will follow your thought processes, so visualize drawing energy in from the atmosphere and into the perineum area, between your genitals and anus. Build strong fires of energy in the sex centres of the first and second chakras and circulate this energy back and forth. Once the energy feels powerful and strong, move it up and continue circulating it from the genital area to the belly area, the first and second chakras. Again, once you feel that the energy is strong, let it flow from the belly to the heart, the fourth chakra, via the solar plexus, the third. Then move the circulating energy on from the heart to the fifth, throat, chakra. You may find it helpful to consciously make sounds, opening the throat and allowing energy to then circulate upwards from the throat to the third eye, circulating between the fifth and sixth chakras.

Finally, visualize the energy flowing between the third eye and the top of the head, the seventh, crown, chakra. Now you should start to feel the energy shoot from the top of your head and a full body orgasm will hopefully begin stirring. Follow the flow of the orgasm. Your breathing patterns may change and with practice you will learn to ride the waves of your orgasm and allow them to keep it going for longer and longer periods of time.

Don't worry if you don't reach orgasm first time round. This is a technique that requires a lot of practice. The breathing exercises alone will reap their own benefits by cleansing your mind of mental blocks and hurtful memories, clearing the path for more positive orgasmic experiences.

BELOW | It may be helpful to do some further research on the chakras so that you will know what you are trying to visualize. Each chakra is distinguished by a colour and a frequency of vibration which will become familiar to you as you practise.

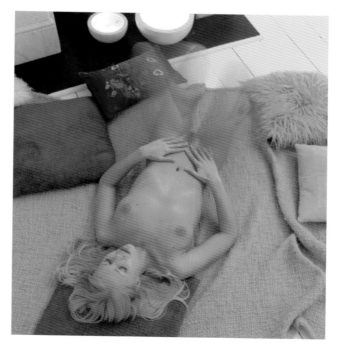

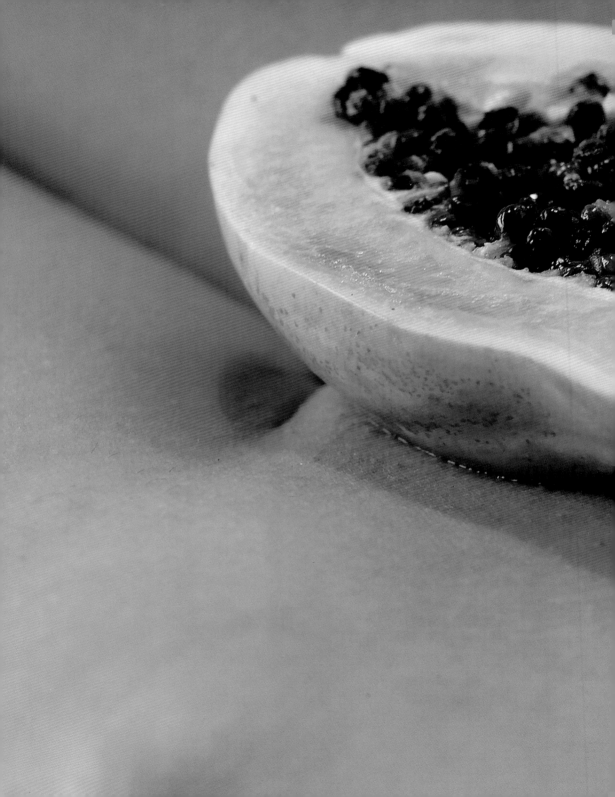

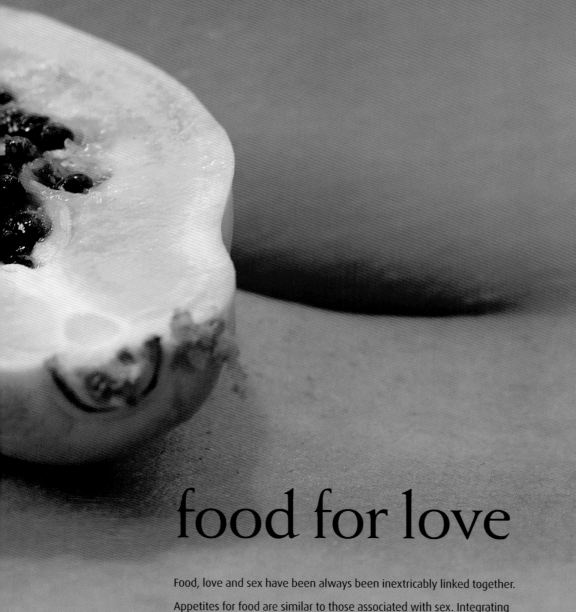

food for love

Food, love and sex have been always been inextricably linked together. Appetites for food are similar to those associated with sex. Integrating food with your lovemaking can lead to explosive results, as you nurture your two most basic needs simultaneously.

food and sex

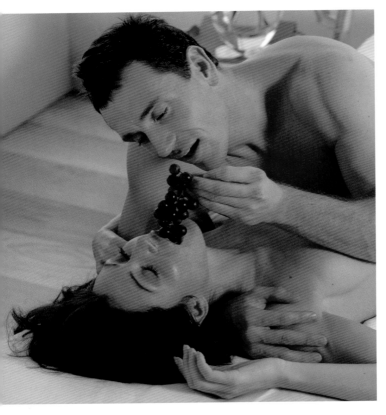

Part of the excitement of courtship is finding out about each other. You can tell so much about the person you are with from the food they buy, the method in which they cook and present it, what they choose from the menu in a restaurant and how they eat it. People with hearty appetites who really enjoy their food often have a healthy appetite for sex as well.

We use our mouths for many different things – talking, kissing, sucking, smiling, laughing, as well as eating – so watching your partner slide the flesh of an oyster into their mouth and imagining the salty, silken texture slipping down their throat can be very arousing. Eating draws attention to the mouth. The tongue, the lips and genitals all have the same neural receptors, called Kraus's end bulbs, which make them supersensitive to stimulation. This is why kissing is such an important part of the prelude to lovemaking.

a lovers' menu

Of course, we eat with our eyes as well as our mouths. The shape of certain foods can be very erotic and can conjure up all manner of suggestive images; a downy peach looks like a voluptuous bottom, oysters and figs are reminiscent of a woman's vulva, and bananas, celery and asparagus are phallic. Some foods just look irresistible – think of sashimi or chocolate cake.

In fact all the senses come into play. The pervasive aroma of truffles is astonishingly sensuous, while the sweet scent of strawberries or mangoes makes the mouth water. Texture is as important as flavour and intrinsically sexy foods include: caviar that just bursts on the tongue; anything that you eat with your fingers from a chicken drumstick to edamame (soya beans); most shellfish from scallops to crayfish, although not anything you have to remove with a pin. The sound of food sizzling stirs the appetites. There is something strangely erotic about the crunch when your lover bites into an apple.

ABOVE | Food and sex are inextricably linked and sharing food with your partner is one of the most intimate things you can do.

WHERE WOULD ROMANCE BE without the element of food? We even use foodie words to describe people we are attracted to: she's a peach, or he's really tasty, scrumptious or delicious. Honey, sugar and my sweet are terms of endearment. The reason that food has always played a part in the rituals of courtship is that both eating and sex are two of our strongest instincts and a combination of both can prove irresistible. Food, like sex, is another way of stimulating the senses. The flavour and taste, the texture and touch, the visual appearance, the aromas and even sound of food cooking, all play a part in its sensual appeal.

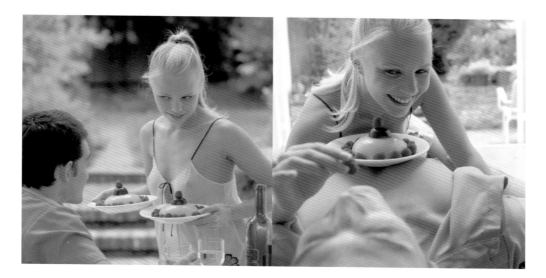

Don't forget that what you drink matters, too. Champagne is a turn-on for most people, cocktails are glamorous and even a mug of creamy hot chocolate after a brisk walk on a windy day can stir the senses. The light sparkling on beautiful crystal glasses adds to the sensuous pleasure of good wine, while many men find the sight of their partners drinking "designer" beer straight from the bottle very arousing. Drinking tequila the traditional way is sexy and fun: place a little salt on the back of your hand between your index finger and thumb and hold a wedge of lime in the same hand, then lick the salt, down a shot of tequila in one and then suck the lime.

saucy snacks

Sex shops sell a range of naughty nibbles, including chocolate body paint and penis-, bottom- and breast-shaped chocolates, combining everybody's favourite aphrodisiac with an element of fun. You can even buy edible underwear.

With a little imagination, you can create your own suggestive dishes. How about setting pink blancmange in shallow, 15cm/6in dishes and, when they're turned out, topping with them with glacé (candied) cherry nipples? Then just try serving them without a sly smile.

sexy cocktails

Why not dress up for cocktail hour? One of you can be the bartender, and the other the Hollywood starlet. Each of these recipes will make one cocktail.

- **slippery nipple** – Stir 1 measure Bailey's Irish Cream with ice. Strain into a cocktail glass and float 1 tsp Sambuca on top.
- **sex on the beach** – Pour 2 measures vodka, 1 measure peach brandy, 2 measures cranberry juice and 1 measure mixed orange and pineapple juice into a cocktail shaker over ice. Shake vigorously, then strain into a tall glass and decorate with a slice of orange.
- **slow comfortable screw up against the wall** – Fill a highball glass with ice cubes, then pour in 2 measures sloe gin and top up with fresh orange juice. Float 1 tsp Galliano on top.
- **bosom caresser** – Dash a little Cointreau over ice in a jug, pour in 1 measure brandy and 1 measure Madeira. Stir and strain into a glass.

ABOVE | Provocative, if not subtle: create your own range of suggestive snacks and find imaginative ways of serving and eating them.

BELOW | Why not try a slow comfortable screw up against the wall – then you'll really need a drink.

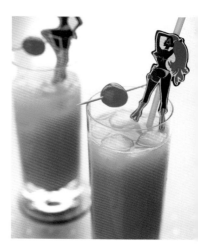

aphrodisiacs

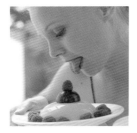

ABOVE | Food can be about more than nutrition.

RIGHT | Any Italian will tell you that spaghetti is one of the sexiest foods around, even if one of the messiest.

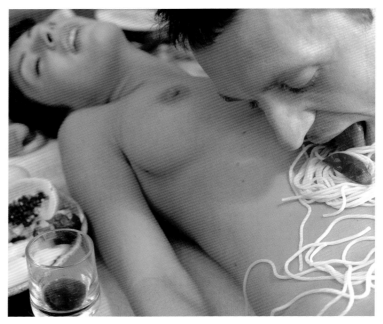

SINCE TIME IMMEMORIAL, men and women have been obsessive in their search for the ultimate aphrodisiac to help flagging libidos, improve their sexual performance and generally enhance the act of lovemaking.

Ayurvedic medicine, which originated in ancient India, so valued the importance of sex that a whole branch of medicine was dedicated to it called "Vajikarana", and there is a wide spectrum of preparations in use around the world that use animals and insects to enhance sexual performance. The Romans ate the penises, wombs and testes of animals such as monkeys, pigs, cockerels and goats, and lizards used to be pulverized and the powder taken with sweet white wine by the Arabs and southern Europeans. The Chinese today often use the genitals of animals and insects to increase the strength of reproductive organs, believing that ingesting

substances with sexual properties will impart those properties to the person consuming them. Snake blood is still consumed in east Asian countries and the gallstones of animals are used in Asian countries alongside ginseng and royal jelly.

chocoholic

Of course, it's debatable whether any aphrodisiacs actually work – there's certainly very little scientific evidence – but most people would draw the line at powdered reptiles and foul-tasting herbs. Fortunately, there is an extensive range of far more palatable options.

On the Richter scale of aphrodisiacs, chocolate is up there among the top three, alongside champagne and oysters. People are passionate about it. The Aztecs brewed cocoa like coffee, and Aztec leader Montezuma is alleged to have drunk up to 50 cups a day so that he could keep going with his harem of 600 women. It may have gained its reputation because the Aztecs believed the cacao pod was a symbol of the human heart. The notorious Marquis de Sade is said to have demanded chocolate cake while imprisoned. Chocolate lovers will gladly eat it before, during and after sex and some even choose it instead of sex. But what is it about chocolate that is so special? It's questionable that it can really affect sexual performance, but it does possess certain stimulating properties. As you swallow it, a chemical called phenylethylamine and the feel-good neurotransmitter serotonin are released in your brain, spreading a feeling of tranquillity. Then, the theobromine in chocolate kicks in to create the high feeling that you have when you are in love. Chocolate also contains other stimulants, such as caffeine, which excite the central nervous system, but all these properties exist in such tiny amounts that you would have to consume vast quantities for it to have any real sexual effect. What is certain is that chocolate contains sugar, which provides energy, and that, combined with its pleasurable texture and flavour, may explain why so many people find it so addictive. For many women, the fact that it is a "forbidden food" is also exciting.

foods for sex

Champagne, of course, like any alcoholic drink, reduces inhibitions, but too much will cause a downturn in your sex life. Oysters, on the other hand, have a long-standing reputation for stimulating the libido. This is undoubtedly much to do with their appearance and texture, but, interestingly, they are extremely rich in zinc, "the sex mineral" essential for the production of healthy sperm and fertility. Scallops also contain high levels of zinc and have a reputation for increasing the sex drive in women. In fact, aphrodisiac qualities have been ascribed to seafood of various sorts, including lobsters and caviar, while Chinese medicine recommends mussels and shrimps for increasing the libido.

Many foods, such as asparagus, morel mushrooms, figs and avocados, have been thought to possess such properties simply as a result of their appearance. Others, such as salmon and pigeon, seem to have been designated as aphrodisiacs because of the living creature's courtship rituals. The reasons for the reputation of still further foods are even more mysterious. The Romans swore by bread, which may have been because eating a lot of it tends to make you want to lie down. However, eating a lot of it also promotes flatulence, which is distinctly unsexy. When tomatoes were first imported into Europe, the French called them love apples for their heart-like shape. Nevertheless, tomatoes are high in lycopene, which is essential for prostate health. The Chinese recommend ginger and this too has a grain of validity in that it promotes healthy circulation, especially to the genitals.

So do aphrodisiacs really work? It seems unlikely, but their placebo effect can work wonders and, as we all know, the most powerful aphrodisiac that exists is the imagination.

BELOW | In different cultures and throughout history, a range of foods have been thought to raise the libido. Certainly some foods have an erotic sensuousness and sharing them with your lover can be very arousing.

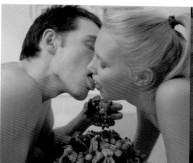
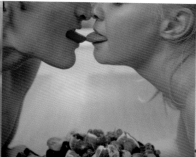
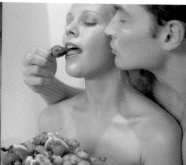

foodplay

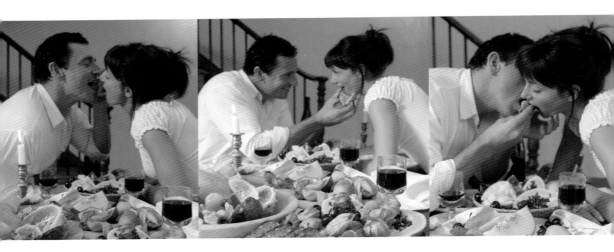

ABOVE | Choose the tastiest morsels and most succulent treats and feed them to your partner with your fingers or your lips.

OPPOSITE | A truly seductive meal can easily turn out to be more than metaphorical foreplay and you may not be able to wait to clear the table.

WHEN PLANNING A PASSIONATE evening with your partner, think of your meal as part of the foreplay to your lovemaking. Never underestimate the importance of food and wine in the enjoyment of a romantic evening. Teasing each other across a candlelit table can be so tantalizing. The cardinal rules for eating before sex are never to eat too much and never to select food that is too heavy. No one wants to make love on a full stomach – their own or someone else's.

Sharing your food and feeding each other is a potent form of foreplay. Having a romantic meal in the privacy of your own home is a wonderful opportunity for you to be outrageous flirts and to act out your seductive desires. You both know what's coming, but so much of the enjoyment is in the getting there.

Set the scene beforehand. Make the table look enticing with a lovely cloth, some flowers and candles, but don't use your best china as it may get swept to the floor in the heat of the moment.

Because no one else is there, you can act out your romantic fantasies and pull out all the seductive stops. Remember all those scenes in movies which you have always wanted to try out?

Well, now here's your chance. Think Jennifer Beals in *Flashdance* or Mickey Rourke and Kim Basinger in *9½ Weeks*, rather than Meg Ryan in *When Harry Met Sally*. It's also a perfect opportunity to tell each other things that you don't necessarily say over the breakfast cereal. In this romantic setting you remind one another just how much you still desire each other. Don't forget the music. It should be romantic, sexy and not too loud, something that is meaningful to both of you.

gourmet sex

The whole process of eating can be incorporated into the art of seduction. Start your sensuous feast with pre-dinner drinks and little canapés as light as butterfly kisses. Next, the appetizer should be a tantalizing treat, promising much more and seducing you with its textures and flavours. The main course is the climax of the meal, satisfying but not satiating your appetite, while dessert is a pause for refreshment.

Playing with the stem of your glass, running your fingertips around the rim and stroking the stem has its own connotations. Locking eyes with your lover over your glass of wine, caressing his or her hand across the table, making soft moans and sighs of pleasure as you enjoy an asparagus tip dripping with butter, even the way you butter your roll, can all create a tremendous sexual tension between the two of you. As the meal progresses and the wine diminishes, you can become bolder, eating off each other's plates or kissing the traces of food from each other's lips. End this wonderful meal by feeding each other delicious morsels of fresh fruit, passing them from mouth to mouth and allowing the juices to flow. Lots of action can take place under the table as well as on top. Kick off your shoes and caress each other's feet and legs.

finger foods

There is always something especially sexy about eating with your fingers, perhaps because we were always told not to do it when we were children. The only places where it is acceptable are fast food outlets, which must be among the least seductive locations on the planet.

If you're not in the mood for a three-course meal, then prepare a mini-banquet of succulent snacks that you can eat with your fingers – or better still, feed each other with your fingers. In fact, why not keep a ready supply of enticing nibbles in the refrigerator for just such occasions?

Include your partner's favourite rude food as well as your own. For the purposes of erotic eating, you can interpret the words "finger food" very loosely. Fruit is a perfect choice. Try wedges of watermelon or slices of mango and then lick the juices that have run over your partner's hands or chin. Bite into a strawberry or lychee and then offer your mouth to your partner.

weekend break

At the other end of the day, treating yourselves to a leisurely breakfast in bed at the weekend is a deliciously indulgent experience. It needs a little advanced planning, otherwise by the time it is ready, the mood will have been lost. The night before, prepare a tray with cups, saucers and plates, knives, spoons, marmalade or jam and, perhaps, a single flower in a small vase. Set the coffee maker ready to switch on and make sure that you have some croissants or rolls to pop into the oven in the morning. Avoid bowls of cereal, both messy and unromantic, and toast, which produces uncomfortable crumbs.

Don't take the newspapers back to bed with you and forget morning television, although some quiet background music could be atmospheric. That way, when you have finished eating, you'll have to think of something else to do.

fruity

Of all the food groups, it is fruit that is most closely associated with sensual pleasure. Grapes, the fleshy fruit, are associated with the ancient gods Dionysus, Priapus and Bacchus, the true connoisseurs of sex and pleasure. Across North Africa and the Middle East, dates are believed to increase erotic potency in men and desire in women. Coconuts are believed in India to increase the quality and quantity of semen. Strawberries and raspberries invite you to feed your lover, piece by piece. But it is fleshy fruits such as papaya, mango, peaches and apricots which spill over into true, and outrageously sticky, sensuality.

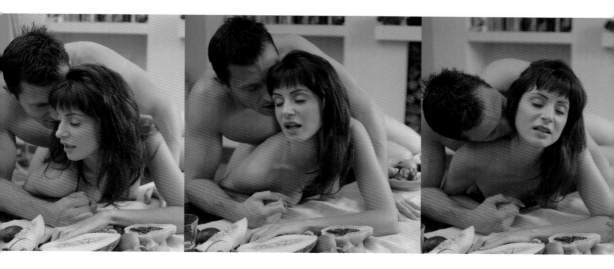

cooking with your lover

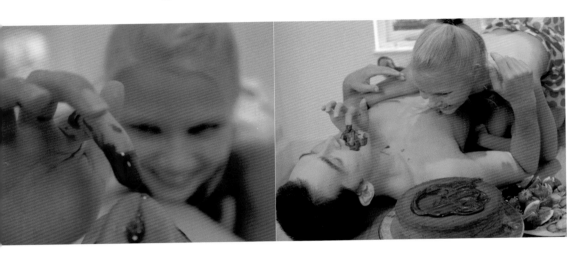

ABOVE | Nothing quite comes close to the taste and texture of molten chocolate.

ABOVE RIGHT | Making a cake to share with your partner can be just as much fun as eating it afterwards.

BELOW | Once the main course is cooking in the oven and the dessert is prepared, it's time to turn up the heat.

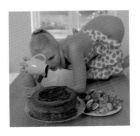

COOKING TOGETHER can bring an extra romantic dimension and sense of intimacy to the whole process of eating. Lots of people don't really enjoy the nitty gritty of food preparation, but when it's done together, you can make it much more fun. Put on some music, open a bottle of wine and get your ingredients together.

Choosing the ingredients that suit your mood at the time adds to the joy of sharing the cooking experience. It's fun to shop together, especially at an outdoor market, where you can handle the produce and ponder over which particular item you think is best. You can linger over plump, bright red tomatoes and let yourselves be seduced by the smell of ripe cantaloupe melons or fresh juicy mangoes.

If you are adventurous, it's a great turn-on to try to cook something totally different. Leave plenty of time for the preparation and have an adventure in the kitchen while you are chopping, slicing and stirring.

This is a wonderful opportunity for some serious love play as well, as you add a pinch of seduction to the list of ingredients. While the chocolate cake is rising in the oven you could be stripping down to your sexy underwear or negligee. For the truly adventurous, why not strip off totally and cook wearing nothing more than an apron? Take Isabel Allende's advice in her book *Aphrodite*: "Everything cooked for a lover is sensual, but it is even more so if both take part in the preparation and seize the opportunity to naughtily shed a garment or two as the onions are peeled or leaves stripped from the artichokes."

man about the house

Recent research has revealed that women are turned on by men who cook and you have only to think of the devoted female following of the many male celebrity chefs on television to see a clear manifestation of this. Women undoubtedly have a more emotional attitude towards food than men, so when a man is wielding a whisk or chopping a chilli, he is not just entering traditional female physical territory, but also her psychological home ground, which can be very alluring.

Another study by the Smell and Taste Treatment and Research Center in Chicago may provide an additional incentive to any men reluctant to enter the kitchen until the meal is on the table. The aroma of different foods as they cook has, apparently, a profound effect on the libido and, in particular, the smell of meat cooking significantly increases the flow of blood to the penis. This fact could make basting the Sunday roast a whole lot more fun.

feasting the senses

Cooking shouldn't be a chore, but it can often seem to be, particularly when it's a routine responsibility. Cooking with your partner can change this, especially if you tackle the task with a new attitude, actively relishing the textures, colours, smells and flavours of your ingredients. Preparing food can be as sensuous as eating it, especially when you are sharing the experience. Try out some new recipes, adding your own special touches, inhaling the aromas and tasting as you go. Does the chocolate mousse need more

orange juice? Dip in your finger and hold it out for your partner to decide. By the time they've finished licking it clean, they will probably have forgotten the question. Waft a spoonful of your newly created sauce beneath their nose, but tantalizingly deny them a taste until they have guessed at least three of the spices that flavour it.

Enjoy sharing the sensations of cooking and encourage each other to be daring in the kitchen. If you've never attempted to toss a pancake, try it and see who can catch it. Ice a cake together – literally, if you like, squeezing your partner's hands and the icing bag at the same time. Messy, but fun. Get out the food colouring and see who can create the most outrageous masterpiece with the mashed potatoes. Food is one of our most basic needs, and we all know how important it is to have a balanced diet, but you can still have a lot of fun together while you are preparing it.

BELOW | Experimenting together and tasting the fruits of each other's labours makes cooking together fun.

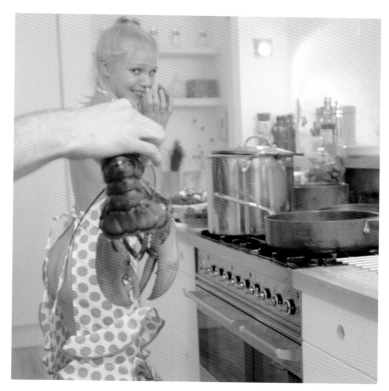

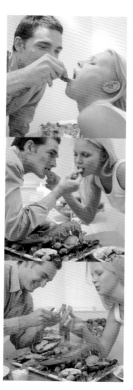

food without plates

THE MOST EROTIC WAY to share food with a lover is when you are both totally naked, so that you can eat from each other's bodies. It's a mutual experience. Where one enjoys the sensation of having food eaten from their body, the other enjoys the application and the subsequent pleasure of eating off their lover's body without using their hands.

What food you use is a question of personal taste. Many people enjoy the cool, silky sensation of cream or yogurt being drizzled over their body before being slowly licked off. Honey is another favourite, especially when massaged into the breasts before being nuzzled off. Smooth peanut butter can be warmed and smoothed over the penis (avoiding the urethral opening). Take your time slowly to suck it and lick it off. If you have a sweet tooth, you may prefer to use vanilla ice cream or strawberry jam. (These might prompt a much more dramatic response, as neurological research has shown that the smells of these two substances increase penile blood flow by anything up to 40 per cent.) Be creative when laying the food across the skin. Use a mixture of flavours, textures, aromas, tastes and temperatures. Cover your lover's naked body with slices of your favourite fruit or vegetables or make patterns with melted chocolate and eat them off.

If you really want to go for it and have a full body banquet, one of you can be the main course and the other the dessert. Don't eat very much the day before, make sure you have everything within easy reach and leave yourselves plenty of time. In between courses, you can have a long leisurely bath together, to be relaxed and receptive for the next course. Be especially mindful when you come to the more sensitive, delicate regions of the body such as the eyes, the vagina and the penis. Avoid any acidic, astringent irritants, such as vinegar, pickles or lemon juice, and particularly never use any form of chilli where it may sting.

BELOW | Asparagus is an age-old sexual remedy for men and there is nutritional evidence that it can assist in regulating hormonal balance. Mushrooms are a good source of the vitamin B complex, while truffles smell fantastic.

BELOW RIGHT AND OPPOSITE | Turn your partner into a banqueting table and feast off their bare body before offering your own for dessert.

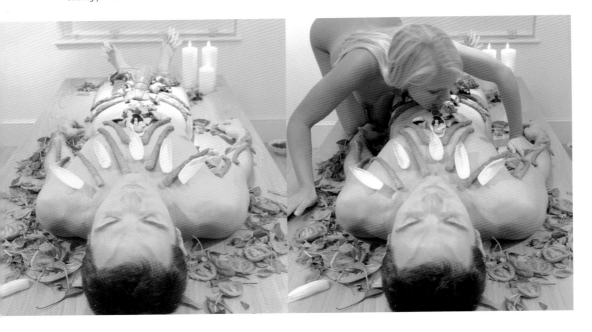

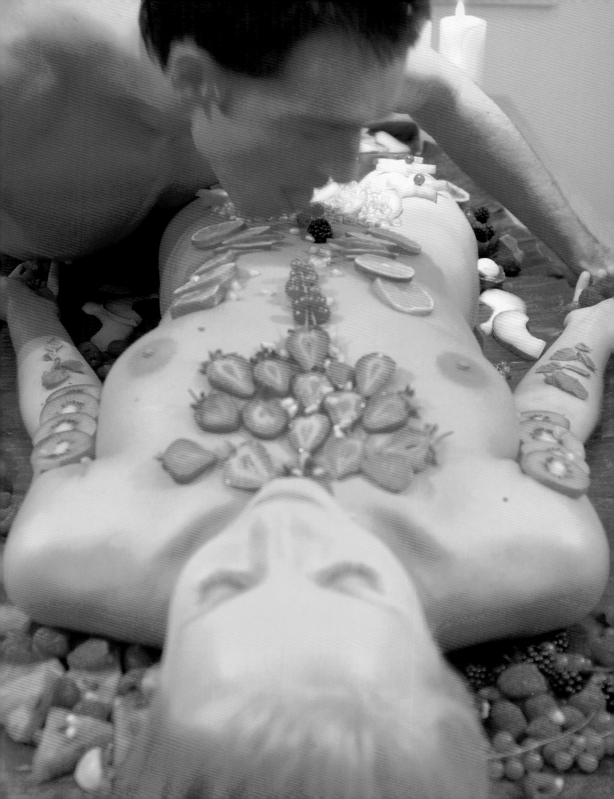

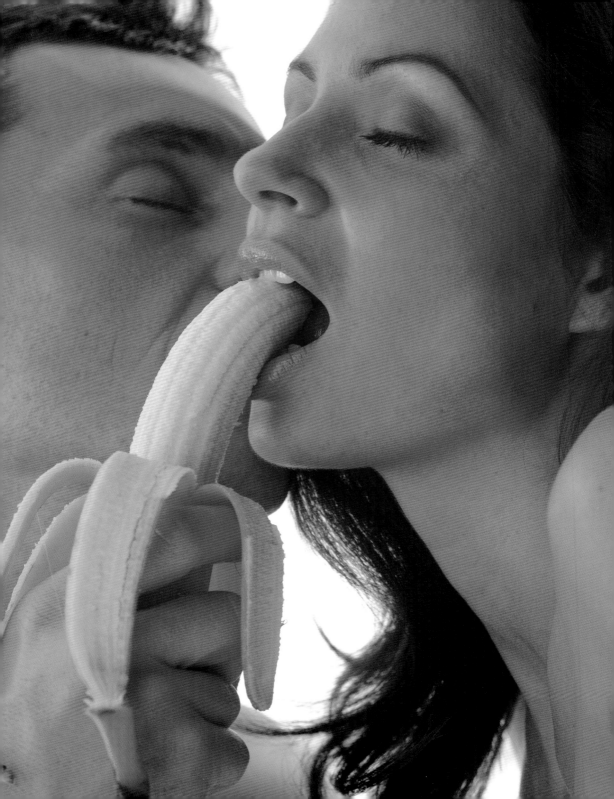

good food, good sex

FOOD ISN'T JUST FOR FUN AND SEX – it helps your body to stay on top of things. Eating well is essential to good sexual health and function. There are many, many reasons for loss of libido and impaired sexual function, but often one of the primary reasons is the balance of our sex hormones. However, this balance is also linked to our metabolic hormones, and these rely on a constant supply of certain nutrients that we provide through our diet.

minerals

Important dietary minerals include iron, zinc, magnesium, calcium, iodine, selenium, chromium, arginine, co-enzyme Q10 and essential fatty acids (EFAs). There are many food sources that are rich in these minerals. For example, chicken and red meat are rich in iron, which is needed for haemoglobin production in blood, essential for arousal, erection and lubrication. Nuts, brown rice, eggs and cheese all contain zinc, from which the sperm's tail is formed, so helping with fertility and sexual performance. Shellfish, dried fruit and dairy produce all contain calcium, crucial for bone growth and cardiovascular health and an essential ingredient for arousal, as it plays a part in sending messages to the nerves, enabling the sensation of touch. It is also needed for the contractions of muscle during male and female orgasm.

vitamins

In helping to maintain physical and sexual health, vitamins such as vitamin A, vitamin B complex (including B_1, B_2, B_3, B_5, B_6, B_{12} and choline), vitamin C and vitamin E all have their own roles.

Spinach, watercress, dairy produce and oily fish all contain vitamin A, which is vital for healthy eyes and strong bones and teeth. It is also an antioxidant required for cardiovascular health. Pulses, nuts, avocados and meat contain vitamin B complex such as B_3, which helps the circulation, allowing more blood to specific areas, such as the penis during erection; B_6, which plays an important role in regulating sex hormone function such as testosterone in men; and choline, which helps with transmission of nerve impulses necessary for boosting libido and energy during sex. Vitamin C helps to boost sex drive and strengthen male and female sex organs and can be found in food such as potatoes, ginger, beetroot (beet), citrus fruit and sprouted beans. Vitamin E is essential for healthy skin and its protective nature makes it vital for sexual health and vitality. It can be found in avocados, spinach, wheatgerm and all leafy green vegetables.

A good basic principle is to always have a balanced diet and to eat small portions regularly. Sex on a very full stomach is never a good idea.

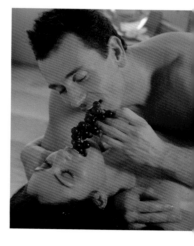

ABOVE AND OPPOSITE | it's the way that you eat it that counts.

BELOW | There are certain elements which are crucial to keep body and soul together, and without which a healthy sex life would be impossible. Nutritionally speaking, fruit and seafood are some of the richest foods.

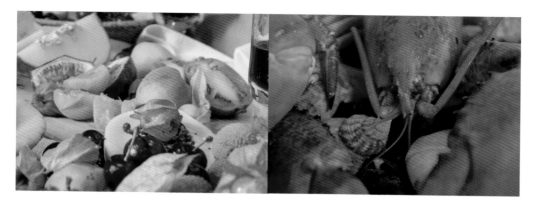

seasons

A long-term relationship is constantly subject to change, with ebbs and flows, ups and downs. As you journey through your lives together your relationship changes and matures, as do the seasons of the year, from the exciting, carefree years of early spring to the more laid back and contented golden winter years. Your sexual needs and desires follow these ebbs and flows, but are the essence of what keeps your relationship youthful and timeless.

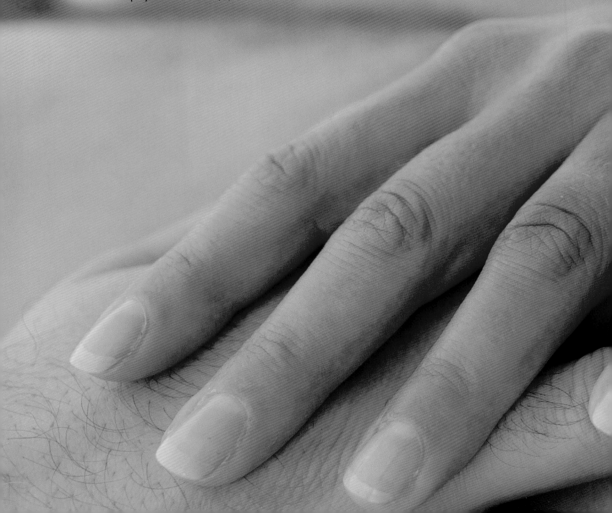

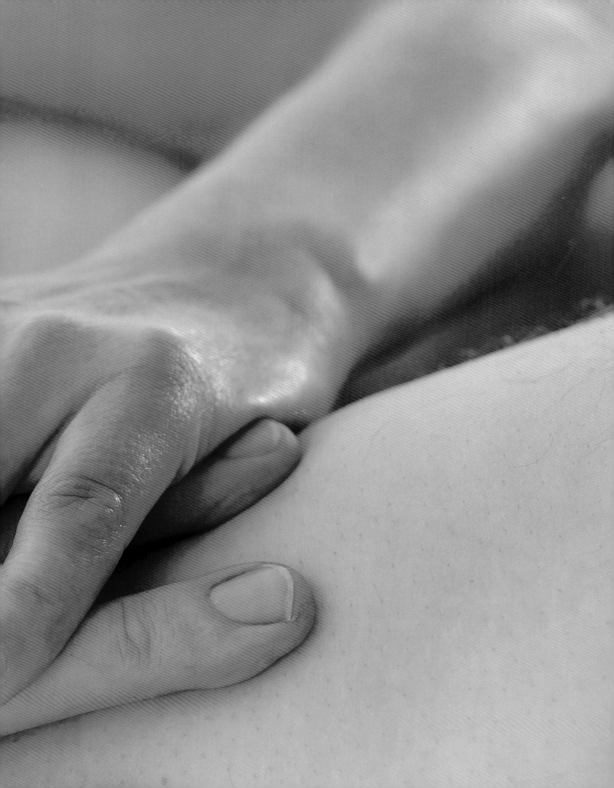

long-term lovers

A RELATIONSHIP CAN BE LIKENED TO THE SEASONS of the year, with spring, summer, autumn and winter each bringing with them their own qualities and climatic changes. Even the strongest relationships tend to be cyclical, with ups and downs, good times and bad. This is worth remembering as you go through your journey together, so that when there are stormy bad times, you can weather them by looking forward to better, sunnier times to come.

spring

The season of spring is the beginning of your relationship with your partner, the first few years when you meet, fall in love, before you decide whether to marry or cohabit. This is often the most carefree time, in which you spend a lot of time getting to know one another and allowing your roots to entwine, building the foundations on which you will grow as a team. With little to tie you, this is often a romantic season in which you feel truly secure in the knowledge that you will cope with anything life throws at you, because you have each other.

Springtime sex lives are exciting and adventurous. You can rarely take your hands off one another and use every spare moment together in making love and being romantic. If things become tougher in the future, it will be this era that you will refer back to. You will be able to

RIGHT AND BELOW | In the springtime of your relationship, you are endlessly fascinated with your lover and want to be with them all the time.

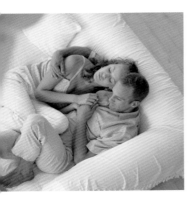

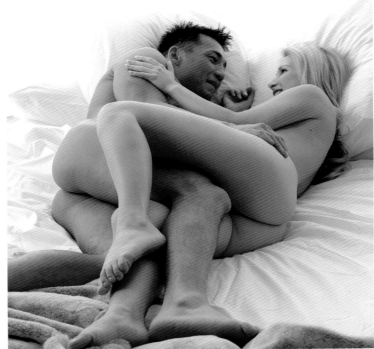

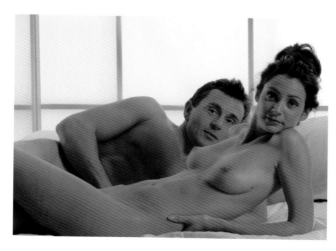
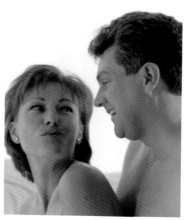

remind each other of how much love you have shared – you are building a scrapbook of memories that you can call on in the future.

summer

The summer of a relationship signifies a settling down period in which you begin to build a nest, find a home together, plan your futures and realize your dreams. Deciding on children will cause you both to re-evaluate your priorities over careers, social lives and sex lives. Sex changes during this season, as the emphasis is upon making love and creating another human being together, rather than having sex just for fun. Having a baby together is one of the most powerful and bonding things any two people can do. With a bit of time both of you will adjust to the changes and enjoy your new roles as mum and dad, providing you don't ignore the fact that you are also still lovers with sexual needs and desires.

autumn

Autumn is represented as the time when the kids fly the nest and lovers return to being just two again. This can be a difficult time for parents who have devoted the last couple of decades to their children. It is difficult to remember what life was like before the children came on the scene, and so it is important that a couple discuss the issues well

in advance. This is a time to plan your future together once again, to start talking about retirement and to make plans to finally fulfil your long-term dreams. Sexually this is a time of rediscovery, confirming each other's sexuality and using the stability and confidence in yourself and each other that you have built over the years to create better sex.

winter

The onset of winter signifies the beginning of another distinct, golden season as you share your retirement and, for many, grandchildren. You can enjoy each other's company with all the stresses and strains of work and dependent children finally put behind you. Most people do not associate senior citizens with sexuality, but in many cases this is an important and precious aspect of a long-standing relationship. You may no longer be swinging from the chandeliers but sex and touch are still important. Although there may be more health challenges to face as you age and libidos may not be what they once were, romance and seduction never age. By continuing to regard each other and your relationship as challenging and fun, you can maintain excitement and indulge each other with the frivolity that the freedom of old age can bring, working together to make your relationship both timeless and ageless.

ABOVE LEFT AND ABOVE | In the summer and autumn of your relationship you can face anything if you keep communicating.

BELOW | The romance doesn't have to fade with the years.

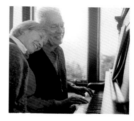

starting a family

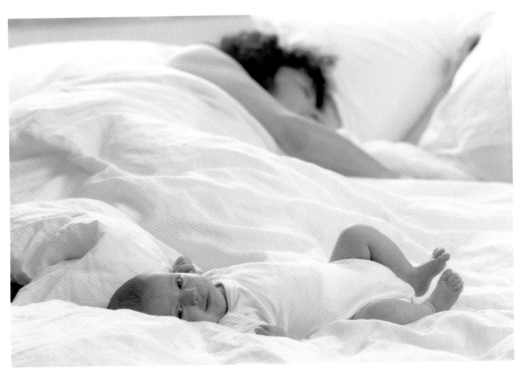

ABOVE | For many couples a long-term relationship is a welcome reprieve from the singles circuit. However, once you decide to start a family, your bed will never be your own again.

FOR MOST COUPLES, the first few years of marriage or cohabitation are an exciting time. You have finally escaped the dating scene and are confident and content that you have discovered the person who makes you happy. This can be a unique time for many relationships where you can concentrate on each other's sexual needs without any other forms of distraction, such as children or responsibility for elderly parents. The next stage for many couples is starting a family. This said, the introduction of a third set of feet in your home brings with it a total rearrangement of your priorities, your social life and, yes, your sex life.

Sex is often the last thing on the minds of new parents, until their baby settles into a routine of sleeping through the night. There are numerous emotional problems that are common to almost every couple during this time. New mothers can become both physically and emotionally exhausted. Many feel their role as a sexual woman has been totally replaced by that of a child-bearer who is constantly cleaning, feeding, bathing and nurturing her new baby, with no time for nurturing herself. Men may feel neglected or even left out of this new regime. These are all very common issues that new parents face as their lives go through one of the biggest transitions. It's important to remember that these changes are occurring to you as a couple and not as individuals and you need to talk about it together.

During your child's early years they will require a lot of your time and attention and it is all too

sex during pregnancy and after the birth

With a normal, healthy pregnancy, there is absolutely no reason why you should not continue to have a normal, healthy sex life, unless advised otherwise by your doctor. You cannot hurt the baby, who is comfortably cushioned in the amniotic fluid. As the pregnancy progresses, man-on-top positions are likely to become uncomfortable, even impossible. Experiment with positions that suit the two of you. "Spoons" is often a favourite and some women favour rear entry positions. It is a myth that lovemaking will bring on a premature labour, although there is some evidence that substances present in semen may encourage labour at full-term.

For reasons of health, women are usually advised not to have penetrative sex for six weeks after giving birth. If an episiotomy scar hurts or the birth itself was very painful, a woman may be afraid that lovemaking will also hurt. Adapting the Extended Sexual Orgasm technique, combined with gentleness and patience, will probably overcome this. If she is breastfeeding, sore or cracked nipples may mean this is definitely not an erogenous zone. This is a difficult time for men as well, who may be tired after waking with the baby in the night if you are taking turns. This is a major life adjustment for both of you – sharing the burden together will unite you.

easy to put your sex life to one side, or neglect the need for time out to be a couple. Try to set aside some time once a week to make a date with each other. Get a babysitter or ask grandparents to take the kids once a week. Use this time to get out of the house and spend some romantic time together discussing issues that have been on your mind, but try to avoid constantly discussing your children. This is a perfect opportunity to talk freely about sex and how you can both work to improve things. If the kids can stay away overnight from time to time it's even better, as you can enjoy each other in a more uninhibited manner.

families today

There are many different relationships and family structures nowadays that work equally as well as the stereotypical married couple. Many couples prefer to remain unmarried, even though they have a family together, and some couples even choose to live apart as they can be a happier unit when they are together by keeping their own space. More same-sex couples are setting up home together and choosing to adopt children or find surrogate mothers or fathers or sperm donors, to help them have their own.

Relationships can be complicated whichever sexual path you follow. Not all couples who get together stay together for the rest of their lives. Often people separate or divorce and begin a life

with a new person. Starting again with someone new, when either you or your partner already have kids from a past relationship, can be tricky as you have to integrate yourself or your partner into a ready-made family. Children are understandably fiercely loyal to both their parents and so often a new partner on the scene can cause problems.

Children of blended families (couples who both have children) and stepchildren will invariably need plenty of reassurance and understanding when a new relationship begins. Any stresses and strains in a relationship will affect its sex life. Ultimately, given time, much joy and happiness can be found in these kinds of relationships.

One of the most important roles of a parent is to make sure that your children become confident and unafraid of sex and their developing sexuality. This can be harder than it seems and much of their attitude towards it will stem from how you react to their questions.

It is very common for children to walk in while you are making love, and you need to prepare for it before it happens or else you may react in a way that you will regret. Try just covering up slowly, without making it appear like you were doing something that you shouldn't. Often children think that sex looks like "daddy was hurting mummy" and so it is important to emphasize that what you were doing was positive, and something that two people do when they love each other.

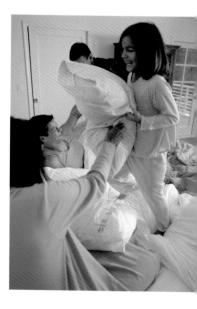

ABOVE | Family life can often be a battle – but making time for a healthy sex life will help maintain the balance in the equation.

middle years

IF YOU HAVE CHILDREN, then sometime you will experience the "Empty Nest Syndrome". One or all of your babies will have flown away – to university, jobs or into marriage – and you are left alone in your house with your partner. This period in your life often creeps up on you and you don't realize the impact until it happens. What was a longed-for dream of more time together may turn out to be a period of incredible emotional emptiness until you get used to the absence of the children and to spending so much time together.

Once you get used to the idea, it can be a very exciting time. If your sex life has been on the back burner for some years, now is the time to get to know each other again and become sexually reacquainted. You have more time and tend to be more relaxed and positive about having sex.

Another aspect of having more leisure time is that there will be more time to exercise. Whilst physically you will be slowing down, this is a great opportunity to take control and become fitter – start going to those yoga classes! This is crucial because as we age, we need to remain active, not only for our health but also for a good sex life.

time of life

It is the period when women may be going through the menopause, the end of their reproductive life. This causes emotional and physical challenges, so talk to your partner about how it makes you feel so he understands the process. Many women find that taking HRT (hormone replacement therapy) can help them through this period of change – lessening the hot

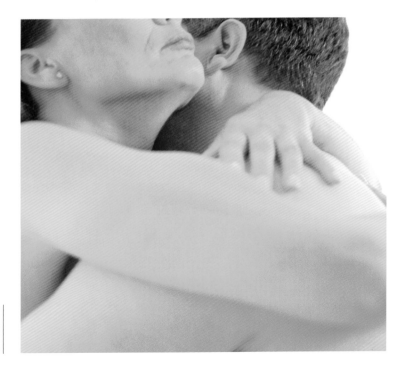

RIGHT AND OPPOSITE | Once the kids have flown the nest, you will have more time to spend alone with each other.

flushes, mood swings and forgetfulness. Sexual desire or libido varies greatly in every woman whether pre- or post-menopausal. Hormone levels determine sex drive and diminished hormone levels undoubtedly interfere with sexual desire. Although oestrogen plays a part, the hormone that has been shown to be most closely associated with sex drive is testosterone. The ovary, although capable of producing oestrogen after a "natural" menopause, may continue to produce significant amounts of testosterone for several years. This is the reason why many women maintain a good sex drive for a considerable length of time. These testosterone levels provide additional benefits to the naturally menopausal woman. Tissues of the body are able to convert some of this circulating testosterone to oestrogen.

When women undergo a hysterectomy where the ovaries are also removed, this benefit may be lost. Some women even find that their sexual desire increases after menopause (if their ovaries are left) as they are free from pain and excessive bleeding.

mid-life crisis

Men also may well be experiencing a slow-down in their sexual response time, taking longer to become aroused as they approach middle age. In fact, both men and women may need more stimulation to become aroused and to orgasm. But, since you will hopefully be able to spend more time together, take advantage of this. Talk to each other about what pleases you. If you have difficulty communicating, or are not able to take that step forward together, then you may well need to speak to a therapist.

It is at this stage that men may have a "mid-life crisis". This can manifest itself in seeking reinforcement in a younger girlfriend or a new motorbike when he normally drives a family car. This is just a glance back at his youth and women often have similar feelings. Patience is required during this time, on the part of both of you. It can be frightening to let go of the younger part of you that you are accustomed to – however, you are exchanging it for the confidence and experience that can only come with age.

looking lively

It is important for both men and women to make an effort to look attractive for their partner and for their own self-respect. Perhaps you can get into the routine of spending an hour or so having a long bath and pampering yourself. Invest in some glamorous nightwear that makes you feel sensuous. Give yourselves the time to feel sexy as adults and not just parents or workers.

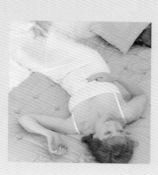

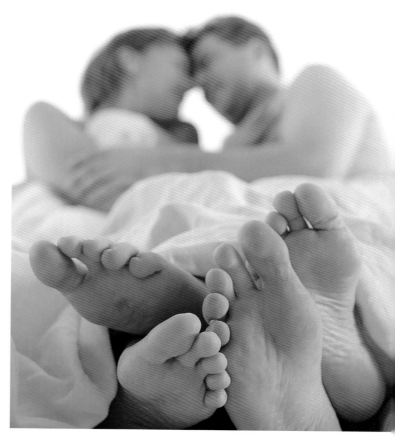

golden years

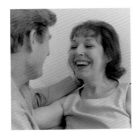

IT IS A MYTH THAT YOU STOP HAVING SEX when you are in your "golden years". Just because you are older, it does not mean that you don't need the same physical and emotional intimacy that you demanded when you were young. Intimacy is an important part of your life at any age.

An active sex life will keep you mentally fit and healthy, and having a good companion whom you can share your life with is said to be the key to living longer. The emphasis on the necessity of regular exercise promoted over the last couple of decades means that older people will be fitter

than ever. Having a positive attitude is crucial for a good sex life. Your body may be aging, but for many, your desires certainly aren't. If you are experiencing problems having erections on a long-term basis, you can ask your doctor for their advice. Older men may need some more stimulation in order to achieve erection – a little manual assistance is sometimes necessary. In these cases oral sex and mutual masturbation can be an enjoyable path to explore together. The time that you make love can be an important factor in later years as well. It is frequently recommended

ABOVE AND BELOW | Companionship has many mutual benefits.

RIGHT | Taking up a hobby, like dancing, with your partner can be one way to rekindle romance.

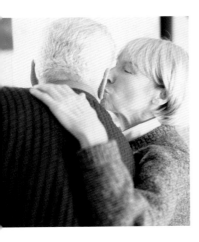

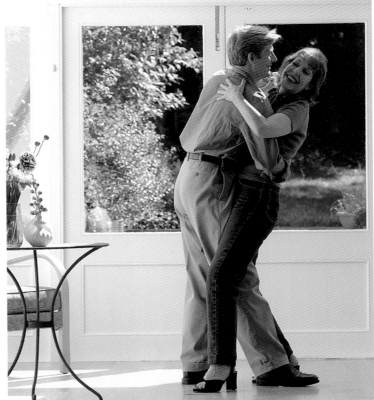

that older adults should try making love in the morning, as older men are more likely to have a firm erection in the morning after a good night's sleep. There are also unexpected advantages for men as you get older; you can delay ejaculation for longer, and your partner will love you for this.

freedom years

By their golden years, women have finished with the menopause and can experience a new sense of sexual liberation. There are some physiological changes of course such as vaginal lubrication, which instead of taking only 15 to 30 seconds when younger can now take up to five minutes. There are plenty of lubricants, and even hormonal treatments that can help. Women who continue to have sex after the menopause finishes will remain fitter and their vaginas will remain more elastic than those women who do not.

A woman's sex drive over the age of 65 is more stable than a man's. In fact a woman reaches her peak in her late twenties or thirties and remains on that plateau until her sixties. A woman of 80 has the same physical potential for orgasm as a woman of 20.

Even if sexual desire has abated, intimacy is still an important part of any loving relationship, regardless of age. Touching and cuddling up together and learning how to massage each other can be extremely sensual. Setting aside time to visit galleries together or to go for long walks – perhaps joining a dance class – can give you that extra contact outside the home that you need. To stay young you have to feel young, regardless of what your body is doing. Being active together, and remaining tactile with each other, will help to keep your relationship as fresh and exciting as in the early days when you had only just met each other.

going it alone

As women tend to live longer than men, the major problem is often having a partner to share their sexuality with. Many older people have to come to terms with the loss of their loved one and one of the important issues is how you deal with the loss of intimacy and sex that was part of a

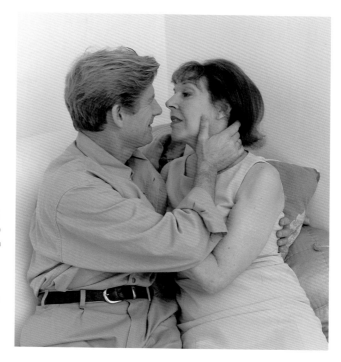

loving relationship. Sexual desire and drive do not die with your partner. Masturbation can be especially helpful in these circumstances and will help you to keep your sexual identity and sexuality alive.

You are never too old to fall in love, and on a happier note, many older people can find new love and companionship in their golden years. This can bring comfort to them, their new partners and their extended families alike.

Society's image of "old people" is that they are too sagging, wrinkly and unattractive to even think about having a sex life. It is up to all of us to resist subscribing to that kind of agism, not just mature people themselves, but also younger generations. As the baby-boomer generation comes of age, attitudes will surely have to change – there are going to be a lot of healthy pensioners out there.

We owe it to our children and those who come after us to claim our sexuality in old age. If we don't do it, how will they?

ABOVE | Mature couples have more time to themselves to rekindle the eroticism of their early relationship.

rediscovery

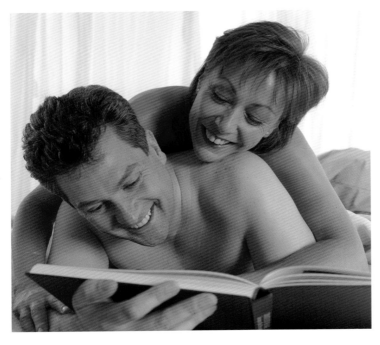

ABOVE | Life is tough and sometimes your sex life can suffer, becoming dull or non-existent. It is time to take action, read a book about sex together and share your laughter.

THERE INEVITABLY COMES A TIME in most couples' lives when the emphasis of their relationship is no longer on sex, and in fact has not been for quite some time. It is easy for this to happen to couples who have been together for a while and have devoted their partnership to their kids, careers, home-building and the multitude of other tasks, whatever their age. Standard patterns and routines somehow appear over the years, often without you realizing it. Sex may be dull, and many feel that they have worn out the possibility of having exciting, exhilarating sensual sex again.

It is never too late to reawaken each other's sensuality. Good sex is the magic ingredient to a great relationship. There is joy in store for some, perhaps discovering orgasm for the first time after a lifetime of frustration and disappointment. To get all your sexual fantasies fulfilled in the later stages

of a relationship can be heartening. The lesson is that it is never too late to start.

Rediscovering your own and your partner's sexuality is a journey through known territory that will invariably lead you to a new destination. Remember a particular place where you both felt passionate – revisit it. If there is a particular song that invokes special memories for you both, play it while you cuddle or massage each other. Perhaps there is one dish or type of wine that reminds you of a particularly memorable evening. Each of these may reawaken the spontaneity that you may have lost over the years, but the main focus should be on setting aside some time for you both to talk and appreciate each other's needs and wants.

The biggest erogenous zone is the brain, so this is a good place to start stimulating each other's sensuality. Talk to each other, avoiding selfless topics such as the children. Visit museums or cinemas together, share interesting extracts from a book, or create meals together in a new style.

practical steps

The following are some hints and tips that couples can incorporate into their relationship to help them to rediscover each other's sexuality, and their own. An understanding of trust and respect is paramount in all loving relationships, and as you age and mature together you need to develop an element of flexibility to allow for personal growth and development. This may involve taking practical steps to nurture, listen and act on one another's needs:

● Talk to your partner about making time for lovemaking and if you lead very busy lives, clear a space in the diary. Don't rush sexual activity and make time for the post-coital cuddles, too.

● You may well both be feeling horny at different times, so that will have to be negotiated. There's no prescribed perfect frequency of lovemaking – how often you do it, or how infrequently – it just has to work for both of you.

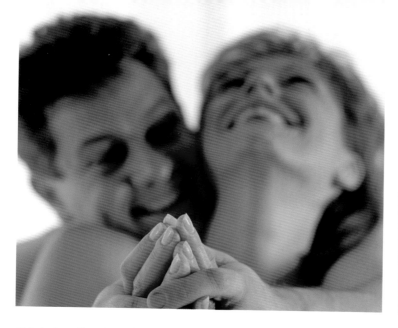

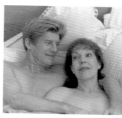

ABOVE | No matter how long you have been together, it is never too late to change things for the better.

LEFT | Trying something new together might end up just being a laugh, but then wasn't that part of the idea?

• Talk about sexual fantasies together and see whether it is possible to carry some of them out. If you find you are falling into a routine, take stock and try something different for a change. "How about trying this today?"

• Many people see sex as a way of making up after an argument, which can be very exciting, as well as an easy way of keeping emotionally close to their partner. But the potential for misunderstanding the real problem that caused the argument in the first place is enormous. Try to understand how you both function emotionally, talk about it and see how you can progress.

• Many people feel that they are not fully satisfying their lover and worry about it. Make yourself feel better by addressing some of the things that concern you and discuss your sexual performance with your partner, asking them how you can make sex better for them.

• Familiarity can breed contempt in a long-term relationship, so try to retain some of the mystery and your own personal privacy. For example, the bathroom can be a great place to shower and bath together but it should also be a private space sometimes. You need to be able to tell each other when you need some privacy and your own separate space and time.

• And lastly, be romantic and thoughtful towards each other. Kiss each other before you say goodbye and when you see each other again. Remember the thank yous and the small pleasantries. Buy each other small gifts or tokens – after all, it's the little things that matter.

keeping the bedroom hot

Here's how to maintain the spice:
• Use soft sexy music, dim lighting and candles or try covering the bed and floor with rose petals to create a more sensual space.
• Reorganize the bedroom every now and again to make a change in the surroundings – perhaps move the bed to a different position or bring in furniture from other rooms.
• Brighten up the room with flowers, or change some of the pictures in the photo frames. You could even buy a new print or painting to hang on the walls.
• Use sexy bed linen, perhaps silk sheets or a new bed-throw of fake fur.

• Experiment using different coloured light bulbs or change your net curtains for lightly-dyed sheer fabric: a change of light intensity or colour can completely alter the ambience of a room.
• If you have a television in the room, try taking it out for a while. A recent study showed that couples were having more sex in the 1950s than they are today, and one of the reasons was because of today's reliance on television for entertainment. By taking it out of the bedroom you will have to be creative and work on entertaining each other in different ways.

long-term tactics

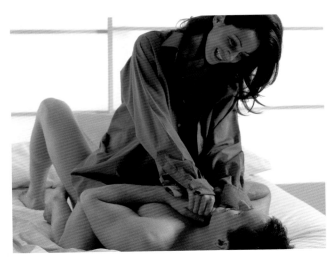

sex appeal

Rediscovering your sex appeal is about building your confidence. If you feel ashamed or embarrassed about your body then you will not be able to go full throttle during sex. If your body image is inhibiting your sex life then you have to take positive steps to do something about it.

Start doing more exercise; take time to dress up, wear sexy underwear. Go out together somewhere smart that requires you both to dress up a bit.

SOME OF THE MOST SUCCESSFUL long-term relationships cite humour and being best friends as the essential ingredients that make it work. Great friendship involves respectful behaviour towards each other, friendly gestures, lots of touching and cuddling and of course good sex. If you can have a great laugh together as well, all the better. A loving relationship should be a mutual appreciation society, to coin a phrase. Respect your differences and remember, you can't change the other person. Only they can change themselves.

Studies show that laughter is seriously good for your health. It lowers blood pressure, reduces stress and boosts your immune system. It also triggers the release of endorphins, chemicals that provide a natural painkiller for the body, and produce that "feel-good factor".

If we all looked at the physical mechanics of the way people make love, the mess they get themselves into, the funny faces they pull when having an orgasm, the fumbling, farting and funny noises that emanate from the bed, no one would ever be able to keep a straight face while having sex. Although sex is seriously fun, it has its ridiculous side. There's a good reason why we say that laughter is the best medicine and this applies equally to your sexual relationship.

buying gifts

Buying each other sexy gifts is another fantastic way of reawakening each other's sexuality. Everyone loves both receiving and giving gifts, especially if they are spontaneous. Men can buy their partner some sexy lingerie or underwear from specialist boutiques. It is important that he buys something that will suit her taste – if in doubt then ask the shop assistant, they are usually only too keen to help! It is important also to buy it in the right context. If he buys it because he secretly wants her to look more sexy, or feels that their sex life is boring and wants to spice it up, she will invariably pick up on this and may feel offended or hurt. A better approach is for him to gently discuss with her beforehand the possibility of spicing things up, saying things like: "I would really love to spend more time with you sexually, perhaps we can try some new things together." Then she will be more prepared for her new gift, and the likelihood is that it will be better received.

More adventurous gifts such as dildos, vibrators and other sex toys must also be handled with sensitivity. If a couple has got into a pattern of rather repetitive and mundane sex and then one springs a vibrator on the other, it may be a bit of a shock, regardless of the intentions. Again, it is important to establish through discussion that you both want to try something new – there's no room here for unilateral action.

sex talk

For some reason couples often find talking about sex together really difficult regardless of how long they have been together. One reason for this may be that although sex is something that you do together, often the experience is pretty personal. During orgasm, for example, individuals often disappear temporarily into their own intense world of pleasure, and even building up to orgasm requires an element of personal concentration.

Another reason couples may find it tricky to talk about sex is fear that they may upset or offend their partner by telling them what they like, and, more importantly, what they do not like. This is especially true for couples in long-term relationships who may have spent years doing it in a specific way that is not necessarily giving one or both of them enough satisfaction.

The important thing to remember is that when you love one another, the need to satisfy and please each other sexually is crucial. All you need to do is approach the subject sensitively, avoiding direct criticism. A good technique is to use the question and answer method. When you are in bed together, spend time trying to rediscover areas of sensuality on your partner's body by asking questions such as "May I touch you here?" or "Can I stroke you there?" The recipient should avoid responding with negative responses such as "No that feels awful." Try "That feels great, but if you do it this way it feels even better."

A tricky situation is when your partner is doing something to you that you really don't like, but are unsure how to deal with it without hurting them. Try focusing on the positive by saying things such as "I like it when you do that but I much prefer it when you do this", or "I love giving you a blow-job and I love the way you taste, but I find it uncomfortable when you thrust too deeply into my mouth, perhaps we could try a different position."

BELOW LEFT | Don't force anything on your partner you feel they won't like.

BELOW | Make a pact to buy each other something you would like them to try: "I have heard that using a vibrator during sex can be really fun, I'm quite keen to try this, what do you think about it?" Even if they are not keen, the door has been opened for a discussion on their sex life.

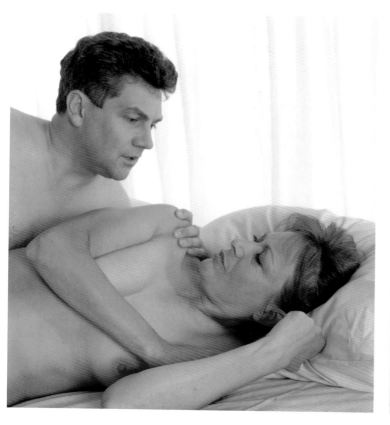

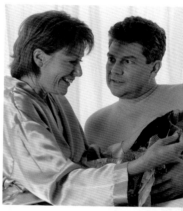

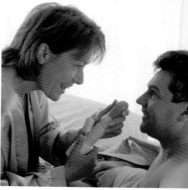

talking and listening

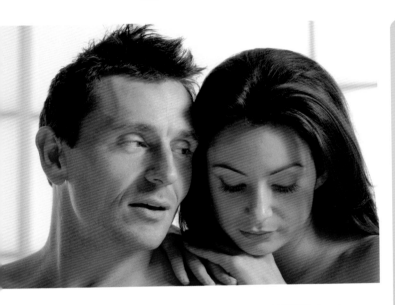

ABOVE | Making a connection with your partner is more than just a physical thing – talking and listening are crucial to keep a relationship strong and healthy. If you stop communicating, things can only get worse.

take turns to talk

Set aside some uninterrupted time to take turns to talk together. The talker should begin by discussing a neutral subject or a recent event, and say how it made them feel, what they found interesting and what they found boring. The listener must work hard to really listen to what is being said to them and avoid commenting or reacting until it is their turn.

Next time you try this, include five more minutes at the end for the listener to repeat back the basics of what the talker had been saying, showing that they have taken on board what has been said. With time the listener will become much more accurate as couples learn to listen more closely, which in turn will help to rebuild the foundations of trust and respect in their relationship.

ONE OF THE MAIN PROBLEMS that couples experiencing difficulty have in common is an inability to talk effectively. Communication is the key to getting what you want out of a relationship. If done with sufficient sensitivity, it can help you to air grievances with one another and to stop one partner doing something that the other feels is annoying, hurtful or aggravating. Communication is a learned skill and blocks often occur from situations that have happened in an individual's past. It is important that each couple works together to find out what their communication strengths and weaknesses are in order to understand what makes them react to each other in the way that they do.

learning to listen

Listening is paramount in successful communication. Often people who do not listen to their partners find themselves cutting in on them, or remaining silent. Inwardly they may be thinking about what they are going to say next, without actually paying attention to what their partner is saying. Listening is one of the most valuable skills that a therapist can teach. Often couples learn this by noting how their therapist listens to each of them when they speak, and the positive effect this has on them. Therapists can encourage individuals to listen more openly and not to feel defensive when their partner is speaking, thus reducing the need to attack. By listening, couples learn to give each other time for self-expression, taking away the bad feeling or resentment that is engendered when we believe we are not being heard.

Some of the listening techniques that counsellors may advise are as follows:
- Give your full attention to your partner when they are talking by focusing on their face and voice.
- If other thoughts intrude into your mind allow them to gradually fade as you gently swing your attention back round to what is being said to you.

- Once they have finished, don't jump in immediately, give yourself a couple of seconds to evaluate what has been said and ultimately make them feel like you are taking stock of what they have been saying to you.
- Listening is not all about being quiet and maintaining eye contact, it is also about encouraging your partner to speak and open up to you. The person listening should try to keep their body language as open as possible by turning towards their partner and not blocking them with gestures. They should keep their face turned towards them and look interested in what they are saying.
- Acknowledgement signals are very helpful, a nod or encouraging "yes" or "okay" all tell the partner that their words have been heard, and although you may not necessarily agree, you are accepting what they are saying. If they pause, use words that will encourage them to elaborate. Phrases such as "That incident must have made you very angry," or "You must have felt very upset when that happened to you," will help your partner to say more about their feelings and emotions.

talking to each other

Talking is also an important skill that therapists will help couples to learn. When a relationship is in its early stages, couples tend to talk a lot together to learn more about one another. As they continue, this talk becomes less and less since they already know each other and so don't feel the need to ask as much. Conversations can become short-lived and stagnant, discussing mundane issues such as "What do you want for breakfast?" as opposed to "How do you feel this morning?"

The worst thing a couple can do when they talk together is attack one another. Often when people feel passionate about something their choice of words is instantly on the offensive and confrontational, making them feel like they are getting their point across but leaving their partner feeling defensive.

The following are some common phrases and constructions that often trigger arguments, and some alternative ways of addressing the issue that may be less explosive.

blame "You ruined my evening when you told everyone that story." Instead of blaming your partner try to describe how you feel: "I felt uncomfortable and didn't enjoy myself this evening."

accusation "You made me feel furious when you forgot to pay the gas bill." Admit to your feelings by saying: "I feel..." instead of "you made me feel..."

nagging "I have asked you hundreds of times to do the dishes." Try a more constructive approach such as "Shall we do the dishes together?"

shouting Try not to raise your voice and point your finger to get your message across. Shouting will evoke an immediate defensive response. Instead, try using a softer tone and less harsh hand gestures.

BELOW | Sometimes we need to go back to school, and unlearn some bad habits.

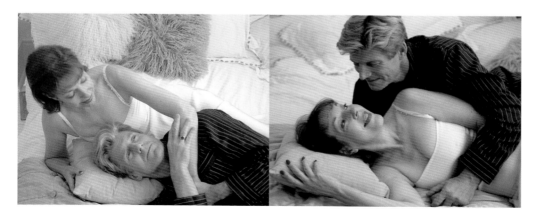

seeking help

COMMUNICATING WITH ONE ANOTHER is one of the most useful tools for ensuring success in a relationship. Sadly, successful communication is not as easy as many people may think. As a relationship progresses and other factors and influences take over such as work pressures and children, many couples find themselves communicating less and less often, unwittingly building barriers that eventually seem impossible to break down.

Therapy and counselling can be a huge benefit here. Many therapists say that a lot of couples come to them thinking that their relationship has already ended and that they have lost faith in their love and are trying therapy as a "last resort". The encouraging news is that all too often this is not the case. The use of sexual and relationship therapy has become increasingly popular as couples are less inclined to settle for an unsatisfactory love life and quite rightly seek to better their alliance on both an emotional and physical level.

The therapist will take time with the couple to re-evaluate the communication skills, find the root of the problem and help them to change their approach to each other so that their conversations become more positive and encouraging. Often communication problems stem from learned patterns picked up as children. A child whose parent was non-communicative or even abusive can carry the emotional effects of this over into their relationship in adult life, often without realizing it. This is a very common problem and once it has been identified, it can be worked through and with the help of the therapist, the couple can begin working on developing more effective methods of communication.

visiting a therapist

The majority of couples who visit a therapist do so because they believe that their relationship is in trouble. Often they are unsure of how bad things

BELOW AND RIGHT | Whatever you do or don't do in bed with your partner, it is crucial to keep the channels of communication open. Masters and Johnson, through their research, popularized the concept of sexual therapy and openly talking about sex.

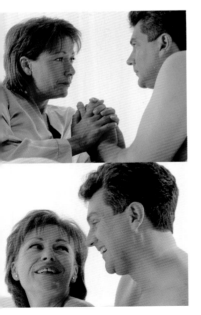

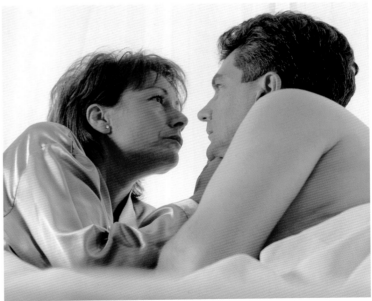

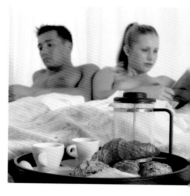

ABOVE | When you wake up with the same person every day, it is hard to maintain any mystery.

BELOW | Try to talk clearly using unthreatening gestures and positive language so you won't start an argument, and remember to listen as well.

are and need an external voice to help them to get back on track. People who no longer feel good about each other or rarely talk except to row have often built up barriers over time that they alone cannot break down.

Relationship support organizations have trained counsellors who will help couples to feel more positive about each other. Choosing and deciding to see a counsellor is often the first and hardest step for any couple experiencing difficulty, and it relies on a real desire from both parties to work together to sort out their problems. Often people are nervous, as they are unsure of what to expect from their first visit. The main purpose of the counsellor will be to provide a safe and supportive environment in which to help you rebuild your relationship. They aim to help you find the external point of reference that you need to see in order to re-evaluate your relationship.

The appointment with the therapist usually takes place in a private room where the couple can relax with the therapist and be guided to talk about their problems. A wide range of approaches and individual techniques are used, so that there is no fixed formula. They look at each individual's past to help provide meanings and answers for problems that may be occurring. They use their interactions and conversations with couples to help highlight or reflect on the roots of some of the problems and they also suggest some practical exercises that couples can try together to take a more active approach towards improving their relationship.

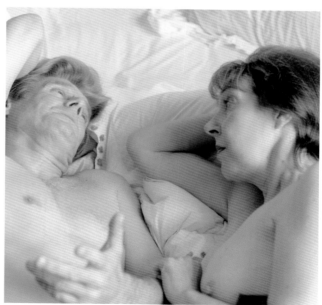

differently abled

BODY IMAGE is one the hardest things that most disabled people have to contend with, whether they have physical or learning difficulties. Other people's attitudes towards them and their own attitudes towards themselves can be a barrier in their social interactions. Other people constantly reinforce a negative attitude and most able-bodied people do not associate sexuality with the physically challenged. This perception has a knock-on effect and can inhibit a disabled person's ability to be sexual. Not only do people with disabilities have to fight the prejudices in society that do not recognize them as sexual beings, but they have to learn to accept themselves and become confident. They have exactly the same needs as able-bodied people.

effects of disability

Many disabled people have limited contact with the outside world, so it can be difficult to meet other members of their peer group. Shyness and a lack of confidence can add to the problem.

One of the most frequently asked questions about disability is whether men in wheelchairs get hard-ons. The answer to this is more often than not yes. Usually a man who has no feeling in the genital area will not be able to get erect from visual stimulation alone, although they can still feel aroused. Direct physical stimulation of the genitals is normally needed in order to get an erection, and here vacuum pumps, injections and implants can be of help.

Those with high-level spinal cord injuries often get reflex erections when their genitals are touched although these are usually not associated with arousal. These reflex reactions usually go down once the touching stops but couples can learn to use these reflex erections by keeping the stimulation going in order to have intercourse. Learning to read their body signals in order to know when they are feeling aroused is a valuable skill as an erection is not always a reliable sign. Other arousal signals are hardened nipples, goose

bumps, heavier breathing and an increased heart rate – much the same as able-bodied people.

Many men who are paralysed, especially those with more serious spinal cord injuries, experience problems ejaculating. Physicians can relatively successfully "milk the prostate" by placing electrodes into the rectum and shocking the nerves in the prostate, but this is somewhat invasive if not a bit dramatic. Some men with serious spinal cord injuries claim that they are able to ejaculate with the help of a vibrator on the penis.

Another common question people have is whether women in wheelchairs can experience orgasm. In 1976 Bregman and Hadley interviewed a number of women with spinal cord injuries. Their findings concluded that their descriptions of orgasm were much the same as non-disabled women's experiences, heartening news considering many non-disabled women have such difficulty achieving orgasm, too. Women with spinal cord injuries may find that the sexual lubrication in their vagina is either lessened or absent, and may find the assistance of extra lubrication can benefit them and help them to achieve orgasm. Also some people with spinal cord injuries report having what are known as para-orgasms, which are different from the genital variety, as they occur from stimulation of other areas of the body. Para-orgasms can be so strong that some women need to be aware of, and monitor, rapid changes in their blood pressure.

Most women with disabilities are able to become pregnant even if they are paralysed from the shoulders down. It is important, therefore, that they continue to use birth control unless they are trying to have a baby.

disability and illness

There are illnesses that can lead to disability of varying degrees, all of which can have a knock-on effect on your sex life. Diabetes, for example, can cause men to lose the ability to have an erection;

BELOW | Attitudes towards disability are slowly changing, and the prejudices of the past are giving way to a greater understanding and fuller appreciation that the emotional and sexual needs of disabled and able-bodied people largely coincide.

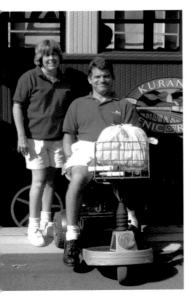

with arthritis, joints become so painful that it is not possible to masturbate or touch yourself. Multiple sclerosis can make you so fatigued that you no longer have the energy to do anything and some sufferers lose the ability to orgasm due to excess nerve damage. With some treatments for other illnesses your libido may be either dulled, or lost altogether. People experiencing these difficulties should consult their doctor who may be able to prescribe alternative treatments to help them. For example, Viagra and apomorphine have helped many male diabetes sufferers and there is some research to suggest that these treatments have positive sexual effects on women too.

practical solutions

Men and women with physical difficulties commonly use vibrators. They can supply the necessary stimulation when a hand is unable to. If your hands cannot grip a regular vibrator then a ball-shaped one is available which may be easier to handle. Also it is possible to get vibrators with longer shafts if it is difficult to reach between your legs. A rechargeable or battery-operated vibrator is usually better if you are incontinent as plug-in models could pose an electric shock risk, although these are pretty outmoded today.

Able-bodied people all too often forfeit better sex because of their inability to communicate their wants and needs to their partner, often relying on their genitals too much for sexual arousal, totally or partially ignoring other sexually sensitive areas. For a disabled person, this is not an option. A disabled person needs to tell their lover how to touch them, where and how to lie with them, what to do with their hands, legs and mouths, how not to hurt them and how to make sure they do not hurt their partner.

Although this may seem clinical and complicated, it doesn't have to be like that. Communication is the key to all great sex, so sexually confident disabled people often make the most wonderful lovers – in many cases they achieve equal, balanced and open relationships, the dynamics of which many able-bodied people could learn from.

learning difficulties

It is not just the physically disabled, but also adults with learning difficulties who have the right to a sex life. Some people may regard those who are mentally challenged as not having the emotional maturity to be able to control their own sexuality. This is a mistaken attitude and one that creates many barriers for a disabled couple. There is usually no good reason why they should not have a healthy sex life, and live fulfilled and independent lives.

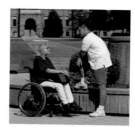

looking after the carers

Most carers are devoted to the people they look after, but caring comes with some hidden agendas, especially when caring for your own relatives at home. The commitment to being a carer can leave very little time for your own needs, emotional, physical and sexual. So it is important for you to try to balance your life and get time off and space to be a sexual being for yourself. Whether you are caring for an elderly parent, disabled child or partner, often you may feel like you are in a constant state of red alert. It can be very exhausting both physically and mentally, so it is imperative that you take time out to care for yourself as well. There are many support groups available to carers, so make sure you get the necessary assistance and advice that is available to you.

getting support

Social clubs and dating organizations offer those with physical and social disabilities the chance to gain confidence, make new friends and potentially, find a partner. It is all too easy to become isolated and feel like an outsider if you do not have any support. There are charities which can offer practical suggestions for meeting, seducing, and having sex with people. They can help you find new ways to experiment, try new positions and combat a lack of confidence.

At times, it must feel as if the obstacles to a normal life are insurmountable, but once you have overcome your own inhibitions and your partner can do the same, then you will be more able to relax, laugh and have some good sex.

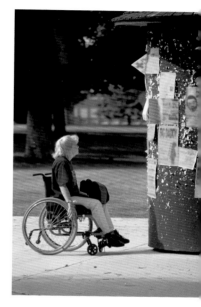

ABOVE | Being confined to a wheelchair is just the most obvious obstacle a disabled person will face.

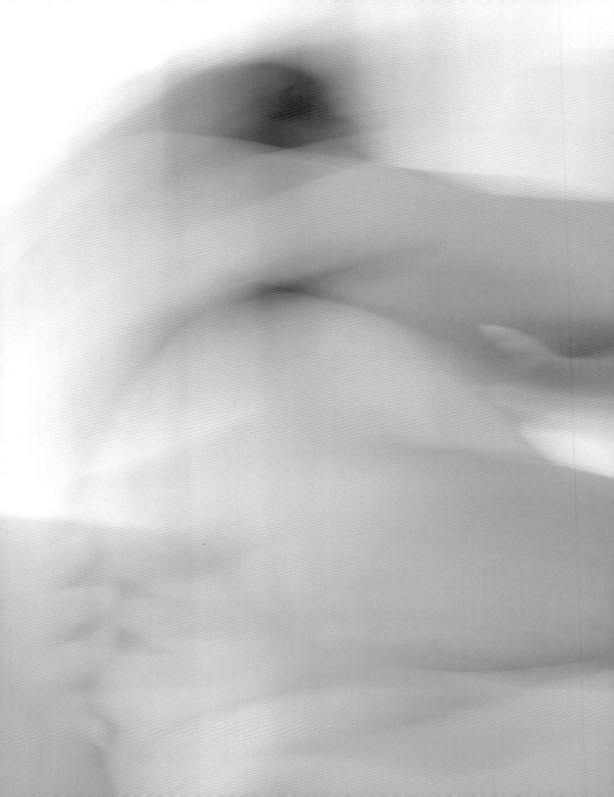

sexual health

Good sex is usually invigorating and energetic and therefore needs to be backed up by a fit body. Eating the right food and taking exercise can help people cope with life's challenges, maintaining energy and vitality in their sex lives. Taking responsibility for contraception and practising safer sex is also important to staying healthy.

bedroom workout

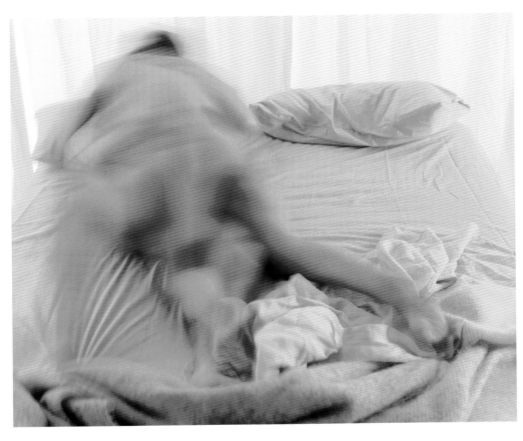

ABOVE | Lovemaking is a workout in itself, but it will be all the more pleasurable – and frequent – if you exercise to keep yourself fit and supple.

GOOD HEALTH MEANS GOOD SEX. Regular exercise promotes energy and stamina. If you are feeling good about yourself and your body, then you can feel good about your sex life, whatever age you happen to be.

There appears to be a direct relationship between being a couch potato and a lack of sexual potency. Research in the USA on a group of middle-aged men who led sedentary lives found that just one hour of exercise three times a week greatly improved their sexual function in terms of frequency, orgasm and satisfaction. Similarly, a

study of women in their forties who exercised regularly revealed that they had more frequent and enjoyable sex than women of the same age who did not exercise.

Sex is, of course, a form of exercise in itself, needing cardiovascular and muscle fitness, so exercise is important for that reason alone. And one of the many benefits of sex is that it is actually a fantastic workout that helps to keep you fit. The average person's heartbeat is around 70 beats per minute, and during lovemaking this can increase to up to 150 beats per minute, about the same as an athlete's heart rate during maximum effort. Really vigorous sex is the equivalent of 15–20 minutes on the running machine, and burns around 200 calories, which is why many people feel hungry after sex. The contractions of your pelvic and other muscles during sex also help to strengthen and tone these muscles.

fitness regime

In order to maintain an active sex life as we age and slow down, it is necessary to supplement our carnal workout with other fitness regimes. Vigorous exercise, such as running or swimming, for half an hour or more, three times a week, helps to keep everyone mentally and physically fitter. Your level of mobility and state of health will dictate the sort of activities that you should do. Whether it is a brisk walk or cycle, or a trip to the gym to use equipment such as the treadmill or rowing machine, all will help to increase your own personal fitness level.

A regular fitness regime not only helps to keep your muscular and cardiac systems healthy but also has many other benefits – helping to lower stress and blood cholesterol levels and reducing the risk of heart disease, high blood pressure, strokes and diabetes. It also increases your muscle and bone strength and your flexibility. These benefits not only help you keep sexually active for longer, but also help you to practise positions that may previously have been too difficult for you to try.

It is never too late to start exercising, although it is better to start a regime before you actually experience problems. People can begin exercising at different levels at any time in their lives. If you are unsure about how much and what sort of exercise you should do, it's a good idea to pay a visit to your doctor for advice, especially if you have any medical conditions or you haven't taken much exercise since you left school.

Exercise programmes are available for everyone – pregnant women, seniors and disabled people alike. Age-related symptoms are often alleviated by increased mobility and activity and many recreation facilities have specialized classes for people who may have mobility problems or

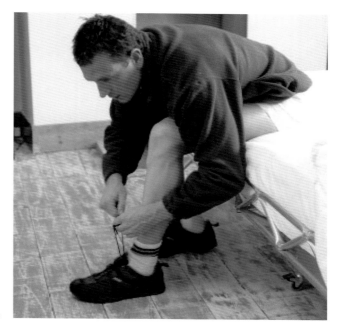

special needs. It is well worth visiting your local gym or recreation facility and talking to a trained professional about the options available and their suitability to your particular needs. Fitness professionals are extremely welcoming and motivating to everyone who is interested in increasing their fitness levels and the chances are that they will give you the utmost support to help you achieve your goals.

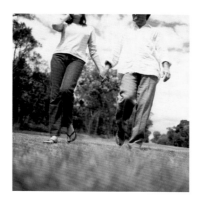

ABOVE | Running is a great way to get fit and increase your stamina and, apart from the cost of a pair of good, supportive running shoes, it's completely free.

BELOW LEFT | There are many kinds of exercise you can try, whatever your age. Just taking a walk in the open air together whenever you can will keep you in shape.

sexercises

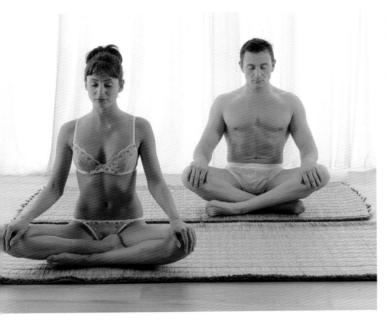

ABOVE | Practising yoga increases suppleness and flexibility, which makes for great sex. PC exercises contract the anal muscles, PC muscle and navel into the body, increasing energy, while strengthening other muscles in the area.

A GREAT SEX LIFE is dependent on good health, and one aspect of keeping well is keeping fit. You will benefit by keeping your heart and lungs strong and your muscles toned.

for her

There are certain exercises that women in particular need to do to keep themselves sexually fit. As they get older, muscles become flabbier if they are not worked and when women hit the menopause, the muscles begin to weaken even more. This also applies to the PC (puboccygeus) muscle. This is the pelvic floor muscle that runs between the legs from the anus to the genitals in both men and women and is the muscle that contracts at a rate of just under once a second during orgasm.

Women who have given birth will probably remember the mid-wife telling them not to forget their pelvic floor exercise. She was referring to the PC muscle, which will have been stretched when the baby was born. There are good reasons for doing the exercises: to avoid problems with bladder control (sneezing and coughing causing leaks, for example) and uterine prolapse in later life. The exercises also help keep a tight vagina for sexual activity. Pelvic exercises are also essential for young women and those who have never given birth, just to keep the muscle toned.

Sexercises were practised in the ancient civilizations of China and India, but it was an American, Dr Kegel, who developed the famous Kegel exercises in the 1950s which are now widely used for pelvic exercising. The quickest way to find your PC muscle is to stop and start when you are urinating, although it is important not to do Kegel exercises during urination. Once you have found it, exercise the PC muscle daily by tightening and relaxing the muscle in turn, starting with 20 times at one session, twice a day. Build up to 60 or so a day and when you have accomplished this, try prolonging the squeeze to five seconds at a time up to 200 times a day.

These exercises can be done while waiting at the bus stop. Even better, while having sex, a woman can squeeze her vagina around her partner's penis and he'll love it. This used to be called Cleopatra's kiss and certain royal courtesans were famous for it. Alternatively, exercise your PC muscle while you are masturbating. One of the results will be to help you and your partner to intensify and prolong orgasms.

for him

If a man has a strong PC muscle, it will help him control the timing of his orgasm, but it won't make his erection any harder. An additional exercise for men is to place a small wet towel on their erect penis and then practise moving it up and down. Once they have achieved this, they can use a bigger towel. This exercise is also excellent for strengthening the muscles of the lower abdomen.

yoga and pilates

Yoga and Pilates are extremely beneficial and holistic forms of exercise for both men and women, young and old. Because sex can require stamina, flexibility and muscular endurance (holding your partner up around your waist for half an hour, for example), both yoga and Pilates will positively help. Making a regular space with your partner to do these exercises every few days will help you to stay relaxed, supple and optimally fit. Doing it together will give you the incentive you need to keep at it.

wall slide

The aim of this exercise is to lengthen the base of the spine without over-tilting the pelvis or tucking it under too far. At the same time it will strengthen the thigh muscles and stretch the Achilles tendon. Stand with your back against the wall and your feet hip-width apart and parallel, 15cm/6in from the wall. Place hands on hips or by your side. Lean back against the wall and breathe in, lengthening through the spine. Breathe out, pull up the pelvic floor and draw your lower abdominals back to the spine (this is also termed zip up and hollow). Slide about 30cm/12in down the wall. Breathe in as you slide up. Repeat eight times.

the full hundred

Lie on the floor, or a comfortable mat or rug, with your knees bent and feet flat on the floor. Your arms should be by your side, palms down. Breathe in and prepare. Breathe out, zip up and hollow. Tuck the chin in slightly and curl the upper body off the floor, at the same time straightening one leg into the air. Reach through the fingertips, lengthening the shoulder blades down the back. Turn out your legs from the hips and flex the feet, lengthening through the heels, so you feel the stretch on the inside of your legs. Squeeze your inner thighs together and engage the pelvic floor. Breathe in for a count of five beats of the arms, then breathe out for five beats, moving the arms as if you were patting the floor. Continue for 100 beats then repeat with the other leg. For beginners, release the head and rest it on the floor.

the half hundred

This is a slightly more advanced version. Breathe in and prepare, breathe out, zip up and hollow. Tuck in the chin slightly and curl the upper body off the floor, or rest your head on the floor. This time bend both knees at the same time while you repeat the movements above. Keep this up regularly, and you will feel an improvement very quickly.

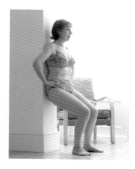

ABOVE | The wall slide will strengthen your legs and stomach muscles.

BELOW LEFT | The full hundred, with straight legs.

BELOW RIGHT | The half hundred, with knees bent.

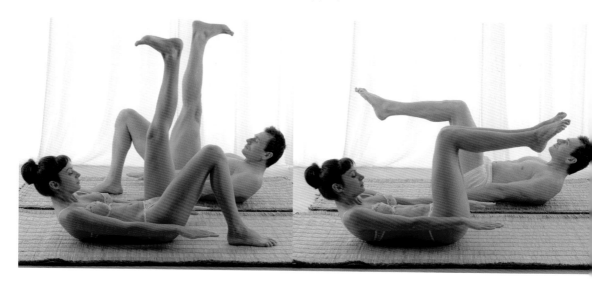

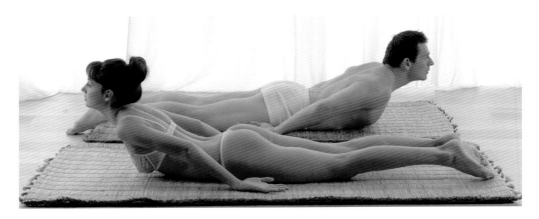

ABOVE | The dart is a gentle exercise that tones all the muscles of the back and neck.

BELOW | Scissors is a Pilates exercise that will improve the condition of your legs and stomach muscles.

BELOW RIGHT | The bridge is quite a demanding pose. Continue with regular practice of these basic exercises, and it will become easier very quickly.

scissors

Lie on a mat, bend your knees to your chest and hold your right leg behind the thigh. Breathe in to prepare. Breathe out and zip up and hollow. Breathe in and straighten both legs in the air, pointing the toes. Breathe out, lengthen and lower the left leg, stopping just above the floor. Breathe in and raise the leg as straight as possible. Breathe out and change legs, crossing over like scissors. This movement will strengthen the abdominals, improve the flexibility of the hamstrings and increase your co-ordination.

the bridge

Begin by lying on your back with your knees bent and your feet flat on the floor close to your body and parallel to each other. Rest your arms alongside your body with your palms facing down. As you

exhale, rotate your pelvis back and push the small of your back into the floor. As you inhale, lift your back off the floor, vertebra by vertebra, starting at the tailbone. Hold the pose for 15 to 30 seconds, or until you feel discomfort. Bring your spine back down to the floor in the same way, beginning with your upper back and stretching your spine towards your heels.

the dart

This position strengthens the back extensor muscles and shoulder blades and works the deep neck flexes. Lie on your front with your arms by your sides and palms facing upwards. Keep your legs together, point your toes and lengthen your neck. Prepare by breathing in, tucking in your chin and lengthening your spine. As you breathe out, zip up your pelvic floor muscles and hollow your

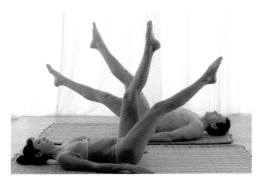

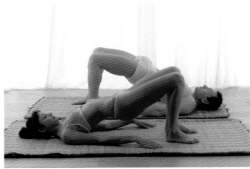

shoulder blades, pulling them down into your back. At the same time lengthen your fingers towards your feet and keep looking straight down at the floor. Avoid tipping your head back but squeeze your inner thigh muscles together, keeping your feet on the floor.

pelvic tilt

This is a marvellous exercise to flatten your stomach muscles and keep you feeling good about your body. Lie on your back, placing your hands on your pelvis with the fingertips on the pubic bone and the pads of your hands resting on the pelvic bones. Breathe in and lengthen through the top of your head. Breathe out and draw up the pelvic floor muscles and pull the lower abdominals back towards the spine, hollowing out your lower stomach (this is referred to as zip up and hollow, which is a requirement for almost all the exercises). Keep your tailbone on the floor lengthening away and do not push into the spine or tuck under the pelvis. You are in neutral position. Breathe in and then relax.

Try this again, with your legs flat on the floor. Lie on your back, lengthening your spine through your head. Your legs should be shoulder-width apart and totally relaxed. Your arms should be by your side with palms facing up. Breathe in to prepare, breathe out and zip up and hollow from the pelvic floor. The tailbone should be on the floor lengthening away. Breathe in and relax.

It is a good idea to start any new exercise regime by attending a class before you try to do it by yourself. Find one that suits you and try to go

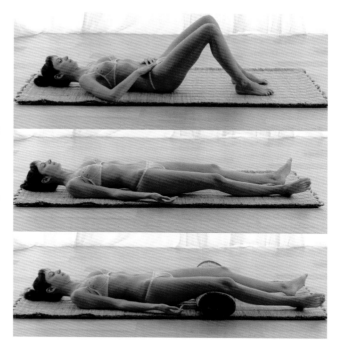

with your partner at least once a week. Once you have learned some of the positions, you can practise at home with the aid of a book or a video. With good teaching, you are unlikely to suffer injuries. Working on some of the postures, like hip openers, will help you to achieve more complex sexual positions that you thought you would never do again. It really is possible at the age of 55 to bend forward, hook your big toes with your fingers and rest your head on your straight knees.

ABOVE | The pelvic tilt helps to build up strength and stamina around the pelvic girdle, vital for an active sex life. If you have lower back problems you can use a cushion or rolled-up mat placed this under your knees, which will release any pressure around the lower back area.

feel-good factor

The body responds to physical exercise by releasing more of the hormone adrenaline. After exercise the come-down after the adrenaline rush makes you feel relaxed and often also increases feelings of arousal, making some kind of fitness regime an excellent idea for people who may have flagging libidos.

The body also releases "feel-good" hormones from the brain called endorphins, the body's natural equivalent to morphine. Endorphins block out pain and make you feel exhilarated, energized, invigorated and generally happy and calm. In other words, they create a perfect physical

and emotional state for lovemaking. As exercise also encourages the flow of blood through all the organs of the body, this can help with arousal, heightened sensation and lubrication. An increased blood flow also helps to make orgasm more intense. In short, the fitter you are, the better the sex.

contraception and safer sex

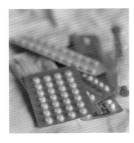

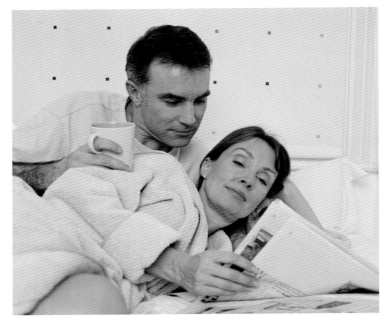

ABOVE | As well as the female pill, new male contraceptives are under development in the form of a transdermal gel and patch that rely on MENT™ (7a-methyl-19-nortestosterone), a synthetic steroid that resembles testosterone but lacks the unwanted side effect of an enlarged prostate.

sex education

A survey carried out for the sexual health charity Marie Stopes International, revealed that one in five parents believed their children would find out about sex for themselves.

Research has shown that one-third of under 16s are sexually active and every year 15,000 girls under 18 have an abortion. It is known that parents who discuss sex openly with their children will have more sexually responsible children who are less inclined to lose their virginity because of peer pressure.

CONTRACEPTION AND SAFER SEX precautions should be paramount to everyone who has sex, not just people who do not want to have babies. Everyone should have been told about the importance of safer sex and should be well aware of the measures that can be taken, but for some reason too many people are still willing to take the risk. As with so many things that are good in life, there is a downside. Just as cake can make you fat and alcohol gives you a hangover, sex can make you sick. And it starts from the first kiss. Even a seemingly innocent little kiss can lead to herpes viruses that never go away.

It is fairly hard to avoid this, but when beginning a new relationship it is important to evaluate what type of person it is that you intend to get intimate with. Never assume that other people are as responsible with their bodies as you are. You have no way of knowing their previous history and, in many cases, infection and disease is passed on unknowingly as many diseases can be carried without showing noticeable symptoms.

When deciding on suitable contraception methods there are a several factors that should be considered: age, lifestyle, health, whether you have children, and whether you may want to have children in the future. The important thing to remember is that contraception is for *everyone*, whether male, female, married or single. When you are in a relationship, contraception should be seen as a mutual project and not the responsibility of the man or woman alone. Bearing this in mind will lead to a more fulfilling love life and a trusting partnership.

No contraceptive is 100 per cent effective but many are close. For extra peace of mind you can always use more than one product – such as the contraceptive pill combined with condoms.

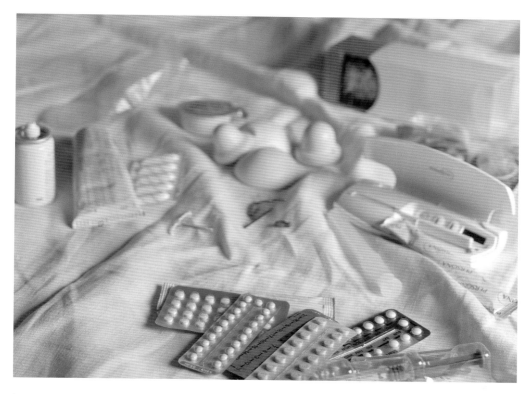

hormonal methods

The contraceptive pill is hormone-controlled contraception, which is either in the form of the combined pill or the progesterone-only pill.

The combined pill combines the two hormones oestrogen and progesterone to prevent the monthly release of an egg from the woman's ovary. If taken correctly, the combined pill is 99 per cent effective.

There is increasing evidence to support the theory that the pill may offer some protection against uterine or ovarian cancer. However, it is not always suitable for women who have conditions such as high blood pressure, circulatory disease or diabetes. Women over 35 who smoke or are overweight are usually advised to use another form of contraception.

The progesterone-only pill is also known as the minipill. The progesterone causes cervical mucus to form a thick barrier which prevents sperm from entering the uterus; it also makes the uterine lining thinner to prevent fertilized eggs from attaching to the wall. The minipill is advised for breastfeeding mothers, older women and women who smoke. This method is 98 per cent effective if taken correctly.

For longer acting contraception, an injection is now available which is 99 per cent effective. It slowly releases progesterone into the body, preventing ovulation. Each injection lasts for 8–12 weeks. Side effects can include continual menstruation or no menstruation at all.

Implanon is a progesterone implant, which acts in a similar way by releasing progesterone into the body. It is 99 per cent effective and lasts for three years, but can lead to irregular periods or even cause them to stop altogether. Hormonal methods do not provide protection against STIs, so should be used with a barrier method.

ABOVE AND OPPOSITE | The variety of contraceptives available on the market today means you do not have to remain with any contraception that does not suit you. Discuss any side effects, likes or dislikes with your partner.

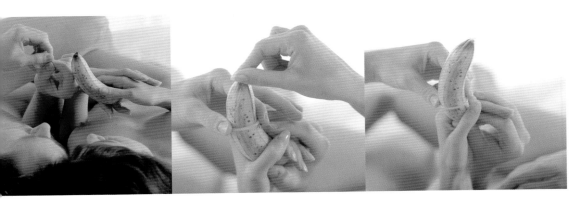

ABOVE | If you or your partner have never used a condom before, why not try putting one on a banana or cucumber before trying the real thing? It is important to exclude the air from the bubble on top, otherwise it may burst later on.

barrier methods

Condoms are the most common forms of barrier method. If used properly they are 94–98 per cent effective, but always make sure they carry an official approval symbol. Condoms are usually made of latex or rubber and work by being placed over the erect penis. They should be placed on as soon as the penis is erect because it can drip semen before ejaculation. Although robust, they must be used with care as they can split or come off. Men must withdraw as soon as they ejaculate and make sure that they do not spill any semen.

Semen has immuno-suppressant qualities. These are important for vaginal penetration as they allow the sperm to enter the vaginal canal without being attacked by the woman's immune system. When sperm is swallowed, stomach acids break down these properties. Little is known about the effects they have in the anal passage. For this reason, it is important to use condoms when performing anal sex, as well as to protect against STIs such as HIV and AIDs. In addition, anal sex without a condom can also result in faecal matter and bacteria becoming trapped in the man's urethral opening, which may not be removed by washing. This can lead to infections in the man, and in the woman if vaginal penetration follows anal sex.

Using lubrication or contraceptive jelly with condoms can also help prevent female urinary tract infections. Make sure you do not use oil-based products, such as petroleum jelly, however, as they reduce the effectiveness of condoms by 90 per cent: water-based lubricants are best.

RIGHT | Condoms have a high rate of effectiveness as contraceptives and also protect against sexually transmitted infections. However, they can tear, burst or simply slip off.

FAR RIGHT | It is always important to take extra care when removing a condom from its packaging to ensure that your nails do not damage it in any way.

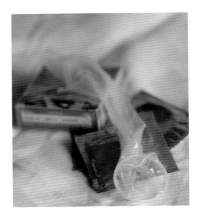

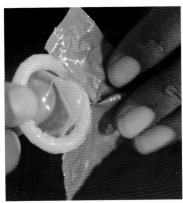

Female condoms are made of quite thin polyurethane plastic. They fit inside the vagina and around the surrounding area to prevent sperm from entering the vaginal environment. If used correctly, they are 95 per cent effective, but it is important that the penis enters the condom and does not get between the condom and the vagina, or it will fail to protect.

The diaphragm or cap is another method of barrier contraceptive that is 92–96 per cent effective. It is a rubber dome that fits over the woman's cervix to prevent sperm from entering the uterus. It must be used in conjunction with spermicidal jelly or pessaries and should stay in place for six hours after sex. Your doctor will be able to measure you for the correct size and teach you how to insert it. This barrier method does not protect you from STIs, such as HIV and AIDS.

The dental dam is a very thin sheet of latex that is laid flat, covering the entire vulva and anal area. It is used in oral sex (anal or vaginal) by both gay and straight couples as a safer sex precaution to prevent transmission of STIs, although the risk can never be completely eliminated.

intrauterine methods

These methods of contraception fall into three categories: the intrauterine device (IUD), the intrauterine system (IUS) and the relatively new Gynefix. They all work in a similar way and are fitted, by a doctor, inside the uterus.

The IUD is a T-shaped plastic device that works by stopping the sperm from reaching the egg and preventing the egg from implanting in the uterus. IUDs can make periods heavier and more painful and are unsuitable for women who have more than one sexual partner as they can increase the risk of infection. Some women's bodies have rejected – and ejected – IUDs, but they have often not realized it until they became pregnant.

The IUS works in a similar way to the IUD, but contains the hormones progesterone and oestrogen, which are gradually released into the body. This system can reduce heavy periods and period pains and is over 99 per cent effective.

Gynefix works in a similar fashion to the IUD and IUS, except it has a more flexible frame. It is composed of a row of copper beads, which bend to fit snugly inside the uterus, and has a fine nylon thread attaching it to the uterine wall, so it is more secure and less likely to be expelled. It can also assist in relieving heavy and painful periods and has been shown to be more than 99 per cent effective as a contraceptive.

All three devices can remain inside a woman for up to five years and doctors teach women how to check for the threads of their IUDs or IUSs to make sure that they are still in place. This is critical and all women fitted with such devices should check regularly. None of them, however, protects against STIs, such as HIV and AIDS. So again, barrier methods are recommended.

old wives' tales

Don't fall for myths that were exploded decades ago; people still do.
- Standing-up positions do not prevent a woman from conceiving.
- Breastfeeding reduces the likelihood of conceiving, but is by no means guaranteed to prevent it.
- Douches have no contraceptive effect and can increase the risk of infection in the woman.
- Jumping up and down after sex is just silly.

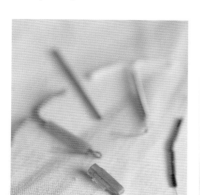

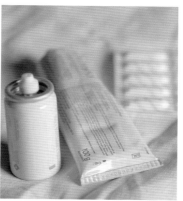

FAR LEFT | IUDs can last for 5–10 years and are a good long-term contraceptive.

LEFT | A variety of spermicides are available in cream or pessary form.

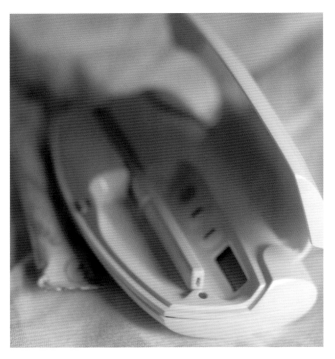

The sympto-thermal method involves taking the woman's temperature at waking every day and plotting the results on a chart. From these temperature changes, the time of ovulation can be calculated, and hence the times when the woman is more, or less, fertile. A special measuring device can be purchased to alleviate the need for complicated documentation.

Hormone testing monitors the levels in the woman's body to tell her which are her fertile days and which are not. A kit will contain disposable urine sample sticks and a hand-held monitor that displays a different colour when she is fertile and when she is not.

Checking dates and the longevity of the menstrual cycle may work better for women who have a regular cycle than those who don't. This method is best used in conjunction with another technique such as monitoring cervical secretions and other hormone-related changes such as breast changes or mood. Cervical secretions change in nature throughout a normal monthly cycle, with dryness directly after the bleeding phase and increased secretions during ovulation.

Many women prefer the natural method, as there are no side effects or chemicals involved. Its success relies not only on the organization and discipline of the couple but also may be affected by age, stress, illness, hormonal treatments, irregular periods and the menopause. Natural methods claim to be 94–98 per cent effective, as long as the instructions are carefully implemented. Once again, this form of contraception does not protect against STIs such as HIV and AIDS.

permanent methods

Male and female sterilization are permanent methods of contraception that some couples opt for if they believe they are sure they do not want children, or they already have all they want. They are not for people who may have doubts, however small, as they are usually not reversible.

Female sterilization is done by a doctor who makes a small incision below the navel to access the fallopian tubes, which are then either clipped, ringed or heat-treated to seal them. This prevents

ABOVE | Using a hormone-testing kit to identify the days when ovulation has occurred is an ideal, though not foolproof, option for couples who don't like the idea of using external methods to control their fertility, through religious or other ethical reasons, medical concerns or simple distaste.

natural methods

Using natural methods of contraception involves identifying the fertile days of the woman's menstrual cycle (the time from the first day of a period until the day before the next period starts) and abstaining from sex during these days or using another form of contraception. The fertile time is the time when she is ovulating (releasing an egg). Although the egg will only live for about 24 hours, sperm in a woman's body can survive for much longer, up to seven days in some instances, so sex a week before ovulation can still result in pregnancy.

Noting the different signs of ovulation can be done by either using a hormone-testing kit, the temperature method or noting dates and cervical secretions. These methods are used as often by those attempting pregnancy as those seeking to avoid it and are more effective if the different methods are combined. If in any doubt about the efficacy of one of these natural methods, a barrier form of contraception should be used as well.

the sperm from meeting the egg. It is a relatively safe procedure that begins to work immediately and is 99 per cent effective.

Male sterilization seals the vas deferens, the tubes that carry the sperm to the penis from the testicles. When a man who has undergone vasectomy ejaculates, his ejaculate contains only semen and no sperm. Sperm continue to be produced but are merely reabsorbed. Unlike female sterilization, vasectomy takes a while to work, as there can often still be sperm in the semen for a few months after the procedure. It is necessary to use other contraceptives until the doctor gives the all clear, and it is then considered to be 99 per cent effective. Neither male nor female sterilization provides protection against STIs, such as HIV or AIDS.

abortion

Many women become pregnant unintentionally and a surprisingly large proportion of these were using contraception of some sort. If you decide on termination, it is important to have a supportive circle of close friends or family to help. The availability of abortion varies from one country or state to another. The important thing to do is seek advice straight away from a reputable doctor or organization. If you do decide to have a termination, then it is best done early, when it's still a relatively simple procedure.

emergency contraception

It is possible to obtain the emergency contraceptive pill over the counter at a chemist's (drugstore) or from your doctor. It is expensive and is not the best method of contraception, but everyone can make mistakes: condoms split or slip off and sometimes people suffer from temporary insanity and don't use anything at all.

This emergency measure must be taken within 72 hours of unprotected sex, in the form of two pills, one 12 hours after the other. The pill may stop an egg from being released, prevent sperm from reaching the egg, or prevent the egg from implanting in the uterus. If a woman vomits up to two hours after taking the pill, then it is important that she takes the second one straight away and then purchases another. New versions of this medication mean that it won't automatically make you feel nauseous.

An IUD can also be fitted up to five days after unprotected sex to prevent pregnancy and can be left in as a longer-term method of contraception, or it can be removed after the next period.

morning after

Emergency contraceptive pills (ECPs) can be taken up to three days after sex. Increased access to ECPs is supported around the world. Women in the UK, British Columbia, France, Belgium, some American states and South Africa can get ECPs directly from trained pharmacists without a visit to the doctor. In Norway, ECPs are available over the counter.

BELOW | Sharing the responsibility for safer sex can increase the sexual trust and enjoyment in a relationship.

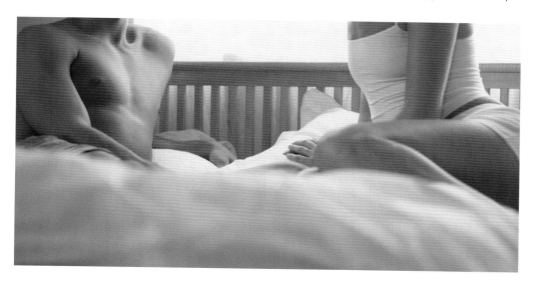

changing needs

THERE ARE VARIOUS FORMS OF CONTRACEPTION for different needs and different times of life. While your body changes throughout your life, one thing is certain: if you are fertile and sexually active, and don't want babies, you need to use some form of contraception. Your doctor, gynaecologist or family planning advisor will be able to give you the best advice for your age and health. Many of the more popular contraceptives are just not suitable for some people. The pill, for example, is not good for smokers. The coil (IUD) is not an ideal contraceptive for women who have not yet given birth and the condom is not 100 per cent reliable. In fact, no form of contraception is 100 per cent reliable, so it is best to have another strategy just in case. For example, if you are on the pill, you should consider using condoms as well.

Couples should decide together about contraception. It is generally women who take responsibility – they are the ones who risk getting pregnant, and they also have a bigger choice of contraception; men are mostly limited to the condom or to having a vasectomy. (The male pill hasn't proved to be a great success.)

Male vasectomy is less risky than female sterilization. It is a big step, so it is wise to think about it very carefully and to consider all the implications. If you do go ahead, and subsequently start another relationship, don't forget that a vasectomy will not protect you from sexually transmitted infections.

When you reach the menopause, don't be fooled into thinking that you cannot conceive. Even if your periods are irregular, you must continue to use contraception until a year after your last period and until you are finally given the all clear, through a hormone test.

infertility

As people age, fertility levels change, most notably in women. Women reach the menopause in midlife, resulting in an inability to have any

BELOW | Couples need to offer mutual support and discuss changing contraceptive needs together.

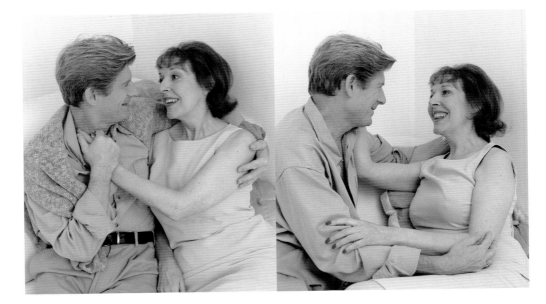

more children. Although men are normally able to father children throughout their lives, their fertility can be affected by problems such as low sperm count or age-related impotence and erectile difficulties. A young, fertile, healthy couple has an approximately one in four chance of conceiving a baby with each cycle. Once the woman reaches the age of 35, the odds of conceiving become greatly reduced, to 10 per cent each cycle. At this stage, some couples seek medical help in the form of hormone treatment or in-vitro fertilization (IVF). Couples trying for a baby need to be in tune with the woman's menstrual cycle, so that they are aware of when she is at her most fertile. The ovaries release an egg each month in the middle of the menstrual cycle, around the 14th day. A woman can be fertile for a few days before and 24 hours after she ovulates. Sperm has a better chance of reaching the egg, however, if it is ejaculated into the vagina 24 hours before the egg is released, as sperm can stay alive in the woman's body for two to three days.

During ovulation, the woman may notice that her mucus discharge is thinner and stringier than at other times. Another way of knowing when the egg is released is by using an ovulation tester kit that detects hormonal changes. An alternative method is to chart changes in the woman's body temperature using a basal body temperature thermometer. When the woman ovulates, her temperature rises by about 0.2 to 0.6 degrees and remains higher until her next period. When she becomes pregnant, her body maintains this increased temperature. (See page 230 for additional information.)

ivf

In-vitro fertilization is a procedure that stimulates egg production through drug and hormone therapy. The growth of ovarian follicles is checked by ultrasound and when the follicles reach the correct size, hormones are administered to cause the eggs to be released. The eggs are harvested using a fine needle guided by an ultrasound image. The eggs are then incubated at body temperature for four to six hours before sperm is added. The fertilized

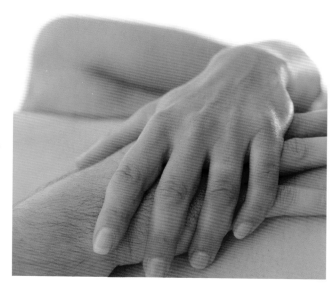

eggs are kept in a culture medium for around two days, before one or more is implanted in the woman's uterus using a fine needle. At present, this procedure is still fraught with difficulties and only around 10 per cent of attempts are successful, making it the least successful method of conceiving artificially. It is often seen as a last resort, not just because of its failure rate, but also because it is fairly unpleasant to undergo.

Another artificial method is used for couples where the man has a low sperm count. This involves injecting a single sperm directly into the ovary via a fine needle. This method has been highly criticized, as there is some evidence that it may increase the likelihood of birth defects. It is also suggested that it interferes with the natural selection process by which only the fittest sperm reach the egg, and that sperm taken from men with a very low sperm count may contain a genetic mutation that could pass on male infertility to future generations.

IVF is expensive, both financially and in terms of the couple's emotions. Couples considering IVF are required to consult a professional expert beforehand to go through their options and get all the and counselling that they will need.

ABOVE | A course of IVF treatment can be an ordeal emotionally, physically and financially, so make sure you go into it together.

fertile ground

Many factors affect the fertility of both men and women. Overeating, smoking, stress and drugs all have a negative effect on sperm production. The correction of mineral deficiencies and eating organic produce are thought by some to improve libido and fertility by up to about 86 per cent.

sexual health

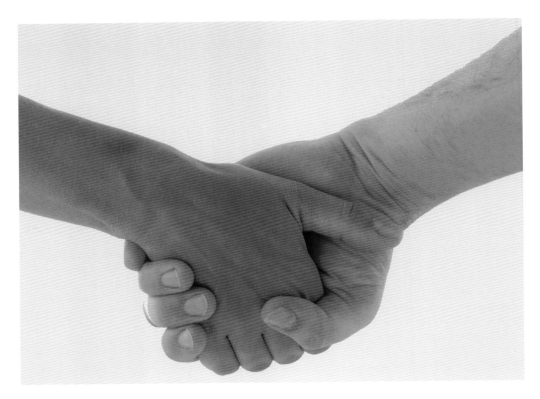

AT SOME POINT DURING YOUR LIFE, your sexual activity is likely to be interrupted and temporarily halted. This could either be as a result of physical illness, such as heart problems or major surgery, or the outcome of psychological challenges involving bereavement, breakdown of a relationship or depression, or a combination. This is equally applicable to both men and women, and it is crucial to get to the bottom of the problem by discussing it with your partner, a doctor or a sex therapist.

men's problems

Men can suffer from performance problems at any time during their life, either in the form of premature ejaculation, erectile dysfunction (failing to get an erection), or an inability to ejaculate. Although erectile dysfunction is more likely to occur later in life, men's penises can let them down even in their teens or early twenties. This can be owing to any number of reasons: anxiety about performance, fear of sex, or even excessive drink and drug use. A vicious circle can occur if, following an isolated incident of impotence, a man is so worried the next time he makes love that it occurs again. In this situation, an understanding partner is essential and a period of sexual abstinence until his normal sex drive reasserts itself will usually solve the problem.

Most men at some point in their lives will have experienced the odd difficulty in "getting it up". Erectile problems are generally considered to be mostly psychological in origin. However, if it occurs regularly, it is wise to consult a specialist. This condition is associated not only with aging, but also with diabetes, surgery for prostate cancer, damage to the nervous system, taking some medication as well as heavy drinking and smoking.

Premature ejaculation (PE) is when a man is not able to control or delay his orgasm. This can be the result of anxiety over his performance, or related to a poor first sexual experience. This condition can contribute to a lack of self-confidence and, if it is a long-term problem, can lead to further difficulties in an existing sexual relationship. If it continues, a doctor or therapist should be consulted. Most commonly PE is the result of persistent learned behaviour, which can in turn be unlearned, and new research shows that in some cases PE is inherited.

Many men find it difficult to talk about their health problems, either with their partners or with a doctor. But it is important to do so. There is the possibility of sildenafil, the "wonder pill" that increases the penis's ability to achieve and maintain an erection once a man is sexually aroused. Every man who is thinking of taking such drugs should have a medical check-up first, as a number of serious side effects have been reported.

Practitioners of complementary medicine have been conducting research on a herbal "Viagra" with, it seems, some degree of success. Ginkgo biloba, the maidenhair tree, has long been used to stimulate the circulation to help treat a number of conditions. There is some anecdotal reportage that daily doses of the herb have led to significant improvements. Herbal practitioners will almost certainly also recommend changes to the diet, probably excluding saturated fats, coffee and alcohol. Smokers will be advised to give up. Acupressure, a Japanese system of applying finger pressure to specific points on the body, has also achieved success for some. Before taking any herbal remedies, you should consult a qualified practitioner. There is no evidence to suggest that alternative methods will work, but any improvement in overall health will help.

women's problems

There are several problems which are common amongst women. Pain while having sex, dyspareunia, may have physical or psychological causes. It can simply be the result of inadequate lubrication, especially with older women. In that case, the remedy is simple, so why not avail yourself of some of the exotic, flavoured gels available from sex shops? If the pain is deep, then it could result from infection or cysts and you should consult your doctor. Psychological problems may vary in severity. Many can be resolved with the help of an understanding partner and a loving touch that stops short of penetration until the woman feels ready. More severe or long-term problems will require professional help.

As with men, women's sex lives will be affected by illnesses such as diabetes, heart disease or high blood pressure. Your doctor will be able to advise you and will almost certainly help you to resume a normal sex life.

BELOW | If one partner is suffering from sexual problems, it is extremely important that the other is both sympathetic and understanding. Keeping the lines of communication open and expressing your love will go a long way towards resolving the difficulty.

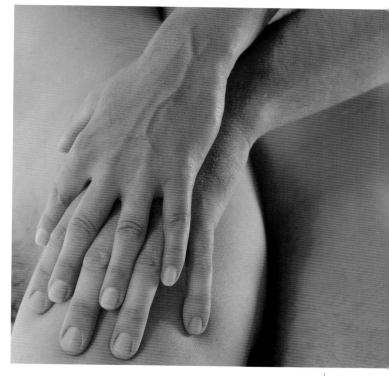

loss of libido and other problems

THE LOSS OF LIBIDO can affect both men and women and presents as a total lack of sexual interest. Sufferers of impotence usually feel frustrated as they still have the desire to have sex, but for one reason or another are unable to perform satisfactorily. To lose the desire to have sex is loss of libido and is just as frustrating but in a rather different way.

People who have a reduced libido tend to take steps to avoid lovemaking by either staying up later to watch television, starting an argument before bedtime or avoiding any form of affection with their partner, often leaving them feeling very confused and rejected.

The causes of low sex drive are often very common things, such as stress, depression, physical illness, overwork or relationship problems. In men, it is a fast-growing problem, owing in part to the strain of today's competitive workplace.

A recent American study showed that 33.4 per cent of women between the ages of 18 and 59

BELOW AND RIGHT |
A temporary loss of libido is very common in long-term relationships. It can be devastating for both partners when it happens, whether caused by emotional or physical problems. However, with the right help, it is usually overcome.

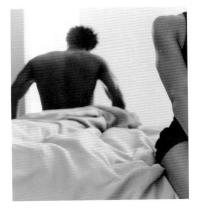

suffered from hypoactive sexual desire disorder (HSDD) or libido loss. The definition is vague because further research showed how varied are the levels of sexual interest among women in general. The causes of HSDD among women are dominated by the menstrual cycle and the stages of their reproductive life and hormone balance.

Many antidepressants such as Selective Serotonin Reuptake Inhibitors (SSRIs), like Prozac, are known to have a negative effect on sexual desire. It is important to continue any medication that you may feel is inhibiting your libido until you have consulted your doctor, who will be able to advise you and offer a possible alternative. Sometimes lack of libido is just a symptom of another problem that can be investigated.

painful intercourse

Sexual intercourse should not be painful, but therapists say that a large number of women suffer for some time before seeking help. Painful intercourse, or dyspareunia, can have a variety of causes from vaginismus (involuntary spasms of the vaginal walls) to lack of lubrication or arousal. The main thing is to take action, not to suffer in silence, as the solution may be simpler than you think. (See page 235 for additional information.)

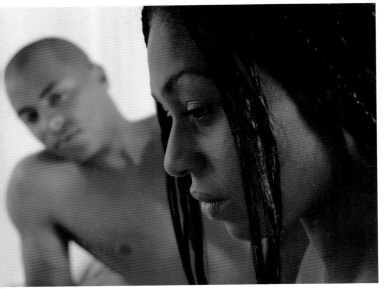

premature ejaculation

One of the most common sexual problems for men is premature ejaculation. It is an inability to control the timing of their orgasms. Some men come as soon as they enter their partner's vagina, others within a few minutes, or within a period that they consider to be far too soon.

Many men experience premature ejaculation at some point, but it is most common in young or inexperienced men. Although no one knows exactly why it happens, most experts agree that the condition is probably psychological, as a result of anxiety about sex and whether they will do it right. Over the years, men generally learn to control their orgasms through experience – by having more sex. And the longer the gap between orgasms, the quicker a man will come the next time round.

If you feel you have a problem, you can train yourself to control your orgasm. Begin by masturbating and bring yourself close to ejaculation. Stop, relax and start again. Repeat until you can't control the orgasm any further. The point here is to learn when you are about to climax, so the more you practise, the more you are likely to be able to delay your orgasm to the exact point at which you want to come. Once you have accomplished this, experiment with your partner. While she is masturbating you, ask her to stop when you are about to ejaculate. Again, stop, relax and start again.

The squeeze technique is another way of achieving the same result. Either you or your partner can squeeze the tip of your penis just before climax. The squeeze forces the blood out of the penis and reduces the erection. Something else which might help is wearing a condom (or even two if necessary) because prophylactics reduce sexual sensation during sex. Alternatively, choose a sexual position in which you find it easier to relax. This is most likely to be one where your partner is on top, taking control.

delayed ejaculation

This occurs in some men who find it difficult to reach orgasm even though they may want to and are receiving the necessary stimulation. The reason

it happens is either physiological – due to diseases such as diabetes or prostatic disease, or certain types of drug therapy – or psychological where some men may have become repressed or inhibited, with a real fear of women or causing pregnancy. Psychosexual therapy can teach men how to overcome the inhibitory behaviour or fears that have become conditioned in them.

retrograde ejaculation

This occurs when men feel the sensation of ejaculation and orgasm but no fluid comes out. Semen is expelled from the testicles but instead of following the contractions and going through the urethra, it travels back into the bladder via the bladder neck. This is relatively common in men who have undergone prostatectomy. Other reasons for its occurrence are disruption of the nervous system caused by spinal cord injury, diabetes, multiple sclerosis and some prescription medications.

erectile dysfunction

During adolescence, young men are frequently embarrassed by how readily – and publicly – an erection occurs. The converse of this is that, with increasing age, it doesn't happen so often, it isn't so firm and it doesn't last so long. By the time this happens, most men should be mature enough to explore other options, from oral sex to a simple change of position.

Alcohol can be the culprit when the spirit is willing but the flesh is weak. Surprisingly, erectile problems as a result of drinking too much – sometimes known as brewer's droop – affect young men more frequently than older men.

Impotence may also be caused by a neurological disorder, where nerve signals are interrupted; problems with the blood flow; hormonal deficiency; diabetes or infection. Not surprisingly, perhaps, men are reluctant to seek help, although many treatments are available. One of the most widely known is Viagra (sildenafil), although this is only effective for one-third of users. Other treatments include vacuum pumps used with a constricting ring, penile implants and urethral injections.

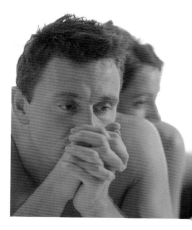

ABOVE | Ejaculation problems can be terribly frustrating but it is important to maintain a perspective on the situation. Sensitivity combined with humour can help, while removing the emphasis from penetration and concentrating on foreplay can divert attention away from the problem and restore confidence.

sexually transmitted infections

THE MAIN CONTRIBUTORS to unsafe sex are drugs and alcohol, which prevent normally sane adults from making responsible decisions. Many sexual encounters and relationships happen when the protagonists are either inebriated or high, which enhances their libido but definitely impairs their judgement and performance.

There have been plenty of awareness campaigns in recent years about the dangers of being infected with the HIV virus and the need to practise safer sex. But HIV is only one of a number of infections that can be caught through engaging in unprotected sex – gay or straight. A passionate situation can develop at any time and it is worth remembering that people with a sexually transmitted infection look just like anybody else and may not say a word about it.

What many people still fail to realize is that many STIs can be contracted without penetrative sex. While condoms will protect you from STIs contracted through exchange of bodily fluids, they will not protect you against herpes, warts, pubic lice and scabies.

With sex between two women, the same principles apply. The use of a dental dam or condoms (if they are using dildos) is recommended as protection against the exchange of bodily fluids. Remember STIs can also be transmitted by sex toys.

As HIV and AIDS first came to public notice there was increased awareness of the need for safer sex, but there is now a developing tendency towards complacency. It is still vital to protect against STIs with condoms and dental dams.

Many people haven't a clue that they have contracted an STI. Sometimes there are no outward symptoms, such as with chlamydia, which may have disastrous effects. However, there are many other infections that do leave their calling card.

signs to look for

If you have any of these symptoms check them out with your doctor:
- Blisters or bumps around the genital area or anywhere from your navel to your knees. Sometimes they are very painful.
- Persistent flu-like symptoms and painful urination.
- Burning or discoloured discharge from the vagina or penis, abnormal bleeding or pelvic pain, pain in the groin, stomach or testicles.
- Yellowing of the skin or whites of eyes, nausea, fever, discoloration of faeces or urine, itchy sores wherever there is hair on the body, itchy genitals, foul-smelling discharge.

If you display any of these symptoms, a trip to the doctor or GU (genito-urinary) clinic, however embarrassing, may be a life-saver or prevent you from becoming sterile. We all know our bodies pretty well, so anything that you think may not be normal should be checked.

human papilloma virus

There are over 50 strains of HPV. Some cause genital warts and the more dangerous ones can cause cervical cancer. HPV is spread by having vaginal or anal intercourse with an infected person. The warts are small painless cauliflower-like lumps that appear on the vulva, vagina, penis or anus. The doctor can successfully remove them, but you do need to take care of yourself and have regular check-ups as condoms are no protection.

BELOW | If you can't face having to tell other partners in person that you have an infection, some sexual health clinics provide a contact slip, which you can send anonymously, and which, in turn, can be presented at any other clinic. The code will let the staff know precisely what they are looking for.

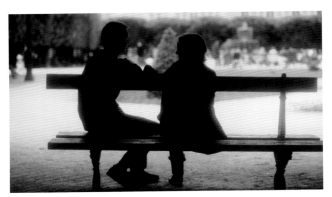

chlamydia

This is the commonest type of STI in the UK and USA. It causes widespread infection in the genital tracts of both men and women, but especially women. It can cause inflammation of the uterine neck, blockage of the fallopian tubes and inflammation of the glands that produce sexual fluids. In men it can cause inflammation of the urethra or tubular part of the testicles and joint or eye disorders in extreme cases. In women it often displays no symptoms but can lead to infertility, highlighting the necessity for regular gynaecological check-ups. If caught in the early stages it is easily rectified with antibiotics. If left, it can cause trachoma, which is a serious eye infection that can lead to blindness and from which 500 million people suffer today.

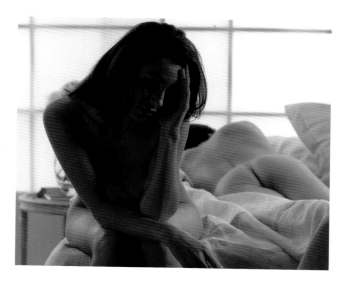

gonorrhoea

This is caused by the passing of bacteria from an infected individual which leads to infection that can spread via the bloodstream. It may not show any symptoms for a while, with an incubation period of two to ten days, and even after this no clear symptoms may present themselves.

Men may find discomfort when they urinate or a whitish-yellowish discharge from the penis. Women may experience a green or yellow vaginal discharge, abdominal pain or disrupted menstruation patterns. If it is left untreated, gonorrhoea can lead to pelvic inflammatory disease (PID), or may close the fallopian tubes, causing infertility.

syphilis

This disease has become more common in men than in women over recent years and the majority of new cases occur in homosexual males. One-third of untreated sufferers die from brain, nerve or heart damage. It has an incubation period of about three weeks and can be treated successfully in its early phases with antibiotics. If it is untreated, a recurring bout can occur up to ten years later. The symptoms usually appear on the skin in rash-like lesions called chancres, which are painless.

genital herpes

This can be a completely symptom-free infection that is passed through genital contact with a partner who has an area of infection. Men may discover blisters on the penis, scrotum or surrounding area (blisters can be found on the navel and upper and lower thighs), which are often painful. Women may discover red bumps, which will turn into painful blisters. These are usually discovered in the labial folds, but can also be present in the cervix, anus or navel. Herpes can also induce flu-like symptoms in both men and women. Herpes has been associated with cervical cancer so if you find you are infected, it is important to follow up treatment with a smear.

hepatitis a, b and c

Hepatitis is an infection affecting the liver, and can be associated with excessive alcohol, drug or chemical consumption or infection by viruses. Hepatitis A is not usually transmitted through penetrative sex, but can be through anal sex. Hepatitis B is passed on via semen, mucus or blood. Hepatitis C is similar to B but is blood-borne so transmission is more common through sharing needles. Hepatitis B and C have incubation periods lasting from six weeks to six months, and may

ABOVE | A trip to your local sexual health clinic is the best way to deal with any fears that you may have about having contracted an STI. No matter how embarrassing it may be for you, you are merely one of thousands of people they help each week.

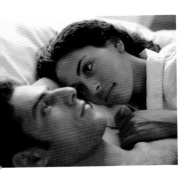

ABOVE | If an infection or other problem is bothering you, it is best to be honest and share it with your partner.

OPPOSITE | Sharing a problem can often make the bonds of your relationship stronger.

show either no symptoms or very severe ones. Symptoms for both include the yellowing of the skin, increased fatigue, darker urine and paler faeces. Unfortunately, as with HIV and AIDS, it is caused by a virus and so there is no cure for hepatitis at the moment, although there are drug treatments available to help control the symptoms.

yeast infections

These are fairly common among women: symptoms usually include itchy genitalia and a dense, clotted whitish discharge from the vagina. Yeast infections are not necessarily sexually transmitted but can be caused by antibiotics and wearing tight-fitting synthetic clothing that does not allow the skin to breathe. Men can suffer from yeast infections too, but it is less common.

Bacterial vaginosis (BV) has similar symptoms but the discharge usually has a fishy smell and is creamier. BV may also cause pain when urinating. Trichomoniasis affects men in their urethra and women usually in the vagina. It can have no symptoms, but a smelly discharge or pain when urinating can be a sign.

pubic lice (crabs) and scabies

These are particularly nasty little mites that are horrendously contagious. Scabies burrow under the skin of an infected individual, causing itchy sores, and crab lice congregate mainly in hairy areas of the body, usually the pubic area. Your pharmacist (druggist) or doctor can advise you on treatment but it is also important to wash all your clothes at a very high temperature. Anything that cannot be washed should be vacuum-packed in plastic for at least two weeks.

hiv and aids

Human Immunodeficiency Virus (HIV) is the primary virus that leads to Acquired Immunodeficiency Syndrome (AIDS). Since the 1980s epidemic, many have died. The reported number of people with HIV in industrialized countries increases each year because of the greater accuracy of diagnosis and decreasing deaths due to antiretroviral therapies. However, many cases are not diagnosed.

The majority of infections first reported are thought to have occurred through sex between men. After an initial reduction in new cases, increasing numbers of diagnoses are now occurring again each year. It is estimated that a quarter of HIV-infected men who have sex with other men have not been diagnosed.

Since 1999, there has been more diagnosis of heterosexual-acquired infection in First World countries, although 80 per cent of cases were infected elsewhere, particularly in Africa. Globally, women are becoming increasingly affected by HIV. Approximately 50 per cent, or 19.2 million, of the 38.6 million adults currently living with HIV or AIDS worldwide are women.

It is important that people are aware of HIV and AIDS, which is spread through exchange of bodily fluids such as semen, vaginal secretions and blood and very, very rarely through saliva. The effect AIDS has on the body is that it gradually breaks down the body's natural defence mechanisms until eventually it is no longer able to fight infection. This results in infected people dying from relatively simple and usually easily treatable infections, such as the flu or, particularly commonly, pneumonia.

The symptoms are often difficult to identify. In the first few weeks, only about half of infected people suffer from flu-like symptoms, such as fevers, tiredness or swollen glands. This is usually when the person is carrying HIV and doctors use combination drug therapies to keep people in this relatively "healthy" phase for as long as possible. If HIV progresses to AIDS, then the individual is liable to get much more ill, with consistently swollen glands, chronic diarrhoea, weight loss, fever and the development of skin lesions.

It is important – vital in fact – that people are constantly reminded of the risk, regardless of their sexuality, as it is still a very real, worrying and distressing problem. The main weapon against AIDS is education and myth-busting. It is not an act of some retributive deity punishing the human race for its sexual actions; it is a disease that can be prevented from spreading. The message is: use condoms.

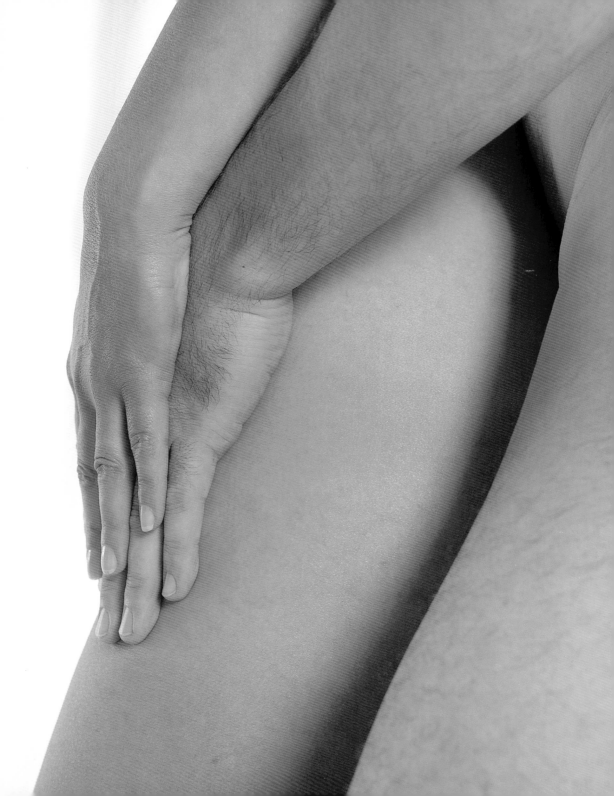

rape and abuse

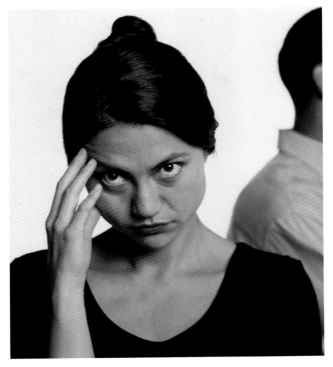

ABOVE | There is no magic formula for recovering from sexual or violent abuse. It is important to remember, however, that time and counselling are great healers. Most important of all, remind yourself that it was not your fault that it happened.

RAPE AND SEXUAL VIOLENCE are far more common than most people think, and anyone can be a victim: young women, old women, men, children – in short, people of all classes and all cultures. Most rape and sexual violence is carried out by men against women. The majority of women who have been raped know their attacker, because they are a current partner, ex-partner, family friend, neighbour or workmate: someone they trust.

why do men rape women?
Rape is not so much about sex as about power and control. For example, the notorious date rapes, of which young women under the age of 25 are the main victims, are carried out by men, often with the use of drugs, such as Rohypnol, which are used to spike drinks. Many of the men questioned do not admit that their behaviour is wrong. All too often, the perpetrators have it in their minds that a woman saying no doesn't actually mean no. She wanted sex, she was gagging for it, they maintain, and feel they deserve something in return for the money and attention they have spent on her.

One of the most common arguments that men raise for forcing themselves on their wives, girlfriends, or dates is that, in the midst of a heavy petting session, when the man is all ready to go, the woman decides she doesn't want to continue. She ends the session, leaving her partner frustrated. However, if a woman says no, it means no. If a woman wants to pull out at the last moment, that is her right. There is absolutely no biological or psychological reason why a man cannot stop.

why do men rape men?
In many countries, male rape has only recently become a crime. In Britain, Home Office statistics for 1997 state that 342 men reported being raped. This is believed to be a huge under-representation of the true figure.

Although there has been less research on the subject than on female rape, and there are far fewer services for male victims, we know that a lot of men won't report being raped. This is also about power. It is prevalent in institutions, particularly prisons, and has only recently been taken seriously by the authorities. Many myths surround male rape: only gay men are raped; men are raped because they are weak; men are strong and should be able to defend themselves against their attackers. Heterosexual as well as gay men are raped and this can make them doubt their sexuality as a consequence.

what to do if you are raped
If you are raped, whether you are a man or a woman, get to a safe place, call the police or a rape crisis centre, or phone a family member or

friend to help. You must see a doctor to have a medical check-up. You will also need medical evidence for any prosecution. Don't change your clothes, don't have a bath or shower, even comb your hair, or adjust anything until you have been examined by the doctor; otherwise you could destroy evidence.

If you have been raped, or sexually abused by a family member, the most important thing to remember is that it is not your fault. Rapists are responsible for their own actions. It is a brutal and humiliating experience and you will need tender care afterwards. Therapy is often a necessity after such an ordeal.

While most rapes are carried out by men who are known to the victim, there are rapes that are completely random. People must be vigilant wherever they are, whether walking down a dark street at night, or in an empty train carriage (coach) or even in a work situation. Keep your wits about you and, if you are planning to travel alone, think carefully about how you are going to get to your destination safely.

Many people feel suicidal, suffer from post-traumatic stress disorder and go into deep depressions when they have been raped. Therapy is probably the best long-term solution after such a horrendous ordeal.

One in four women will experience rape or attempted rape, and most will not report it to the police. The legal definition of rape varies from country to country, but if a man has sexual intercourse with a person who at the time does not consent to it, that it is essentially rape. It is defined as the non-consensual penetration of the vagina or anus by a penis. Forced oral sex and the penetration of the vagina or anus by a foreign object are, at the very least, serious sexual assault. Touching and other kinds of unwanted sexual contact is also sexual assault.

abuse

This is an extreme form of control. While mostly carried out by men against women or children, it happens within gay relationships and violence by women against men appears to be on the

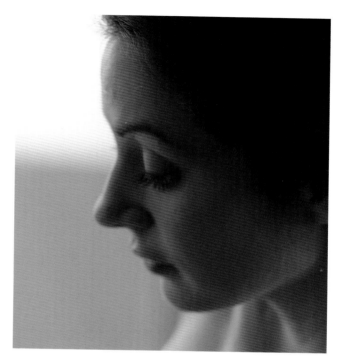

increase. The abuse can be both emotional and physical. A partner can be hit, kicked or beaten, humiliated in front of other people, threatened with death, or made to perform sexual acts that they do not want to do: in effect, rape. Even the silent treatment, in which one partner refuses to communicate, is a form of abuse.

Being abused can cause depression, anxiety and illness, as well as injury. In many cases it can lead to homelessness and, in extreme cases, it results in murder. Many abusers don't understand the meaning and effect of emotional and verbal abuse, and need to be educated about what respectful behaviour towards a partner means. Many victims lose their self-esteem, and may even lose all control of their actions and lives.

Nobody should have to put up with it, so if you are being abused, seek help. Most people are acutely embarrassed by abuse and its consequences, but it is crucial that you seek the help of a professional to guide you through this time.

ABOVE | After a traumatic experience, don't suffer in silence, however ashamed or frightened you feel. Find someone you can trust, who will support you and find out about which organization to contact for help should you wish to.

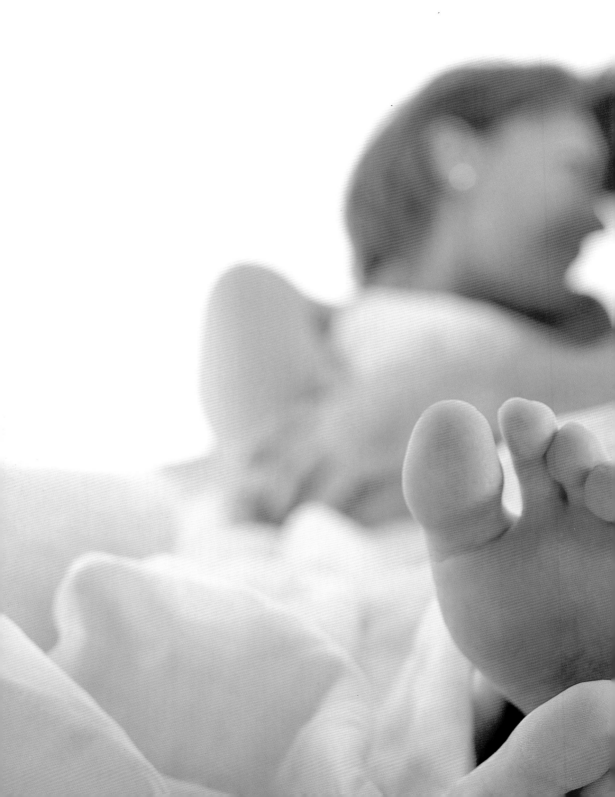

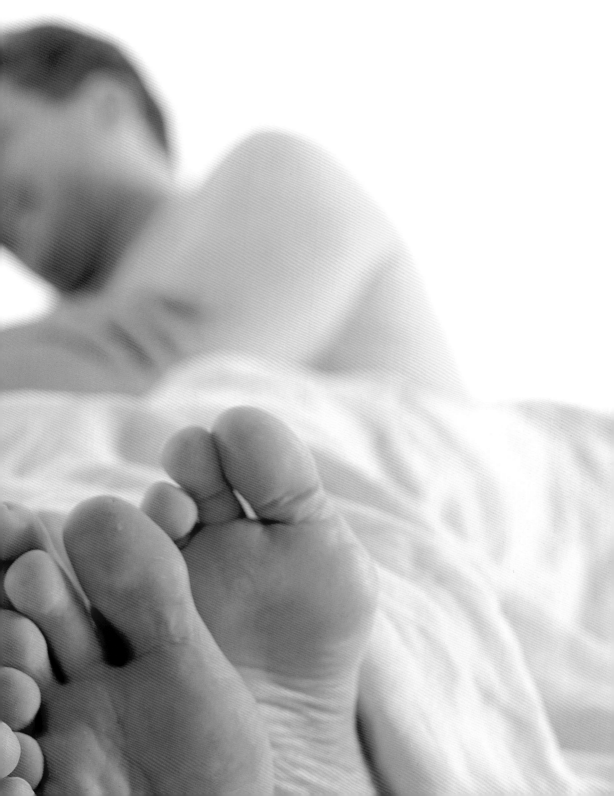

glossary

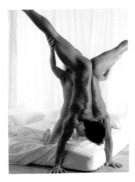

A spot The anterior fornex erogenous spot is the G spot's neighbour. Located about one-third of the way down the front vaginal wall.

adrenaline A hormone released after exercise which can increase the libido.

anal Relating to the anus, as in anal sex.

anal beads A string of beads placed up the anus and pulled out at the point of orgasm.

aphrodisiac An experience or substance that stimulates or enhances sexual desire.

B/D Bondage/discipline.

BDSM Bondage discipline and sadomasochism – the elements of dominance and submission.

bisexual A person who feels sexually aroused by both sexes.

blow job Oral sex done on a man; fellatio.

body modification Altering your body with tattoos, piercings and corsets.

bondage Sexual arousal by physical restrictions, such as handcuffs and rope restraints.

bottom The submissive half of a bondage duo. The dominant half is known as the top.

buggery Anal intercourse.

butt plug A diamond shaped or flared implement that is inserted up the anus and is usually made of silicone or plastic. It is used to create a feeling of fullness.

CAT Coital Alignment Technique – an intercourse technique where you roll rather than thrust.

cervical cap Birth control device that covers the cervix and acts as a barrier to prevent the sperm from entering.

cervix Opening of the uterus.

chakras Described in Tantric sex. These are the seven points in individuals, which are believed to regulate different types of energy.

chlamydia A sexually transmitted infection that affects both men and women. It often displays no symptoms but can lead to infertility, highlighting the importance of regular check-ups. If found early it can be treated with antibiotics.

circumcision A small operation which is performed by either a doctor or a religious expert to remove the foreskin of the penis. It is usually performed for either medical reasons such as phimosis (a tight foreskin), for reasons of hygiene or for religious reasons.

clitoris The only organ in the human body whose sole function is pleasure. This little organ is located at the top of a woman's vulva. It is covered with a clitoral hood and becomes erect when the woman is sexually aroused.

cock ring A penis ring made of either rubber or leather that fits around the base of an erect penis to maintain an erection for longer by trapping blood in the organ. Never wear one for more than 20 or 30 minutes.

condom A latex sheath that fits snugly over the penis is the most commonly used form of barrier contraception.

Cowper's glands Small structures near the urethra inside the base of the penis, involved in the secretion of pre-seminal fluid.

crabs A sexually transmitted infection in the form of lice which inhabit the pubic hair.

cross-dressing When a member of one sex finds sexual gratification in wearing the clothes of and mimicking the opposite sex. NB: cross-dressers are by no means always gay.

cum Slang term for male ejaculate.

cunnilingus Oral sex on a woman. "Cunnus" is Latin for vulva and "lingere" is Latin for lick.

diaphragm Contraceptive barrier method which holds spermicidal jelly against the woman's cervical opening.

dildo Penis-shaped object, which can be inserted into the vagina or anus for sexual stimulation. Not to be confused with a vibrator, which is similar in structure but is battery operated and vibrates for extra stimulation.

dildo harness A device that can be worn with a dildo attached, allowing hands-free thrusting.

doggy style A sexual position where the woman is on all fours and the man enters from behind.

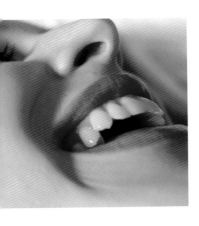

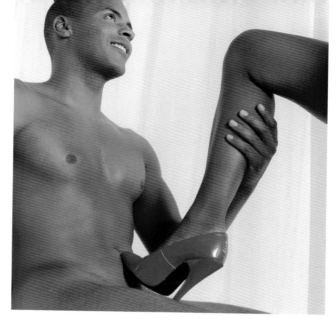

dom Dominatrix or dominator.

double dildo A dildo that can be used at both ends by two people at the same time.

double penetration A penis or dildo in the vagina and anus at the same time.

ectopic pregnancy When the developing embryo implants in the fallopian tubes and not the uterus. If not caught quickly it can lead to maternal death.

ejaculate The white fluid which usually accompanies male orgasm.

endorphins These are the body's feel-good hormones, neuro-transmitters which have a wide range of functions. They help regulate heart action, hormone function, the perception of pain and the mechanisms of shock from blood loss and are thought to be involved in some way in controlling emotion, mood and motivation. Exercise, sex and chocolate are thought to stimulate production.

felching Licking male ejaculate out of either the anus or vagina.

fellatio Oral sex for the male; a blow job.

fetish A specific object or body part that an individual eroticizes for sexual gratification.

foreskin A flap of skin that extends from the shaft of the penis and over the head to maintain moisture and provide protection. In the circumcised male it is removed.

French kiss A mouth-open, tongue-twizzling kiss!

frenulum Located below the glans or head of the penis, on the side that faces away from the body, when erect. This is an extremely sensitive area.

frottage Simulating sex with your clothes on.

full hundred A Pilates-based exercise which you perform 100 times.

G spot Named after Ernest Grafenburg who claimed that an area on the roof of the vagina is potentially sexually stimulating for some women.

gender dysphoria When a person of a specific sex wishes to be of the opposite sex.

genitals Sex organs.

glans The head of the penis.

golden shower Urinating on your partner as a means of sexual stimulation.

gonad A sex gland.

hermaphrodite An individual who is born with both the male and female sex organs. This is usually caused by an excess of the hormone androgen during pregnancy.

herpes A virus that can affect either the mouth or genitals. It forms a rash and can cause flu-like symptoms. Once infected, it remains in the body, usually in a relatively harmless dormant state. It is important to use barrier methods of contraception such as condoms if you are aware that you are a carrier, but especially if you are not 100 per cent confident that your partner is not.

impotence When a man is unable to get an erection on a regular basis.

IUD Formerly known as the coil, an interuterine device is fitted into the uterus and prevents conception by stopping the egg implanting in the uterus wall.

Kama Sutra An Indian classical book on the technique and art of love and lovemaking.

Kegel exercises Squeezing and contracting your puboccygeus muscle. These help to make you more aware of sexual sensation and some say that they can result in more intense orgasms. Especially useful for women to regain genital strength after childbirth.

Kinsey average The amount of time researcher Alfred Kinsey estimated it took for the average male to reach orgasm during intercourse.

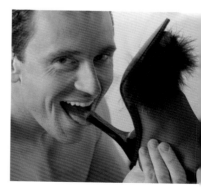

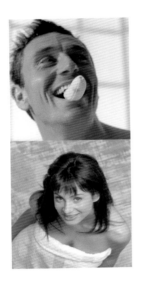

kundalini Derived from the Sanskrit word "kundal" meaning coiled up, which is normally represented as a coiled or sleeping serpent in Vedic and Tantric texts. An awareness of the presence of this energy within the human body was considered by the sages and saints to be the highest knowledge.

labia minora The inner lips of the vagina that are attached to the clitoris. Pink in colour and thinner than the outer lips (labia majora).

lesbian A woman who prefers sexual relationships with other women.

libido The desire that drives us to have a sexual relationship with another person.

lingham Sanskrit for penis, a definition used in Tantric texts.

maithuna A skill men use to suppress their orgasm in Tantric sex.

masochist A person who welcomes pain and finds sexual gratification in receiving it. Also known as a "bottom" or submissive.

masturbation Stimulating your own genitals to achieve sexual gratification.

merkin A wig made specifically for the pubic region, held on with glue.

missionary position The man and woman have sex in a horizontal position facing one another with the man on top.

monilia A vaginal yeast infection (candida albicans) that can be painful and cause thick discharge together with intense itching.

mons pubis The fleshy mound on top of the vulva that pubic hair grows from.

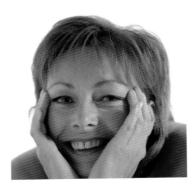

Montgomery glands Small bumps on the nipples.

morning after pill Emergency contraception that comes in the form of two pills taken 12 hours after each other. Can be used up to 72 hours after unprotected sex.

mula bandha or root lock – a yoga position concentrating on the pelvic floor muscles.

nipple clamps A clip that is placed on the nipples during sex play. They come with varying degrees of pressure and are often used in BDSM.

nocturnal emission A wet dream, common in boys during puberty.

nonoxynol-9 Ingredient of most contraceptive foams and gels that changes the pH of male sperm and renders it infertile.

nonspecific urethritis An infection of the urinary tubes that is pretty common.

orgasm The sensations that ripple through your body at the climax of sexual excitement.

orgasmic platform The vulva and the first third of the vaginal passage where there is a concentration of nerve endings.

papervine A drug injected into the penis, which makes it hard and erect.

Pelvic Inflammatory Disease (PID) A bacterial infection that causes inflammation of the female sex organs, usually the fallopian tubes.

pelvic tilt An exercise to keep the muscles of the pelvis in trim.

perineum Sensitive area between the anus and the male or female genitals.

pessaries Spermicides in the form of small bullets which are inserted into the vagina.

Pilates A gentle form of exercise for the body inspired by Joseph Pilates.

polyamory Individuals who have a committed sexual relationship with more than one partner.

pranayama This is a breathing technique practised in yoga.

precum The fluid that leaks from an erect penis during sexual excitement. Its properties deacidify the urethra so that ejaculate has a greater chance of impregnating the female.

prepuce The foreskin of the penis.

priapism Named after the Greek God of male reproductive power Priapus, this is an often painful affliction that causes a "trapped" erection, i.e. one that will not go down. It is often necessary to seek medical assistance to prevent permanent damage.

Prince Albert A male genital piercing that goes through the urethral opening of the penis, coming out on the underside of the shaft.

prostate The gland that is responsible for a portion of the male ejaculate, it contracts seconds before orgasm. Located on the floor of the rectum.

puboccygeus (PC) muscle This holds the pelvic floor together.

rape Forced sex on either a male or female. A serious criminal offence that results in tremendous psychological damage to its victims.

rimming Kissing and licking the anus.

safe word Used in bondage, this is a prearranged expression that the bottom uses to tell the top to either stop, or ease up.

safer sex It is important to take precautions against STIs, but there is no such thing as safe sex.

Sanskrit The ancient Indo-European literary language of India.

scissors A Pilates-based exercise holding the legs in the air and making a scissor action.

serotonin The neuro-transmitter and hormone 5-hydroxytryptamine (5-HT) which is found in many tissues, especially the brain, the intestinal lining and the blood platelets. Serotonin is concerned with controlling moods and levels of consciousness.

S&M Sexual scenarios where individuals act out submission and domination fantasies.

smegma Build-up of thick pungent substance

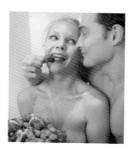

underneath the foreskin or clitoral hood.

sodomy Generally understood to mean anal penetration.

soixante-neuf (69) Where a couple perform oral sex on each other simultaneously.

spermicide A cream, gel or pessary that will kill sperm on contact, often added to condoms.

STI Sexually transmitted infection. Also known as STD (sexually transmitted disease) or, less commonly nowadays, VD (venereal disease).

swinging Husband-and-wife-swapping, often involving group sex or specific parties where couples swap and have sex with other partners.

switches People who participate in BDSM and alternate, being either the "top" or the "bottom".

Tantra A number of Hindu and Buddhist writings giving religious teaching and ritual instructions.

thrush A vaginal yeast infection caused by either candida or monilia fungus. Penile thrush can also occur in men but is less common.

tipped uterus A uterus that points towards the back as opposed to lying parallel to the spine. Can cause problems in conception.

top The master, mistress or dominator in BDSM.

toxic shock syndrome (TSS) A rare but potentially lethal infection associated with using tampons.

tubal ligation Permanent female sterilization, which involves surgically sealing the fallopian tubes.

urethral sponge Cushioned area that protects the urethra during intercourse.

vibrator An electrical vibrating device used most commonly by women for masturbation. Can be used vaginally or anally.

voyeurism A fetish involving individuals achieving sexual stimulation from watching other people undress or have sex.

vulva The external female genitalia.

wall slide An exercise to strengthen the thigh and stomach muscles.

yeast infection Fungal infections that particularly afflict moist areas such as between the toes, the vagina and penis.

yoga An ancient and holistic form of exercise suiable for all ages.

yoni The Sanskrit word for a woman's vulva, a term often used in Tantra.

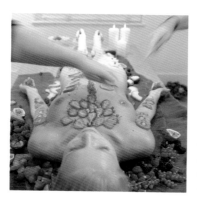

bibliography

Allende, Isabel, Aphrodite: The Love of Food and the Food of Love (Flamingo, UK, 1998)

Allison, Sadie, Tickle Your Fancy (Tickle Kitty Press, USA, 2002)

Alman, Isadora, Doing It (Conari Press, USA, 2001)

Anderson, Dan, and Berman, Maggie, Sex Tips for Straight Women from a Gay Man (2nd edn, Thorsons, UK, 2002)

Blank, Joani, Still Doing It: Women and Men over 60 Write About their Sexuality (Down There Press, USA, 2000)

Burton, Sir Richard, The Kama Sutra of Vatsyayana and the Phaedrus of Plato (Kimber Editions, 1963)

Cattrall, Kim, and Levinson, Mark, Satisfaction: The Art of the Female Orgasm (Thorsons, 2002)

Comfort, Alex, The Joy of Sex (5th edn, Mitchell Beazley, UK, 1996)

D'Argy Smith, Marcelle, The Lover's Guide: What Women Really Want (Carlton Books, UK, 2002)

Davies, Dominic, Gillespie-Sells, Kath, Shakespeare, Tom, The Sexual Politics of Disability: Untold Desires (Cassell, UK and New York, 1996)

Delvin, David, The She Complete Guide to Sex and Loving (Ebury Press, UK, 1985)

Dennis, Wendy, Hot and Bothered (2nd edn, Grafton, UK, 1993)

Easton, Dossie, and Hardy, Janet W, The New Bottoming Book (Greenery Press, USA, 2001)

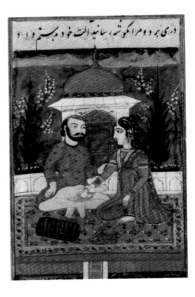

Friday, Nancy, My Secret Garden (Quartet Books Ltd, UK, 1975)

Hooper, Anne, Massage and Loving (Unwin Hyman Ltd, UK, 1988)

Joannides, Paul, Guide To Getting it On (2nd edn, Vermilion, UK, 2001)

Kriedman, Ellen, Light His Fire (Judy Piatkus Ltd, UK, 1990)

Lacroix, Nitya, Love, Sex and Intimacy (7th edn, Lorenz Books, UK, 2002)

Lacroix, Nitya, Tantric Sex: The Tantric art of Sensual Loving (2nd edn, Southwater, UK, 2000)

Lawson, Michael, The Better Marriage Guide, (Hodder & Stoughton Ltd, UK, 1998)

McConville, Brigid, My Secret Life: Sexual Revelations from Long-term Lovers (Thorsons, UK, 1998)

Paget, Lou, How To Give Her Absolute Pleasure (2nd edn, Judy Piatkus Ltd, UK, 2001)

Paros, Lawrence, The Erotic Tongue (2nd edn, Arlington Books Ltd, UK, 1988)

Powling, Suzy, and Thoburn, Marj, The Relate

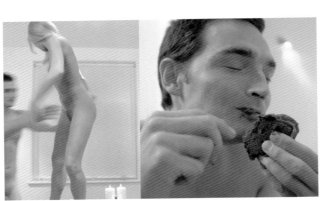

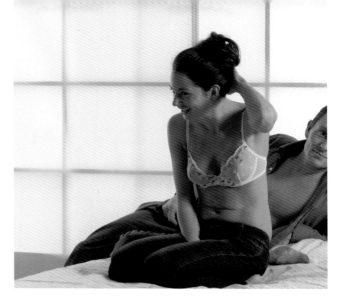

Guide to Loving In Later Life: How To Renew Intimacy And Have Fun In The Prime Of Life, (2nd edn, Vermilion, UK, 2000)

Quilliam, Susan and Relate, Staying Together: From Crisis to Deeper Commitment, 2nd Edition, Vermillion, UK 2001

Reyes, Alina, The Butcher (3rd edn, Minerva, UK, 1992)

Youngson, Dr Robert, The Royal Society of Medicine Health Encyclopedia, (3rd edn, Bloomsbury Publishing Plc, UK)

articles

Campbell, Carolyn, Speed Dating: A New Form of Matchmaking (Discovery Health Channel website)

Crisp, Charlotte, Talking Dirty (Cosmopolitan, May 2002), p.145

Goleman, Daniel, Language of Love (New York Times, February 14th 1995)

Guerra, Fred, What is Semen Made From? (JakinWorld.com Science Corner)

Hill, Amelia, Women to Get Sex Toys on the NHS, (The Observer website, September 29th 2002)

Kaylin, Lucy, The Porning of America (GQ, August 1997), pp.166–170

Keyishian, Amy, The Complete Guide to Your Clitoris (Cosmopolitan, May 2002), pp.137–140

Mauro, Jim, Keeper of the Flame (Smoke, vol 11, no.2), pp.84–91

O'Connell, Sanjida, Follow Your Nose (Guardian Unlimited, September 27th 2002)

Stewart, Fiona, R U RDY 4 THS? (iVillage.co.uk, September 5th, 2002)

Vincent, Sally, Everybody's Doing It (The Guardian Weekend, August 10th 2002)

Whitfield, John, The Sweet Smell of the Immune System (Nature News Service, March 7th 2002)

websites

www.cliterati.co.uk
The website that admits that women like sex too.

www.tantra.com
The resource for Tantra, sex and the Kama Sutra.

www.tantra.org
Church of Tantra and the text of the Kama Sutra.

www.tantraworks.com
Vatsayana's contribution.

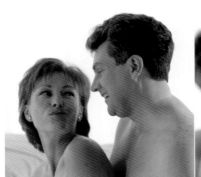
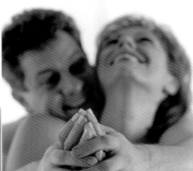

useful addresses

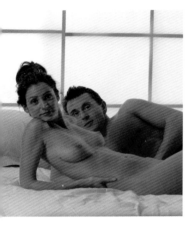

American Counseling Association

5999 Stevenson Avenue, Alexandria, Virginia 22304

(800)347-6647

www.counseling.org

The Association to Aid the Personal and Sexual Relationships of People with a Disability (SPOD)

286 Camden Road, London N7 0BJ

020 7607 8851

www.spod-uk.org

Auckland Rape Crisis

09366 7213

rapecrisis.org.nz

British Association for Sexual and Relationship Therapy (BASRT)

National charity with a list of therapists.

PO Box 13686, London SW20 92H

020 8543 2707

www.basrt.org.uk

The British Columbia Coalition of People with Disabilities

204–456 West Broadway, Vancouver,

British Columbia, Canada V5Y 1R3

(604) 875-0188

www.bccp.bc.ca

British Pregnancy Advisory Service

08457 30 40 30

www.bpas.org

Dateable International

Social organization for people with disabilities.

7830 Wisconsin Avenue, Bethesda, MD 20814

(301) 656-8723

www.dateable.org

Education for Choice

Information about abortion, professional training and education.

2-12 Pentonville Road, London N1 9FP

020 7837 7221

www.efc.org.uk

fpa (formerly the Family Planning Association)

2-12 Pentonville Road, London N1 9FP

helpline: 0845 310 1334

www.fpa.org.uk

Marie Stopes International

Sexual and reproductive health information.

www.mariestopes.org.uk

www.mariestopessouthafrica.co.za

www.mariestopes.org.au

National AIDS Helpline

0800 567123 (24 hours)

NHS Direct

0845 4647

www.nhsdirect.nhs.uk

Outsiders

Enabling the disabled to express their sexuality.

www.outsiders.org.uk

Rape, Abuse and Incest National Network, USA

National Sexual Assault Hotline 1.800.656.HOPE

www.rainn.org

Rape Crisis Federation Wales and England

Unit 7 Provident Works,

Newdigate Street, Nottingham NG7 4FD

0115 900 3560

www.rapecrisis.co.uk

Relate – the relationship people

The UK's largest and most experienced relationship support organization.

Herbert Gray College, Little Church Street,

Rugby, Warwickshire CV21 3AP

0845 456 1310

www.relate.org.uk

Relationships Australia

PO Box 313, Curtin ACT 2605

02 6285 4466

relationships.com.au

Survivors UK

Resources for men who have experienced any form of sexual violence.

020 7357 6222

www. Survivorsuk.co.uk

World Health Organization

Avenue Appia 20, 1211 Geneva 27,

Switzerland

(+ 41 22) 791 21 11

www.who.int

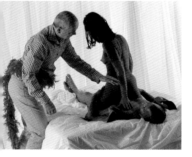

index

A

abortion 226, 231
abuse 243
AFE (anterior fornix erotica) zone 68–9
AIDS 120, 230, 240
al fresco 148–9
alcohol 20–1, 105, 187
anal sex 108, 109, 120–3
Ananga Ranga 162, 166–71
  positions 172–3
anorgasmia 69
anus 30, 37, 38, 39, 154
aphrodisiacs 188–9
Arbuthnot, F. F. 163

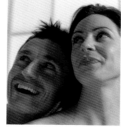

B

bathing 17, 29, 34, 57, 150
bed versus floor 101
bedroom workout 220–1
bisexuality 59
biting 170–1
blind dates 21
blow jobs *see* fellatio
board games 131
body language 22–3
body manipulation 126
body modification 135
body odour 17
bondage 132–3, 157

brain function 46, 65, 137
Brauer, Alan 159
breasts 38–9
  checking 43
bridge exercise 224
bulbourethral glands 32
bulbs of vestibule 37
Burton, Sir Richard 163

C

cancer 34, 35
caps 229
cervix 40
chakras 175, 178
Chicago, Judy 40
chlamydia 239
chocolate 188–9
circumcision 29
Cleopatra's kiss 222
clitoris 37, 43, 46
cocktails 187
coitus 78
  Ananga Ranga 172–3
  coital alignment technique (CAT) 158–9
  kneeling positions 98–101
  man on top 82–5
  rear entry 90–5
  side by side 102–3
  sitting positions 96–7
  standing positions 104–5
  venues 144–5
  woman on top 86–9
Comfort, Dr Alex
  The Joy of Sex 213
coming out 60–1
condoms 21, 120, 141, 226, 228–9
contraception 32, 226–33

Cowper's glands (bulbourethral glands) 32
crabs 240
cunnilingus 109, 111, 116–19

D

dart exercise 224–5
Darwin, Charles 22
dating 20–1, 24–5
diaphragms 229
dildos 120, 140–1
disabled people 216–17
doggy style *see* rear entry
domination 133
Dubberley, Emily 72

E

ejaculation problems 69, 236
emails 25, 43
embracing 167
emergency contraception 231
epididymis 32, 35
erectile dysfunction 31, 234, 237

erogenous zones 52–3
erotica 126–9
exercises 222–5
  bedroom workout 220–1
exhibitionism 157
extended sexual orgasm (ESO) 159
eye contact 22, 23

F

faking orgasm 69
fallopian tubes 40–1
family life 202–3
fantasy 73, 136, 155, 156–7
feathers 150–1
fellatio 31, 65, 109, 111, 112–15, 181
female body 36–45
fetishes 134–5
fingers 53
first impressions 16–17
flirting 18–19, 22–3
flowers 24, 43
food 57, 131, 186–7

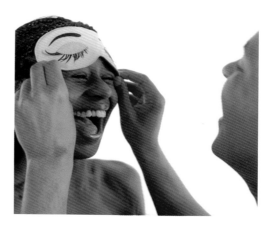

aphrodisiacs 188–9
cooking together 192–3
nutrition 197
seduction 190–1
without plates 194–5
foreplay 46, 50–1, 138, 164, 167
Freud, Sigmund 64
Friday, Nancy
    My Secret Garden 136
fruit 191

G

G spot 46, 68–9
men 30, 33
women 68–9
gay sex 60–1, 120, 121
genital herpes 239
gifts 25, 43, 210
giving head *see* cunnilingus
gonorrhea 239
Grafenberg, Dr 68
Grammer, Karl 19
grooming 16–17, 205, 210

H

hair pulling 171
health 34–5, 222, 226, 238–40
    bedroom workout 220–1
    sexual health 234–5
hepatitis 239–40
Hite, Shere
    The Hite Report 213
HIV 120, 230, 240
hormones 17, 29, 30, 32, 33, 37
HRT 204–5
human papilloma virus (hpv) 238

I

ice cubes 151
infertility 232–3
instep 53
Internet 25, 154–5
intrauterine contraception 229

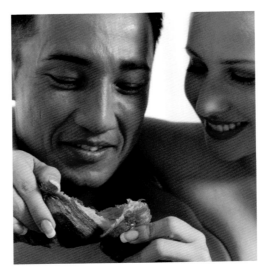

J

Johnson, Virginia 213

K

Kama Sutra 57, 129, 162–5, 166,
    170, 172, 181
Kegel, Dr 159, 165, 222
Kinsey, Alfred 213
kissing 48–9, 51
    techniques 168–9
Kleinke, Chris 19
kneeling positions 98–101

L

labia 36, 43
laughter 155, 210
legal restrictions 123, 148
letters 25, 43
libido loss 236–7
lips 48
listening 214–15
long–term relationships 200–1,
    208–11
    family life 202–3

middle age 204–5
old age 206–7
love balls 138, 141
lubricants 73, 141, 228

M

male body 28–35
Malla, Kalyana 162, 166,
    172
man on top 80–5
massage 54–5, 150, 152–3
Masters, William 213
masturbation 64, 109,
    120, 137
    men 70–1
    together 74, 154
    women 72–3
meeting places 20–1
menopause 204–5, 232
merkins 155
middle age 204–5
midnight feast game 131
missionary position *see* man
    on top
mons pubis 36
morning after pill 231

N

natural contraception 230
navel 52
neck 53
nipples 39, 65
nutrition 197

O

O'Connell, Helen 37
O'Keeffe, Georgia 40
old age 206–7
old wives' tales 229
oral sex 64, 108, 110–11,
    131, 181
orgasm 64–5, 69
    energy orgasms 183
    men 67
    multiple orgasms 158–9
    suppressing 182
    women 66–7
out of the bedroom 144–5
    al fresco 148–9
    quickies 146–7
ovaries 41

P

paddles 133
painful intercourse 234, 236
party games 130
pelvic floor muscle 33, 41,
    165, 222
pelvic tilt exercise 225
penis 28–9, 34, 46
    clitoris 37

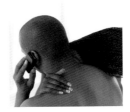

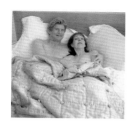

size 31, 35
people watching 23
perineum 30, 37, 38, 43
pheromones 17
philosophy 162–5
phone calls 24–5, 43
Pilates 41, 223
pill, contraceptive 227
pillow talk 58–9
pornography 128–9, 155
post-coital pleasure 56–7
pregnancy 203
premature ejaculation 69, 234, 236
professional help 59, 212–13
prostate gland 29, 30, 32–3, 46, 68
puboccygeus (PC) *see* pelvic floor muscle

Q

quickies 146–7

R

rape 242–3
rear entry 90–5
rectum 33
    hygiene 121, 141
restraint 156–7
Reyes, Alina
    The Butcher 128
rimming 154
romance 46–7
rubbing noses 48

S

sado–masochism (S&M) 126, 133
safer sex 226–31
safety considerations 105, 141
Sanskrit 164
scabies 240
scissors 224
scratching 170
seduction 46–7, 190–1
self-examination 34, 35, 38–9
semen 29, 30, 35, 32
seminal vesicles 32
sensuality 127, 150–1
Sex and the City 140
sex education 226
sex games 130–1
sexual communication 58–9, 65, 78, 109, 210–11
    professional help 212–13
sexual health 234–5
sexual signals 22–3
sexually transmitted infections 238–40
side by side 102–3
sight 46, 127
simultaneous orgasm 69
sitting positions 96–7
smell 46, 127
smiling 22, 23
sodomy 123
soixante–neuf 111
sound 127
spanking 133
sperm 28, 29, 30–1, 32
spoons *see* side by side
squeeze technique 67
standing positions 104–5
sterilization 230–1
strangers game 131
strap-on dildos 120, 141
submission 133
swinging 154, 157
syphilis 239

T

talking 214–15
talking dirty 50, 51
Tantric sex 51, 64, 67, 159, 162, 174–5
    orgasms 182–3
    positions 176–81
Taoist sex 159
taste 46, 127
temptation 46–7
testicles 29, 32, 34, 35
text messaging 24–5, 43
thrusting 94
toes 52–3
tongue 48, 108
touch 127
toys 138–41
trying something new 154–5

U

U–spot 69
undressing 51
urethra 29, 38
uterus 40

V

vadavaka 177
vagina 37, 40
vaginismus 69
vas deferens 32
Vatsayana, Mallanga 162–3, 172
vibrators 138, 140
vitamins 193
voyeurism 154, 157

W

wall slide exercise 223
watersports 135
Wedekind, Claus 17
wet dreams 31
whipping 126
woman on top 86–9

Y

yab–yum 179
yeast infections 240
yoga 223

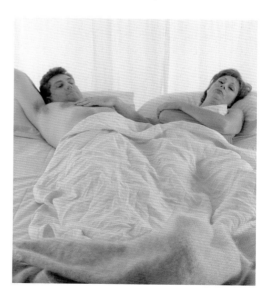

acknowledgements

I would like to say a special thank you to my two colleagues: firstly Clare Spurrell, a budding writer and adventurer who has contributed greatly to the book both in research and editorially, and secondly Tessa Swithinbank, who is a writer and very close friend who has also been a great support and contributor to this book. I would also like to thank Ruth Thomson, Tannis Taylor, Jonathan Hart, Emily Dubberley from cliterati.co.uk, Lynn Warner, Robert Page from *The Lovers' Guide*, Trilby Fairfax, Simon Parritt from SPOD, Robert and Lynn Watson from Dateable, Dr Jane Roy from Relate and all my other

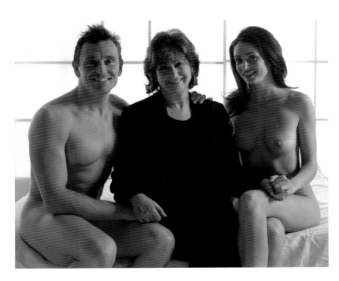

pals who were kind enough to talk to me about their sex lives and fantasies, my editor, Katy Bevan and copy editor Sarah Brown, the photographer John Freeman, his assistant Alex Dow, and make-up artist Bettina Graham. And for using their bodies to illustrate the text, Katy and Nathan, Helen and Armani, Tino and Jennifer, Steve and Barbara, Jessica and Kitt, and Justin and Abigail. Marie Stopes provided the items for contraception. Sh! Women's Erotic Emporium, Coco de Mer and

Myla were very kind to lend us underwear, toys and other paraphernalia for photography. The staff of Ann Summers were extremely informative during the days of my initial research. Thanks to The Terrence Higgins Trust, Stonewall, and Peta Heskell, director of the UK Flirting Academy, www.flirtcoach.com. I would also like to say sorry to anyone I may have forgotten in the dash for deadlines – sincere apologies.

Finally I would like to dedicate this book to all of the men in my life who in their own way have helped me write this book: my father and greatest supporter, Jessel, followed by my many relatives, and much-loved friends past and present: Dominic, Stuart, John, Gil, Charlie, Robert, Roger (who insisted that I mention him) and to B.K. my inspiration.

Thanks to the following for the loan of gorgeous props for photography:

The Cloth Shop
290 Portobello Road, London W10 5TE
020 8968 6001

Coco de Mer
23 Monmouth Street, London WC1
020 7836 8882
www.coco-de-mer.co.uk

Ganesha London
3 Gabriel's Wharf, London SE1 9PP
020 7928 3444
www.ganesha.co.uk

Myla
77 Lonsdale Road, London W11
08707 455 003
www.myla.com

Sh!
39 Coronet Street, London N1 6HD
020 7613 5458
www.sh-womenstore.com

The White Company
No 8 Symons Street, London SW3 2TJ
0870 900 9555
www.thewhiteco.com

NOTES

NOTES

NOTES

NOTES

NOTES

NOTES

NOTES

NOTES